DEVELOPING SPORT EXPERTISE

The development of an athlete from basic performance to elite level of accomplishment is a long and complicated process. Identifying and nurturing talent, developing and fine tuning sport skills, and maintaining high levels of performance over the course of a career require many thousands of hours of training and, increasingly, the input and support of expert coaches and sport scientists.

In this fully revised and updated new edition of the leading student and researcher overview of the development of sport expertise, a team of world-class sport scientists and professional coaches examine the fundamental science of skill acquisition and explore the methods by which science can be applied in the real-world context of sport performance. This book surveys the very latest research in skill acquisition, provides a comprehensive and accessible review of core theory and key concepts, and includes an innovative "Coach's Corner" feature in each chapter, in which leading coaches offer insights from elite sport and critique contemporary practice in sport skill development.

With new chapters offering more material on key topics, such as instruction and observation, and expert visual perception, the second edition of *Developing Sport Expertise* is invaluable reading for all researchers and students in the areas of expertise in sport, skill acquisition, motor control and development, sport psychology, or coaching theory and practice.

Damian Farrow holds a joint appointment with Victoria University, Australia, and the Australian Institute of Sport as Professor of Sports Science. His extensive research activity is designed to support Australian coaches seeking to understand factors critical to developing sport expertise, particularly perceptual-cognitive skill and practice methodology.

Joseph Baker is with the Lifespan Health and Performance Laboratory at York University, Canada. Joe is the author of more than 100 peer-reviewed articles and four previous books. His research considers the influences on optimal human development, ranging from issues affecting youth development to barriers and facilitators of successful aging.

Clare MacMahon is Discipline Leader of Sport Science and Head of Motor Learning and Skilled Performance in Health Sciences at Swinburne University of Technology, Melbourne, Australia. Her research focuses on cognitive aspects of movement skills, including learning and retaining complex perceptual-cognitive skills such as sport decision making.

DEVELOPING SPORT EXPERTISE

Researchers and coaches put theory into practice

Second edition

EDITED BY DAMIAN FARROW, JOSEPH BAKER, AND CLARE MACMAHON

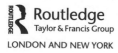

LONDON AND NEW YORK

First published 2007
by Routledge

This edition published 2013
by Routledge
2 Park Square, Milton Park, Abingdon, Oxon OX14 4RN

Simultaneously published in the USA and Canada
by Routledge
711 Third Avenue, New York, NY 10017

Routledge is an imprint of the Taylor & Francis Group, an informa business

British Library Cataloguing in Publication Data

A catalogue record for this book is available from the British Library

Library of Congress Cataloging in Publication Data
Developing sport expertise : researchers and coaches put theory into practice / edited by Damian Farrow, Joe Baker and Clare MacMahon. – 2nd ed.
p. cm.
1. Sports sciences. 2. Physical education and training. I. Farrow, Damian, 1970-
II. Baker, Joe, PhD. III. MacMahon, Clare.
GV558.D48 2013
613.7′1–dc23
2012040417

ISBN: 978-0-415-52523-7 (hbk)
ISBN: 978-0-415-52524-4 (pbk)
ISBN: 978-0-203-11991-4 (ebk)

Typeset in Melior and Univers by Prepress Projects Ltd, Perth, UK

CONTENTS

1 INTRODUCTION

DAMIAN FARROW, JOSEPH BAKER, AND CLARE MACMAHON

PART I: EXPERT SYSTEMS

2 OUTLIERS, TALENT CODES, AND MYTHS

JOSEPH BAKER AND STEVE COBLEY

Coach's Corner
Eddie Jones

3 HOW GOOD ARE WE AT PREDICTING ATHLETES' FUTURES?

JÖRG SCHORER AND MARIJE T. ELFERINK-GEMSER

Coach's Corner
John Keogh

FIGURES

TABLES AND BOXES

TABLES

BOX

CONTRIBUTORS

Bruce Abernethy is with the University of Queensland, Australia, where he is concurrently Professor of Skill Acquisition and Motor Control within the School of Human Movement Studies and Deputy Executive Dean and Associate Dean (Research) within the Faculty of Health Sciences. He also holds a Visiting Professor appointment at the University of Hong Kong, where he was the inaugural Chair Professor of the Institute of Human Performance from 2004 to 2011. A first-class honors graduate and university medalist from the University of Queensland and a PhD graduate from the University of Otago, New Zealand, Professor Abernethy is an International Fellow of the US National Academy of Kinesiology, a Fellow of the Australian Sports Medicine Federation, and a Fellow of Exercise and Sports Science Australia. He is the author of a large number of original research papers on skill acquisition and co-author of the texts *The Biophysical Foundations of Human Movement* and *The Creative Side of Experimentation*. Along with his students and collaborators Professor Abernethy has conducted a number of research projects on the characteristics of expertise and on the development of expert performance in sport, including projects funded by the Australian Research Council (ARC), the Australian Sports Commission, the Australian Football League, and Cricket Australia. In an earlier life, Bruce Abernethy played first-class cricket for the New Zealand province of Otago and as an Australian schoolboy was a national-level 800-meter runner.

Joseph (Joe) Baker, PhD, is Associate Professor and Head of the Lifespan Health and Performance Laboratory in the School of Kinesiology and Health Science at York University, Toronto. He has held visiting researcher/professor positions in the Carnegie Research Institute at Leeds Metropolitan University, UK, Victoria University and the Australian Institute of Sport in Australia, and the Institute of Sport Science at Westfälische Wilhelms-Universität Münster in Germany. His research considers the varying influences on optimal human development, ranging from issues affecting athlete development and skill acquisition to barriers and facilitators of successful aging. Joe is a past President of the Canadian Society for Psychomotor Learning and Sport Psychology and the author/editor of four books, two journal special issues, and more than 100 peer-reviewed articles.

Sian L. Beilock, Professor of Psychology at the University of Chicago, Illinois, is one of the foremost experts on the psychology behind performance under stress. Using her findings concerning why we sometimes fumble under pressure, Dr. Beilock also develops practice strategies and psychological techniques to ensure optimal performance when it matters most. Dr. Beilock received a BS in Cognitive Science from the University of California, San Diego, and PhDs in both kinesiology (sport psychology) and psychology (cognitive neuroscience) from Michigan State University. Her research is supported by the National Science Foundation (CAREER Award) and the US Department of Education. In 2011, she received the Spence Award for Transformative Early Career Contributions from the Association for Psychological Science. In addition to publishing articles on stress and performance in top research outlets (e.g., *Science, PNAS, Psychological Science*), Dr. Beilock has written a best-selling book entitled *Choke: What the Secrets of the Brain Reveal about Getting It Right When You Have To* (Simon & Schuster, 2010; http://sianbeilock.com).

Gary Bernard is the Chief Executive Officer of the Professional Golfers' Association (PGA of Canada) in Acton, Ontario, and a PGA Class "A" Professional, as well as a Class "AA" member of the PGA of Great Britain and Ireland. Prior to assuming this position, he was the Director of Education (2004–2009) and, previous to this, he was a PGA National Education Trainer (1999–2003) and helped to develop a complete revision of the existing national education and professional development program for the PGA of Canada. As National Regional Coach for Golf Canada (1999–2001), he was charged with the responsibility for identifying, recruiting, and training the best junior golfers in Canada. Gary is a past Chair of the National Allied Golf Associations of Canada (NAGA), having served in this capacity from July 2011 to July 2012. Gary is a student of the game of golf, education and leadership theory and practice. He lives with his wife, Nancy, in Mississauga, Ontario.

Ralf Brand has been an active basketball referee in Germany's first league for more than 12 years. He is also Professor for Sport and Exercise Psychology at the Faculty of Human Sciences at the University of Potsdam, Germany. He was trained in physical education and psychology and received his PhD with a dissertation on the topic of referees and stress. Among other positions, he has served as a board member of the German Association of Sport Psychology and recently as the Managing Editor in Chief of the *German Journal of Sport Science*. Ralf has received research grants from national and international funding agencies and has authored more than 20 peer-reviewed research articles in both German and international journals, more than 10 peer-reviewed book chapters, and four books within the past five years.

Steve Cobley is Senior Lecturer in Skill Acquisition and Sport Psychology within the Faculty of Health Sciences at the University of Sydney, Australia. His research interests focus upon the developmental factors that constrain learning, performance, and attainment. Steve is also a joint editor of a recent book entitled *Talent Identification and Development in Sport: International Perspectives* (Routledge, 2011). Steve has also done a range of applied work in sport performance and sport coaching and is a Chartered Sport and Exercise Psychologist with the British Psychological Society.

Jean Côté, PhD, is Professor and Director at the School of Kinesiology and Health Studies at Queen's University, Kingston, Ontario. His research interests are in the areas of sport expertise, children in sport, coaching, and positive youth development. Dr. Côté holds a cross-appointment as a visiting professor in the School of Human Movement Studies at the University of Queensland, Australia. He has published several influential papers that have impacted both research and policy in sport.

Neil Craig is a veteran of 321 games with South Australian Football League clubs Norwood, Sturt, and North Adelaide. He was a State of Origin Captain and coached Norwood from 1991 to 1995. His association with the Adelaide Crows football club began in 1997, where he was the Fitness Coach during the Premiership years before his appointment as Assistant Coach in 2001. Neil was appointed as Senior Coach midway through the 2004 season and has taken the Adelaide Crows to consecutive preliminary finals in 2005 and 2006. Before his involvement with Adelaide Football Club, Neil was a Sport Scientist (physiologist) with the South Australian Sports Institute and worked closely with the successful Australian track cycling team. Neil is currently Director of Football Performance at the Melbourne Football Club in the Australian Football League.

Scott Draper is Head National Coach for Tennis Australia and is a qualified high-performance coach. Scott obtained a career high International Tennis Federation (ITF) ranking of 42 during his singles career, coached Lleyton Hewitt at the 2007 Australian Open, and won the 2005 Australian Open mixed doubles title with Sam Stosur whilst simultaneously competing at the Victorian Open Golf Championship (his first as a professional). Scott transitioned fully to professional golf and toured on the Australasian PGA Tour 2005–2009. He has written his autobiography, *Too Good: The Scott Draper Story*, which details the highs and lows and what he has overcome on the journey.

Patrick (Pat) Duffy, Professor at Leeds Metropolitan University, UK, is a respected leader and facilitator in sport coaching. His recent work has involved the translation of policy objectives and sound technical principles into frontline programs in athlete and coach development across six countries (England, Ireland, Northern Ireland, Scotland, Wales, and South Africa) and a wide range of sports' governing bodies. Pat is currently Vice-President (Europe) of the International Council for Coach Education (ICCE). He is also Chairman of the European Coaching Council, the group which led the creation of the European Framework for the Recognition of Coaching Competence and Qualifications.

Marije T. Elferink-Gemser, PhD, is Assistant Professor at the Center for Human Movement Sciences, University Medical Center Groningen, University of Groningen in the Netherlands. In addition, she recently accepted a position as Associate Professor specializing in sport talent at the HAN University of Applied Sciences in Arnhem and Nijmegen, also in the Netherlands. Her main interest lies in the field of performance development towards expertise in children. Her studies are characterized by their longitudinal design, focusing on multi-dimensional performance characteristics of both the youth athletes and their environment.

Karl Erickson is a PhD candidate in Sport Psychology at the School of Kinesiology and Health Studies at Queen's University, Kingston, Ontario, under the supervision of Dr. Jean Côté. His research interests focus on coaching and athlete development in youth sport. In particular, Karl's work examines the processes and development of coaching effectiveness. Karl's graduate research has been externally funded by the Coaching Association of Canada (CAC) and the Social Sciences and Humanities Research Council (SSHRC) of Canada. More practically, Karl is heavily involved in coaching both basketball and rugby at a number of different levels.

Damian Farrow holds a joint appointment with Victoria University, Melbourne, and the Australian Institute of Sport as a Professor of Sports Science. Appointed as the inaugural Skill Acquisition Specialist at the AIS in 2002, Damian is responsible for the provision of evidence-based support to Australian coaches seeking to measure and improve the design of the skill–learning environment. He has worked with a wide range of sub-elite and elite-level AIS programs and national sporting organizations including the AFL, Cricket Australia, Tennis Australia, Netball Australia, and the Australian Rugby Union. A former physical education teacher and tennis coach, Damian's research interests center on understanding the factors critical to developing sport expertise with a particular interest in the role of perceptual-cognitive skill and practice methodology. He is also the co-author of three general interest sports science books: *Run Like You Stole Something*, *Why Dick Fosbury Flopped*, and *It's True: Sport Stinks*.

Jason Gulbin currently works as the Head of Discipline for Athlete Pathway Development at the Australian Institute of Sport. He has completed a BEd in Post Primary Physical Education at Ballarat University and a PhD at Griffith University Gold Coast. Since 1998, Jason has worked as an applied sports scientist in the area of talent identification and development and has led the national talent identification initiatives at the Australian Institute of Sport (AIS) since 2000. He also squeezed in the Program Manager role for the Australian Women's Skeleton team from 2005 to 2010 and was a member of the Australian Olympic team at the 2010 Vancouver Games. Jason has a broad range of research interests and has published collaboratively in the areas of athlete profiling, exercise-induced muscle damage, biochemistry, genetics, and talent identification and development. Jason was awarded the Australian Public Service Medal in 2011.

Tricia Heberle is currently the Hockey Australia High Performance Director, having commenced this role in November 2012. Prior to this, Tricia was working for hockey in the role of National Network Manager, a position that saw her interface extensively with the State Institute and Academy of Sport network, and, specifically, with hockey pathway programs and the coaching network that sits within each state and territory. Tricia's professional career, the various transitions she has made, and her approach to her new role have all been shaped over 30 years in high-performance sport. She has operated as an elite AIS athlete, a professional coach at national and international levels, and, in more recent times, as a high-performance consultant with government and as an administrator/manager. Tricia's experiences both within Australian sport and in the United Kingdom, where she spent four years, have provided her with great insight into the importance of, and the need for, structured athlete development models and a considered approach to long-term athlete development.

Nicola J. Hodges is an Associate Professor with the School of Kinesiology at the University of British Columbia, Canada, where she studies motor skill learning and correlates of expert performance. She has contributed to the understanding of processes involved in learning from observation and instruction and practice behaviors for elite performance.

Hernán E. Humaña is Assistant Lecturer in the School of Kinesiology and Health Science at York University. Professor Humaña coached the Canadian beach volleyball team at the Atlanta 1996 and Sydney 2000 Olympic Games, obtaining third and fifth place finishes respectively. He also coached the York University women's volleyball team for 10 years and was twice selected as Coach of the Year by Ontario University Athletics. Coach Humaña is the proud father of Melissa Humaña-Paredes and Felipe Humaña-Paredes, both varsity volleyball players at York University.

Patrick Hunt coached over 350 games representing Australia and was Head Coach of the Canberra Cannons in the Australian National Basketball League in 1981. He was one of the initial coaches of the Australian Institute of Sport (AIS) basketball program and has been with the AIS from its inception in 1981, being Head Coach of the men's program from 1983 to 1992. An internationally renowned presenter and coach educator, Hunt has delivered coaching presentations around the globe. Based at the Australian Institute of Sport (AIS), Hunt was Manager of National Player and Coach Development for Basketball Australia and Head Coach of the National Intensive Training Centre Program from 1993 to 2008. In 2009, Patrick was appointed to the new position of Applied Technical Advancement Coach working with the AIS Olympic and world championship caliber coaches. In 2010, Patrick was appointed President of the FIBA World Association of Basketball Coaches.

Robin C. Jackson is a senior lecturer, researcher, and practitioner in Sport Psychology. He gained his PhD on choking in golf from the University of St Andrews, Scotland, and has held posts at the University of Glamorgan, Wales, Brunel University, London, and the University of Hong Kong. Currently, Robin leads the MSc Sport Sciences courses at Brunel University. His main consultancy role was as psychologist and performance analyst for Great Britain Wheelchair Rugby, spanning two Paralympic Games, three European championships, and a world championship. His research focuses on the attentional processes underlying choking in sport and the role of routines in self-paced skills.

Eddie Jones was a small mobile hooker who represented Randwick, New South Wales, and the Australian Barbarians before hanging up his boots and concentrating on his career as a teacher and school principal. Jones began his coaching career at Randwick Rugby Club in Sydney before taking over the Japanese national team in 1996. Jones then accepted an offer as Head Coach of the ACT Computer Associates Brumbies from 1998 to 2001, winning the Super 12 in 2001. Eddie was Coach of the Year two years running at the annual Super 12 awards. He coached the Australian Barbarians in 1999 and the Australian "A" to victory over the British and Irish Lions in 2001. Jones was National Coach of the Qantas Wallabies 2001–2005, making the 2003 World Cup final before losing to

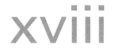

xviii

England in extra time. Since that time, Eddie has coached the Queensland Reds in 2007, Saracens in 2008–2010, and Suntory in 2010–2012, and is currently Head Coach of the Japanese national team.

John Keogh is Rowing Canada Aviron's Senior Women's Coach. Based at the National Training Centre in London, Ontario, he oversees women's high-performance crews, including the 2010 and 2011 World Championship silver-medal women's eight. A former national team athlete in Australia, Keogh began his coaching career in Australia at the college, club, and state levels. In 2004, he took on the role of Talent Development Coach in Great Britain – a role within the World Class Start Talent Identification Scheme with responsibility for identifying and developing athletes from the start of their careers to the podium performance stage. In 2007, Keogh assumed the position of Performance Development Coach and was a member of the British Olympic rowing coaching staff in 2008 in Beijing before joining the Canadian national team program in early 2010.

Noel P. Kinrade is a Lecturer in Sport Psychology, Coaching and Research Methods at Brunel University, London. Having graduated from Sheffield Hallam University in 2003, where he studied for a BSc (Hons) Sport and Exercise Sciences degree, he continued his academic career at Brunel University, completing his PhD in 2010. Noel's research focuses on skill failure under pressure, otherwise known as "choking," more specifically examining the attentional processes that underpin this phenomenon during decision-making tasks in sport.

Timothy D. Lee, PhD, is a Professor of Kinesiology at McMaster University in Hamilton, Ontario. He has published more than 80 papers on the topics of motor control and learning in peer-reviewed journals and edited books, as well as co-authoring *Motor Control and Learning: A Behavioral Emphasis*, and authoring *Motor Control in Everyday Actions*. Tim has served as an editor for the *Journal of Motor Behavior* and the *Research Quarterly for Exercise and Sport* and as an editorial board member for the *Psychological Review*. His research has been supported by numerous grants, including operational funding by the Natural Sciences and Engineering Research Council of Canada. Tim is a member, past President and Fellow of the Canadian Society for Psychomotor Learning and Sport Psychology. He also holds memberships in the North American Society for the Psychology of Sport and Physical Activity, the Psychonomics Society, and the Human Factors and Ergonomics Society. Tim is an avid golfer, hockey player, and student of blues music. He lives with his wife, Laurie Wishart, in Ancaster, Ontario.

Clare MacMahon is Discipline Leader of Sport Science and Head of Motor Learning and Skilled Performance in Health Sciences at Swinburne University of Technology, Melbourne, Australia. Trained in Psychology and Kinesiology in Canada and the US, she has also been a visiting researcher at the German Sport University in Cologne and the University of Münster. Clare is well-published in the cognitive aspects of motor and sport performance and has specifically examined decision making and training in sport officials. She is actively involved with leadership roles in scientific societies and networks nationally and internationally and also links with the applied side of sport through local and national sporting organizations. Her research focuses on cognitive aspects of movement skills, including learning and retaining complex perceptual-cognitive skills, such as sport decision making.

Sue L. McPherson is a Full Professor in the Department of Physical Therapy at Western Carolina University, North Carolina. Sue conducts motor behavior research in physical therapy and has continued to conduct research examining the tactical development of athletes and the nature of expertise in a variety of sports. Sue currently teaches Motor Behavior and Research Methods/Statistics in the Doctor of Physical Therapy (DPT) degree program and Biostatistics in the Masters in Health Sciences program. She also serves as a research consultant for faculty in the College of Health and Human Sciences. Finally, her tennis background includes 10 years of experience as a tennis teaching professional and coach.

Rich Masters is Professor and Assistant Director (Research) in the Institute of Human Performance at the University of Hong Kong. He holds both a BA (Hons) and an MA in Psychology from the University of Otago, New Zealand, and a DPhil in Experimental Psychology from the University of York, England. His work in implicit motor learning has gained attention in a broad range of disciplines, including sports science, rehabilitation, movement disorders, psychology, speech sciences, and surgery. Rich is a greying weekend warrior with children who may someday be superstars and a partner who already is!

Stuart Morgan earned a PhD in Sensory Neuroscience at Swinburne University, Melbourne, and has been a sports scientist for several national and Olympic teams and high-performance sport programs in Australia over the past 12 years. He currently works at the Australian Institute of Sport, where he specializes in data analytics and computer science research for performance analysis. Stuart pioneered developments in computerized notational analysis, machine-learning techniques for team sport analysis, and immersive 3D video technology for understanding tactical skill and decision-making. He serves as a board member of the International Association of Computer Science in Sport and collaborates internationally with research groups in computer science in sport.

Derek Panchuk is a Lecturer in Skill Acquisition in the School of Sport and Exercise Science at Victoria University, Melbourne. He has been in Melbourne for the past four years since completing his PhD at the University of Calgary, Alberta, in 2008 under the supervision of Joan Vickers. Derek's research interests lie in exploring the underlying factors that influence attention control and motor performance particularly when interacting with other individuals. His current research is focused on examining the relationship between attention control and fatigue and determining whether exercise can improve cognitive function in healthy and unhealthy individuals across the life span.

Jae T. Patterson is an Associate Professor in the Department of Kinesiology and Director of the Motor Skills Acquisition Laboratory at Brock University in St. Catharines, Ontario. Jae received his doctoral degree in Human Biodynamics from McMaster University in Hamilton, Ontario, in 2005. His current research interests include identifying and understanding the practice factors facilitating motor skill acquisition in athletes who have experienced multiple concussions. In his spare time, Jae enjoys spending time at his log cabin in the woods on Lake Huron with his two children (Daulton and Fynn), dog (Macy), and wife (Jennifer).

Henning Plessner, PhD in Psychology, is Professor for Sport Psychology and Director of the Institute of Sports and Sports Sciences at the University of Heidelberg, Germany. Among others, he has held visiting researcher/professor positions at the New School University, New York, and the University of Leipzig, Germany. The focus of his research is on judgment and decision-making processes in various applied settings. Henning is Vice-President of the German Society of Sport Science and the author/editor of three books, three journal special issues, and more than 50 peer-reviewed articles and edited book chapters. His interest in officiating has its origin in more than 20 years' experience as a gymnastics judge at all national levels.

Norma Plummer has an impressive netball playing and coaching history. A former Victorian State Playing Captain Coach and Australian Captain, she retired from the court in 1981 but continued her coaching career from the bench as Head Coach of the Melbourne Netball Club, now known as Melbourne Phoenix. Norma's national coaching appointments have included being the Head Coach of the Australian All Stars Team – Australian "B" Team – World Youth Cup Coach in 1996, and 2000 winner of both World Youth Cup Series. From 1999 to 2003, Norma was Head Coach of the AIS/Australian 21/U Netball Program before accepting the position as the Australian National Coach in 2004. Norma completed her term as National Coach in 2011, coaching the team to a dramatic

World Championship title against New Zealand. She is currently Head Coach of West Coach Fever Franchise competing in the ANZ National Netball League.

Markus Raab is Director and Professor for Psychology at the Institute of Psychology at the German Sport University, Cologne. He has worked at the Center for Adaptive Behavior and Cognition, Max Planck Institute for Human Development, at the Free University of Berlin, and the University of Heidelberg. He has a PhD in sport science, as well as a PhD in psychology, and has received awards from the European College of Sport Science (ECSS), the European Association of Sport Psychology (FEPSAC), the German Sport Psychology Association (ASP), and the German Olympic Sports Confederation (DOSB) for his research. His work is published in six books, in numerous chapters, and in papers in reviewed journals. His main areas of interest cover judgment and decision making in sports and beyond, embodiment as well as motor learning and motor control.

Adam Sachs has worked for a range of government and non-government organizations across the sport and recreation sector for more than 20 years. His various roles have provided him with valuable insight and experience in managing the issues or challenges which impact sporting organizations in areas such as sport development, coach education, venue and event management, and high performance. A former elite athlete and coach, Adam was employed by Volleyball Australia as High Performance Manager for eight years, incorporating the Athens 2004 and Beijing 2008 Olympic Games. He is currently employed as Gymnastics Australia's (GA) High Performance Manager, a post which he also held in the lead-up to the Sydney 2000 Olympic Games. In his role with GA, Adam is responsible for the strategic direction of GA's high-performance system, which incorporates everything from talent identification to the selection and preparation of Australia's Olympic teams. His role also requires him to work closely with a range of high-performance system partners towards the development and delivery of integrated national pathways, which enable athletes and coaches to progress towards their goal of podium finishes at events that matter.

Diane M. Ste-Marie, now a Full Professor at the University of Ottawa, Ontario, completed her BEd at McGill University, Montreal, and moved on to do her graduate studies at McMaster University in Hamilton, Ontario. Both her master's (MSc human biodynamics) and doctoral studies (PhD cognitive psychology) concentrated on the cognitive processes of memory and perception. The Natural Sciences and Engineering Research Council of Canada supported her research on memory biases in sport judgments. More recently, research funding through the Social Sciences and Humanities Research Council has allowed her to investigate the importance of self-regulatory processes associated with observational learning, specifically observation of the self. Within her observational learning

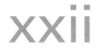

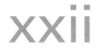xxii

research, Diane also explores the functions of observational learning used by athletes, coaches, and sport officials. Diane's interest in these research issues arose from her own experiences as a competitive gymnast, gymnastics coach, and gymnastics judge.

Geert J.P. Savelsbergh is Professor for Youth and Sport, Head of the Motor Control Group at MOVE, and Visiting Professor in Perceptual-Motor Development and Learning at Manchester Metropolitan University, UK. From 1991 to 1996, he was Research Fellow at the Royal Netherlands Academy of Arts and Sciences and in 2008 he received an honorary doctorate from the Faculty of Medicine and Health Sciences at the University of Ghent, Belgium. His research interest is the visual regulation of movement in sport, motor control, and learning. He has published over 150 papers in international peer-reviewed scientific journals and is the editor of the journal *Infant Behavior and Development* and an associate editor of the *International Journal of Sport Psychology*. He has co-supervised 19 PhD projects and currently supervises 14 PhD projects in the Netherlands, Brazil, Belgium, Spain, the UK, and South Africa. He has a special interest in ball games such as football, tennis, cricket, and golf. At present he is working on book entitled *Athletic Skills Model for Optimal Talent Development* with the coaches of Ajax Amsterdam.

Jörg Schorer, PhD, is a Research Associate at the Institute of Sport Science at the Westfälische Wilhelms-Universität Münster, Germany. His research interests are not only within the field of talent identification and development but also in expertise in sport, perceptual motor skills, and sport psychology.

Joan N. Vickers is a Professor in the Faculty of Kinesiology at the University of Calgary, Alberta. She received her doctorate from the University of British Columbia in the areas of cognition, eye movements, and motor behavior. Her research program specializes in the study of gaze control and visual attention in motor behavior. Her main discovery is the "quiet eye" (Vickers, 1996), which has been shown to be characteristic of elite performance in many motor areas, including sport, law enforcement, and surgery. The "quiet eye" has been featured in *Golf Digest*, on *Scientific American Frontiers* with Alan Alda, and has also been featured on CNN and the Discovery Channel, in *The Wall Street Journal*, *The New York Times*, and many other outlets.

Juanita Weissensteiner is a Senior Research Consultant with the Athlete Pathway Development section at the Australian Institute of Sport. A physiotherapist by background, a former university convener, and lecturer in Sports Science/ Coaching, Juanita's main interest in research is utilizing multi-factorial, multi-disciplinary, and pluralistic methods for examining the dynamics of athlete

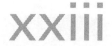

development. Juanita's doctoral dissertation (the University of Queensland/ Cricket Australia, 2008) explored the development of expertise specific to batting in the sport of cricket and featured a complementary mix of qualitative and quantitative research methods across multiple sports science disciplines (psychology, skill acquisition, anthropometry, sociology/pedagogy, biomechanics, and motor control). Along with Dr. Jason Gulbin, Juanita is a partner investigator and academic supervisor for a current Australian Research Linkage project entitled "Improving determinants of Australian sports talent identification and development: a multi-disciplinary approach," which features notable academic and industry experts and sporting partners the Australian Football League (AFL), Cricket Australia, and Tennis Australia.

Hayley Wickenheiser is a four-time Olympic medalist and regarded as the best female ice hockey player in the world. Chosen for the Canadian women's national team at the age of 15, she has since led the squad to six gold medals and three silver medals at the Women's World Hockey Championships. As an Olympian, she earned a silver medal at the 1998 Winter Olympics in Nagano, Japan, and has won a gold medal in three consecutive Olympics, including one at home at the 2010 Winter Olympics in Vancouver. Hayley is a straight-A student who is completing her kinesiology degree while preparing for the next Olympics in Sochi, 2014, and eventually plans to go to medical school.

Tom Willmott is the Head Coach of New Zealand's Winter Performance Park & Pipe Programme, employed by Snowsports New Zealand, supporting athletes and coaches in the Olympic freeskiing and snowboarding disciplines of halfpipe and slopestyle. Tom coached the New Zealand Snowboard Team at the 2006 Torino and 2010 Vancouver Winter Olympics and is currently gearing up for Sochi 2014. Spending six months of the year in the northern hemisphere and six months in the southern hemisphere has meant that Tom has not experienced a summer since 1997; however, two springs per year and plenty of winter allows him to enjoy various outdoor pursuits in his spare time, including ice climbing, mountaineering and whitewater kayaking. Tom received a Bachelor of Science in Sports Coaching (Honors) from the University of Wales in 2001 and a master's in physical education from the University of Otago, New Zealand in 2009. In 2012, Tom graduated from High Performance Sport New Zealand's Coach Accelerator Programme.

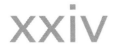

PREFACE

The impetus for the first edition of this text came from an applied workshop convened by the three of us at the Australian Institute of Sport in 2005. This meeting brought together coaches, athletes, researchers, and applied sports scientists to share information under the banner of Applied Sport Expertise and Learning. Researchers at this workshop were asked to consider the following questions when preparing their presentations:

1 What does your research tell us about the development of talented/elite athletes, coaches, and officials?
2 How can the information from your research be used to optimize training and performance?
3 Do your research findings have any application to talent identification programs?

Since the publication of *Developing Sport Expertise: Researchers and Coaches Put Theory into Practice* in 2008 substantial progress has been made, both theoretically and practically, regarding many of the domains examined in the text. Technology has continued to evolve such that testing, measurement, and training approaches not possible in 2008 are now mainstream. Similarly, many countries continue to invest significantly in the development of their sporting talent in the search for more Olympic gold, through talent identification and development systems. Public interest in expertise, and more specifically in sport expertise, has never been greater, thanks to some successful popular psychology books such as Malcolm Gladwell's *Outliers* and Daniel Coyle's *Talent Code* among others. These authors have captured not only the general public's interest in developing sport expertise but, not surprisingly, that of sports coaches and administrators as well as academics from other disciplines. This second edition serves to fill a gap in the available literature that presents accessible theory and practical recommendations from the experts producing the research and actually working in this exciting domain. In filling this gap, we have updated chapters from the first edition and added some new chapters. As a result, the current edition represents a summary of the issues in applied sport expertise research that have particular relevance at the present time.

As with the first edition, the second edition of this book is quite different from other texts on sport expertise. In the current text, the researchers have presented their work in a manner that is applicable not only to scientists, but also to administrators, sport managers, coaches, and athletes. Moreover, current top-level coaches have reviewed and commented on the researchers' findings (see the Coach's Corner segment of each chapter), and present real world application of the concepts discussed. These coaches have been drawn from around the world and represent some of the finest professionals working in sport today. They work with a variety of sports and athletes at developmental, sub-elite, and elite or Olympic levels.

Given the focus on marrying research and application, this book is designed for the progressive coach and athlete who are motivated to adjust their coaching or training programs so that they are making the most out of current research on optimal training and development. It examines sport skill at a macro level (understanding sport development systems, talent, and programming), as well as at a micro level (addressing contemporary issues around the design of training, use of technology, the provision of demonstrations and feedback, and the development of perceptual-cognitive skills). It also includes an understanding of what skill means and how it is acquired for the non-athletic, but equally influential, participants in sport, namely coaches and officials.

Damian Farrow, Joe Baker, and Clare MacMahon

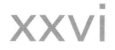

ACKNOWLEDGMENTS

The editors would like to thank all the sport expertise researchers for their contributions to this text. Similarly, we thank all the coaches who provided their insights into the topics presented.

We would also like to thank the Australian Institute of Sport for supporting the Applied Sport Expertise and Learning Workshop in 2005, which provided the stimulus for the development of the first edition of this book.

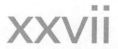

PERMISSIONS

Figure 4.2 Image courtesy of the Australian Sports Commission: http://www. ausport.gov.au

Figure 5.2 Reprinted with the permission of Edizioni Luigi Pozzi (Italy), publisher of the *International Journal of Sport Psychology*.

Figure 5.3 Reprinted with the permission of Edizioni Luigi Pozzi (Italy), publisher of the *International Journal of Sport Psychology*.

Figure 5.4 Photo courtesy of Clare MacMahon.

Figure 7.2 Photo courtesy of Amanda Rymal.

Figure 9.2 Photo courtesy of Tom Willmott.

CHAPTER 1

INTRODUCTION

DEVELOPING EXPERTISE IN SPORT: ENHANCING THE COACH–SCIENTIST RELATIONSHIP

DAMIAN FARROW, JOSEPH BAKER, AND CLARE MACMAHON

Some of the best films of all time tell the story of how an athlete "made it". Recent examples, such as the Academy Award-nominated films *Moneyball* (2011), *The Blind Side* (2009), and *The Fighter* (2010), reflect the nuances of athlete development as well as our continued interest in stories about this process. We want the inside scoop on how the Oakland Athletics came to dominate baseball in 2002, or how Michael Oher and Micky Ward overcame considerable obstacles to develop into outstanding athletes in American football and boxing respectively. We are fascinated with how seemingly ordinary beginnings lead to extraordinary accomplishments for many athletes.

Sport scientists have always had a special attraction to research pertaining to motor skill development and sport expertise, particularly research that tries to understand the differences between athletes during development and on the playing field. Although discussions about the role of environmental influences versus innate characteristics can be traced back to ancient Greece, it was not until the nineteenth century that the scientific study of human skill acquisition began. Francis Galton is generally recognized as the first to examine the varying influences on attainment in sport (rowers and wrestlers) as well as the first to use the phrase "nature versus nurture" to describe the sources of individual differences. This distinction has come to dominate scientific (as well as non-scientific) discussions of why some athletes excel when others do not.

A significant portion of the scientific work on human skill acquisition and achievement was based on the conclusion that biology was the limiting factor to expertise and achievement. Consider, for example, one of the longest and most ambitious

1

studies of human achievement, Lewis Terman's *Genetic Studies of Genius*. This study, which tracked over 1,500 high-IQ children across their lifespans, was based on the notion that IQ (believed to be a genetically determined measure of cognitive ability) would predict achievement. Although the results of this study did not support the relationship between IQ and achievement, it stands as a good example of the perspective that has dominated scientific thinking off and on over the past 100 years. Similarly, research in physical education and kinesiology during this time was dominated by the search for a "general motor ability," which would underpin performance in all sports tasks – a concept now largely dismissed.

Over the past 20 years there has been increasing attention given to the contributory role that experience and practice have in explaining achievement. This environmentalist perspective is based on the idea that individuals start as a *tabula rasa* (blank slate) with no innate traits or characteristics and that all forms of learning and behavior result from interactions with our environment. Perhaps the strongest proponent of this perspective over the past two decades has been the psychologist K. Anders Ericsson, who has examined performers in a variety of domains, arguing that the differences between performers is attributable to what he terms "deliberate practice" (see Chapter 2 for more on this concept), with biological factors playing a negligible role.

Over the same time span, coaches have also had a strong interest in motor skill development and sport expertise. The key difference between the knowledge acquisition of the coach and the scientist is generally that the coach's view is one "from the inside," based on experiential knowledge. Coaches have long been primarily responsible for the skill development of their athletes. Failure to develop skill in their athletes is usually cause for the coach to be replaced. Unlike the scientist, the coach's view of nature versus nurture has not changed much over this time. That is, coaches maintain a firm belief that they can improve the skills of their athletes through tried and tested training methods while acknowledging that a healthy dose of good breeding does not hurt either!

Despite the prominence of extreme views in the history of science, many researchers share the coach perspective and agree that both environmental and biological factors are important. This is perhaps reflective of the scientific process taking its course and is further facilitated by the sporting and coaching experiences of many scientists. Consequently, the attention to the role of training and practice more recently has been valuable for emphasizing the role of optimal experiences in the process of athlete development. For instance, recent questions include:

- can the difference between successful and unsuccessful athletes be explained entirely by training experiences?
- are there early indicators of "talent" that can be used to predict future success?

2

- why do skilled performers sometimes fail?
- what is the most appropriate form of training/practice for developing athletic skills?
- can we improve athletes' and officials' specific skills (e.g., cognitive skills such as perception and decision making) through focused training interventions?

CLOSING THE THEORY TO PRACTICE GAP

Importantly, it seems that, more than at any other time in history, there is a need for rapid translation and application of sport science research into the daily practice of coaching and athlete training. Although applied scientists in the fields of physiology, psychology, and motor learning have developed a significant literature detailing (a) the factors that distinguish expert (i.e., elite) performers from their less successful counterparts and (b) the experiences that may facilitate the development of these qualities, there is often a considerable gap between cutting-edge research and real world application, particularly in the sport coaching environment. Even when research *is* eventually applied, there is often a considerable time lag, and thus it is no longer "cutting edge" from a research perspective.

There are several reasons for the gap and time lag between research and practice in sport expertise. Researchers and coaches generally follow the same processes in their work, both seeking solutions to problems using the methodological approaches at their disposal. However, the cultures and contexts of research and sport coaching are very different, leading to substantial barriers. First, researchers often seek to put evidence behind basic effects using controlled and rigorous testing protocols. These may lead to "obvious" findings, with coaches feeling they are well ahead of the research curve and that research simply tells them what they already knew. When research is of a more complex nature, it may come with many caveats and conditions for when techniques work and do not work; it may be less clear cut and of a riskier nature, with too many nuances to convince a coach of the value of application. In this case, coaches are less willing to wade through the complexity if there is no guarantee of results or if it will take up time and resources. There may also be competing findings, and consequently the path to application is clouded, as we present in this book (more about this later). This is compounded when the main venue of communication for this research is academic journals where the work needs to be framed relative to its contribution to our understanding of basic processes, which makes it more difficult for coaches to access and engage with. Finally, the traditions and culture of sport may be difficult to overcome, particularly when research identifies successful results from practice approaches that go against long-held views. For instance, coaches may feel they must give a lot of instruction, that practice should be free of mistakes, and that athletes must be kept moving as much as possible while completing high numbers of repetitions. Several chapters in this book counter these views. As we know from research on the development of coach expertise, some of the long-held views that research would call "myths" of skill development may come from being trained by mentor coaches and limited engagement with current research.

This book is designed to address these barriers by having leading researchers from around the world provide an accessible synopsis of their research programs and what their research results mean to coaches working with future or current elite performers as well as to athletes, coaches, and officials striving to improve their own performance. We specifically recruited researchers who we know are world leaders in their areas and able to communicate their findings in accessible ways and, most importantly, to make clear links to application. This means that this book does not water down the complexity of the research and, as mentioned, presents views that may compete with each other. It also means that application is a primary goal, not merely an afterthought.

Having coaches (and an athlete) respond to these synopses is also an important part of overcoming the gaps and lags between research and application. All of the authors selected for the Coach's Corner segments are successful and highly respected, and, while they are also forward thinking and generally open to expertise research, we encouraged them to be critical of whether the research discussed had real world application. As alluded to, professional coaches generally evaluate the costs and benefits of research application on two criteria: How much is it going to cost to implement? For how long and how significantly will it improve performance? (For example, see Chapter 12.) One of the key purposes of the coach contributions to this text is to provide insights and critical views about the research, based on extensive experience, sometimes even road testing the training or research discussed. This allows readers to consider both the research and its application and to make more informed decisions about the relative importance of this content in specific programming.

This second edition is divided into five parts. Since the previous edition, considerable attention has been given to the notion of sporting talent, particularly by popular science writers such as Malcolm Gladwell and Daniel Syed, who argue that the concept of "talent" is outdated and irrelevant to understanding the development of exceptional performance in sport and other domains. To this end, chapters in Part I, "Expert systems," consider the emerging literature on the role of proper training (Baker and Cobley, Chapter 2), the research examining the identification and development of sport talent from the perspective of the researcher (Schorer and Elferink-Gemser, Chapter 3), and the national talent development system (Gulbin and Weissensteiner, Chapter 4). This part highlights the complexity of defining talent, modeling elite performance systems, and testing and selecting

4

athletes, all with the goal of creating elite performers. When the three chapters are considered together, Part I addresses the micro (individual athlete), meso (the actual training activities of athletes), and macro (skill testing, selection systems and developmental pathways) ways that elite performers develop. They also highlight the multi-dimensional nature of skill development (i.e., environment and supportive others), even the frustration of defining and understanding who is a talented athlete, an age-old issue in sport expertise research.

Part II, "Expert officials and coaches," focuses on the development and strategies used by expert coaches and officials. In Chapter 5, Henning Plessner and Clare MacMahon examine expertise in sport officials; in Chapter 6, Jean Côté, Karl Erickson and Pat Duffy review work examining how expert coaches develop. Plessner and MacMahon point out the multiple and sometimes unique demands of sport officials. The research in this area is in many ways less developed than that with regard to athletes, yet often draws on many similar concepts. Similar to the chapter that follows by Côté and colleagues, the definition of an expert official is often confused with the level of athlete whose competitions are being officiated. Plessner and MacMahon also consider skills that can be difficult to capture, yet central to officiating efficacy, such as communication. Côté's chapter provides some points about coaching that are particularly relevant for this book. First, the chapter describes the different sub-domains in which coaches must acquire knowledge, such as physiology, conditioning, and general biomechanics. The intention of this text is to communicate the skill acquisition knowledge in an accessible way to coaches that will aid this development and knowledge base. Second, the chapter contrasts the formal and informal pathways that lie beneath coach training, and gives examples of each in university study and mentorship. Both of these pathways still necessitate ongoing knowledge gain and some can argue this is particularly the case for mentorship pathways if there is a reliance on mentoring at the expense of other contemporary information. With the time lag between research findings and applied practice, replicating coaching methods of a mentor can compound the problem of applying outdated methods. Again, this book serves to address this danger, making the knowledge accessible.

Part III is entitled "Contemporary coaching approaches." The provision of demonstrations, instructions and feedback, and the organization of the practice setting are the key tools at the disposal of a coach for developing their athletes' skills. This part describes some of the more recent research-based recommendations for the design of coaching practice. We hope this section will challenge coaches to consider their current approaches and reconcile what they feel works with what applied research currently suggests to be the most effective methods of skill development. Importantly, although the synopses provided by the contributing researchers and coaches are plainly stated, we leave you to consider your position on many of the topics.

Chapter 7, by Nicola Hodges and Diane M. Ste-Marie, focuses on the role of observation in coaching practice. They highlight the need to examine who is being observed and the content and timing of demonstrations, as well as the skill of the learner. Following this, Jae Patterson and Timothy Lee (Chapter 8) discuss research from the field of motor learning, examining methods to improve the organization and design of practice. They address the myth of the repetition and emphasize the importance of thinking in practice. Our final chapter in this part (Chapter 9) by Rich Masters describes his extensive program of research examining how implicit training methods can improve learning and maximize athlete development. In contrast to Patterson and Lee, Masters emphasizes preventing learners from thinking too much. An obvious challenge for both researchers and practitioners in this section is how to reconcile the work of Patterson and Lee with that of Masters. Some reconciliation of this is evidenced in the Chapter 9 Coach's Corner, where Tom Willmott discusses his use of random practice as an implicit training approach with his snowboard athletes.

Part IV, "Expert athlete processes," considers the perceptual and cognitive elements of skilled athletic performance. In Chapter 10, Jackson, Beilock, and Kinrade uncover why expert performers are not immune to "choking." They illustrate ways in which pressure-filled situations change how individuals think about and attend to skilled performance and, importantly, offer the practitioner a range of strategies to inoculate their athletes against such effects. Their discussion of avoidance behavior on the part of performers and coaches can also be used as a stimulus to consider the broader implications of avoidance behavior in the context of theory and practice, for instance, researcher avoidance of differing scientific paradigms from which to examine a research question and coach avoidance as a barrier to the uptake of contemporary research findings. In Chapter 11, Derek Panchuk and Joan Vickers discuss the growing body of research on experts' gaze behavior (the concept of "quiet eye") and how training eye movements may improve performance. Damian Farrow and Markus Raab (Chapter 12) update their chapter from the previous edition summarizing current understanding of decision-making skill and how it can be improved through appropriate training with a particular emphasis on some emerging technologies. Chapter 13, by Stuart Morgan and Sue McPherson, examines research on the differences between skilled and unskilled performers in their use of tactical information and the new methods available for coaches and practitioners to better understand how to utilize this information to enhance performance.

Part V, "Expert commentary," consists of two chapters written by two leaders in sport expertise research. Bruce Abernethy (Chapter 14) and Geert Savelsbergh (Chapter 15) offer an international perspective on the current issues facing sport expertise theory and practice. They specifically focus on some issues that run through the chapters and unanimously highlight, through some clever analogies, that the route to both understanding and developing expertise is a long one. They challenge us all to consider the coach–scientist, theory–practice connection through their musings on the questions "Can research inform practice?" (Abernethy, Chapter 14) and "Can practice inform research?" (Savelsbergh, Chapter 15).

SOME CONCLUDING THOUGHTS

As has been highlighted earlier in this chapter, good research is usually the product of a collaborative team, with complementary skills, pursuing a common goal in a methodical fashion. The same can be said for elite sports performance. So it is perhaps not surprising (or plainly obvious) that the most successful applied sport expertise research endeavors involve a strong collaboration between a scientist and coach. As detailed in Table 1.1, there are elements of communication between coaches and scientists that, if considered more carefully, could improve the translation between research and practice. Like all successful relationships there is a need for give and take from both sides.

When coaches are first exposed to research it is important that they observe how researchers qualify their findings and literature. For instance, motor learning research has a long history of theoretically driven, laboratory-based research that has focused on the behavior of untrained university participants learning and performing simple motor tasks. The disparity between theory and practice as it relates to sport expertise could not be more stark. Expert sport performers usually have a strong underlying level of intrinsic motivation and have practiced complex motor skills for extensive periods of time (over years rather than hours or days) in

Table 1.1 Key issues coaches and scientists identify in collaborations: improving coach and scientist interactions

Coach says	Scientist says
Scientists need to think like coaches (i.e., urgency/performance). Research cannot take too much time away from training	Coaches need to follow through with newly adopted scientific suggestions (give it time to work). Good research can be integrated into a training program but does often cost time and resource
Scientists need to be able to adapt/apply their concepts with critical information, e.g., what does the coach really need to know? Can the information be conveyed simply?	Coaches need to be open minded about what the application/intervention may look like, i.e., it may differ from traditional approaches
Scientists need to spend time understanding the nature of the applied setting before offering to apply their expertise	Coaches need to know how to ask good questions of scientists

a variety of applied settings. Hence, coaches are justified in expressing concern at the relevance of laboratory-based work with novices for their participants. Equally, though, and evidenced throughout this text, applied sport expertise researchers have bridged this gap and developed approaches that satisfy both scientific rigor and applied practice. It is also important to note that applied scientists still value and rely heavily on the knowledge generated by the theoretically driven, laboratory-based work. Consequently, the applied scientist adopts a translational role between theorist and practitioner.

An important underlying element that has contributed to the gap between theory and practice in the field of sport expertise relates to the research topics considered. Put simply, many of the research foci or areas considered in sport expertise have been issues traditionally regarded as falling under the role of the coach. For instance, in reviewing the chapters in this book, talent identification and selection, demonstrations, practice design, instruction, and coaching decision making are all typically handled by the coach. Consequently, coaches needed additional convincing of the value sport expertise research could add to their programs relative to other sports science disciplines such as physiology or biomechanics that are perceived to provide more specialized content. It is the view of the editors that this leap of faith by coaches has occurred recently for a number of reasons. The role of the coach is so multi-faceted (see Chapter 6) that it has become all but impossible for coaches to keep pace with the evolution in sport expertise content. Furthermore, from a coach's perspective, the quality of applied sport expertise research has continued to improve thanks to factors such as measurement technology allowing more *in situ* examination of performance and a tighter coupling between the questions that coaches and scientists are interested in answering.

In summary, there are clear barriers between sport expertise research and its application. Despite this, as evidenced in the remainder of this book, coaches and scientists in sport expertise are now working more closely than ever before. One thing coaches and scientists always agree on is that the journey to expertise is a long one and is often more mundane than typically depicted by Hollywood. However, through the collaborative effort between scientists and coaches, we are confident this book can provide some shortcuts and excitement along the way.

KEY READING

Baker, J., Cobley, S., and Schorer, J. (eds.) (2012) *Talent Identification and Development in Sport: International Perspectives*. New York: Routledge.
Davids, K. and Baker, J. (2007) 'Genes, environment and sport performance: Why the Nature–Nurture dualism is no longer relevant', *Sports Medicine*, 37: 961–980.
Ericsson, K.A., Krampe, R.T., and Tesch-Römer, C. (1993) 'The role of deliberate practice in the acquisition of expert performance', *Psychological Review*, 100: 363–406.

Gladwell, M. (2008) *Outliers: The Story of Success*. New York: Little, Brown and Co.

Sands, W.A., McNeal, J.R., and Stone, M.H. (2005) 'Plaudits and Pitfalls in Studying Elite Athletes', *Perceptual and Motor Skills*, 100: 22–24.

Simonton, D. (1994) *Greatness: Who Makes History and Why*. New York: The Guilford Press.

Syed, M. (2010) *Bounce: Mozart, Federer, Picasso, Beckham and the Science of Success*. New York: Harper Collins.

Williams, A.M. and Ford, P.R. (2009) 'Promoting a skills-based agenda in Olympic sports: The role of skill-acquisition specialists', *Journal of Sports Sciences*, 27(13): 1421–1432.

Wulf, G. and Shea, C. (2002) 'Principles derived from the study of simple skills do not generalize to complex skill learning', *Psychonomic Bulletin Review*, 9(2): 185–211.

PART I

EXPERT SYSTEMS

CHAPTER 2

OUTLIERS, TALENT CODES, AND MYTHS

PLAY AND PRACTICE IN DEVELOPING THE EXPERT ATHLETE

JOSEPH BAKER AND STEVE COBLEY

> It is only through work and strife that either nation or individual moves on to greatness. The great man is always the man of mighty effort, and usually the man whom grinding need has trained to mighty effort.
>
> (Theodore Roosevelt)

The past 10 years have brought increased interest in the concept of "talent," particularly from those trying to build a case that it does not exist. For example, an extremely influential 2006 piece in *Fortune* magazine claimed "talent has little or nothing to do with greatness" (a notion that author Geoff Colvin expanded into the *New York Times* best-selling book *Talent Is Overrated: What Really Separates World-Class Performers from Everybody Else* in 2008), whereas popular authors such as Malcolm Gladwell (*Outliers*, 2008), Matthew Syed (*Bounce*, 2010), Daniel Coyle (*The Talent Code*, 2009), and David Shenik (*The Genius in All of Us*, 2010), among a rapidly expanding group of others, argue that the explanation of "outliers" – those whose performance is clearly superior to others in the domain – is the result of time spent in a very focused and effortful form of training called "deliberate practice." These authors propose that, instead of talent, differences between performers in any domain of endeavor result from time spent in this unique form of practice.

Although much of the discussion in this area, at least among the popular press, has been grounded in circular arguments and/or over-simplification of sometimes very subtle research findings, this chapter summarizes the evidence about the role of practice, training, and experience in the development of expert performers.

WHAT DOES THE RESEARCH TELL US?

To a greater or lesser extent, all of the popular books listed in the opening section of this chapter are based on a concept developed by the cognitive psychologist Anders Ericsson. The concept, "deliberate practice," is the result of decades of studying the value of different forms of training to the acquisition of cognitive and motor expertise. Before examining this concept a little deeper, let us consider the evidentiary foundation it is built upon.

In the late 1800s, one of the earliest studies of the value of practice was conducted at Indiana University by William Lowe Bryan and his graduate student Noble Harter. They were working on the development of telegraph skill. Their research – and much of the research over the past 100 years examining the accumulated effects of prolonged practice and the rate of learning – showed that performance increased according to a power function, whereby rapid improvements in skill happened during the initial hours of practice but were reduced over time and learners were required to invest progressively more hours to accrue progressively smaller improvements. This finding, better known as the "power law of practice" (Figure 2.1; also known as "the law of diminished returns"), has been demonstrated in numerous domains – everything from learning to roll cigars to learning to read words printed upside down. Collectively, this body of evidence highlights the crucial role of practice in developing the elite performer in sport and other domains.

In 1973, the future Nobel Prize-winning economist Herbert Simon and his colleague William Chase went further. Their classic study of chess expertise focused on the perceptual-cognitive differences between grandmaster and lower-level (i.e., master and novice) chess players. They found that differences among these skill levels were attributable not to a superior memory capacity but rather to the ability to organize information in more meaningful "chunks." For Simon and Chase, this finding led them to consider whether the differences among players was simply the end-result of a greater amount of time spent training and playing chess. In their examination, they concluded "there appears not to be on record any case (including Bobby Fischer) where a person has reached grandmaster level with less than about a decade's intense preoccupation with the game."

This statement, based on a simple investigation with three participants (one novice, one master and one grandmaster), has become the "10-year rule of necessary preparation," a general criterion for expertise in domains ranging from running to tennis, mathematics to music. Over the past 40 years, evidence has continued to amass to support the position that, in fields where the distinguishing characteristics between experts and non-experts involve the ability to process domain-specific information, these differences have more to do with training than innate abilities.

14

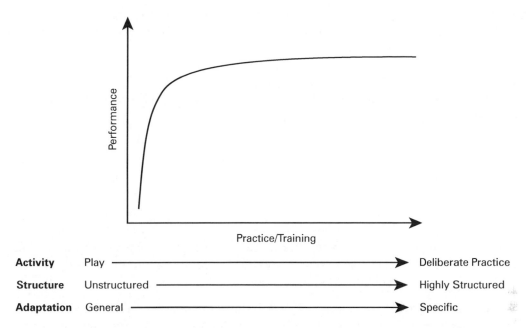

Figure 2.1 Typical relationship between training and performance, indicating rapid increases in performance at the onset of training and decreased improvements with additional training.

In cognitive science, the work of Simon and Chase prompted some researchers to adopt environmentalist (i.e., nurture rather than nature) perspectives on the acquisition of highly skilled performance. The deliberate practice framework created by Ericsson and his colleagues is one of these perspectives. Over the past two decades, Ericsson has steadfastly defended his position that individual performance differences in any domain can be accounted for by the amount and type of practice performed. Likewise, he pronounced the role of genes in determining individual achievement as minimal and that this role could be circumvented by the performance of optimal amounts of quality practice. In a review of studies on skill acquisition and learning, Ericsson concluded that, with few exceptions, level of performance was determined by the amount of time spent performing a "well defined task with an appropriate difficulty level for the particular individual, informative feedback, and opportunities for repetition and corrections of errors."

The deliberate practice perspective extends Simon and Chase's work by suggesting that it was not simply training of any type that differentiated individual performance, but the engagement in what Ericsson refers to as "deliberate practice." For example, a swimmer can spend their time doing length after mindless length of the pool or they can attentively train the specific aspects of performance where they are weak – focusing on stroke improvement, doing intervals at near race pace, that sort of thing. By definition, deliberate practice is the type of training athletes do that is not very much fun, requires hard work, and does not lead to instantaneous rewards – the payoff is in the long run. Up to this point, examinations of learning had generally focused on the total quantity of exposure; the theory of deliberate practice brought the issue of training quality back to the forefront of learning and expertise research.

Data from a series of studies by Ericsson and his contemporaries examining skilled musicians support the relationship between number of hours of deliberate practice and level of performance. They found that expert-level musicians spent in excess of 25 hours per week in deliberate practice activities (i.e., training alone), whereas less successful musicians spent considerably less time in deliberate practice (e.g., amateurs spending less than two hours per week). These notable disparities in weekly training accumulate to become enormous differences after years of training. Expert musicians accumulated over 10,000 hours in deliberate practice by age 20, while amateurs had accumulated only 2,000 hours at the same age.

So far, this relationship is not new; it is still the same positive relationship between training and improvement. What is different is the type of training that constitutes this optimal type of practice. For instance, when learning basketball skills, early attempts to perfect the specific movements of the free throw may constitute deliberate practice; it requires mental and physical effort, there are no immediate rewards, and it is probably not much fun because there is little success. However, once this skill becomes well learned, this type of training is no longer deliberate practice and, instead, the learner needs to move on to something that requires the same intense effort and has the same relevance for improving the current level of performance as free throw practice did during the early stages. According to the theory, continually modifying the level of task difficulty so that it matches current performance levels allows the learner to prevent plateaus and perpetuate adaptation to higher amounts of training stress and, therefore, higher levels of performance.

Much of athlete training comes down to the optimal maintenance of training stress. A great deal of what we know about the human body's response to stress comes from Hans Selye's *General Adaptation Syndrome*. According to Selye, the body has a three-stage response to stress (in our case, training stress). When the body is functioning normally and all systems are in balance, we are in *homeostasis* (Greek for "remaining the same"). Introducing a training stimulus promotes some sort of physical or psychological response. The first phase of this response is *shock*, easily identified in sport by the acute muscle soreness and performance decreases connected with the onset of a new or different training stimulus. During this phase, the body is moved out of normal functioning and must adapt to the new levels of stress. The second phase is *adaptation* and during this period the body adapts to the training stimuli and re-attains homeostatic function. These adaptations can be

16

positive, as when the body reorganizes its functional components to produce a superior, more capable operating system, or they can be negative, as when a physical injury or mental overload occurs. In the third phase, *staleness*, physiological adaptations are no longer being made and performance may again decrease unless training stimuli are modified. During this stage, the athlete has adapted to the previous level of physical or mental stress and training at this level no longer disrupts homeostasis. The duration of the period from shock to staleness is determined primarily by the intensity of the training stress presented in phase one. High levels of stress require greater amounts of time to achieve adaptation. The commonly used approach of periodization (i.e., organizing the training year into different periods to attain different objectives) is intended to prevent athletes from reaching or spending too much time in the third stage (staleness) by varying training schedules so that new training stimuli are presented at the end of the adaptation phase. If there is too long a time between when adaptation occurs and when new training stress levels are introduced, maximal training effects are compromised. On the other hand, if the time is too short, coaches and athletes run the risk of incurring injuries or over-training syndrome. This notion of balance between training and recovery is at the very heart of Ericsson's theory of deliberate practice.

Although it was developed through research with musicians, researchers have also applied deliberate practice theory to a wide variety of sports, ranging from karate to distance running, figure skating to basketball. Although these studies have found good support for the notion that time spent in high-quality training is a good way to distinguish those at the top of their games from those at lower levels, they have encountered some problems in applying Ericsson's original definition of deliberate practice. Most notably, athletes at all levels consistently report that their practice activities are very enjoyable and intrinsically motivating, contrasting with a key component of the definition of deliberate practice activities (i.e., that they are not fun).

Based on these difficulties there is some concern among sports scientists about exactly what forms of athletic training constitute deliberate practice. In Ericsson's original work, only practice alone was seen as meeting the requirements for deliberate practice. In studies of deliberate practice in sport, there are few, if any, training activities that meet the original criteria set out by Ericsson and his colleagues in 1993. Some researchers have argued that, given the unique requirements of sports performance, all relevant forms of training could be considered deliberate practice. The rationale for this is that even training that is lower in intensity may have a critical role in promoting positive performance adaptations. For instance, long, slow distance runs would not be considered very effortful to an elite distance runner, yet this type of training is a staple of their program. This is also important in team sports, where both individual and team practices are beneficial to increasing various aspects of performance. Ericsson's position has also been criticized for not considering the specific needs of athletes at different levels of development.

PLAY VERSUS PRACTICE IN ATHLETE DEVELOPMENT

As a result of these criticisms, developmental sport scientists have begun differentiating between the concepts of "deliberate practice" and "deliberate play" (i.e., unstructured, play-oriented activities done in the absence of supervision and corrective feedback), a concept advocated by Jean Côté and his colleagues. Deliberate play is grounded in the notion that, during early development, athletes require intrinsically motivating activities that "plant the seeds" of future expertise while concurrently developing important components of skill. Research is beginning to emerge regarding the importance of this approach. For example, studies have illustrated the value of deliberate play on the development of tactical game intelligence and creativity of athletes in team sports.

Collectively, research from both the deliberate play and deliberate practice perspectives emphasizes the use of appropriate training at the appropriate time. Deliberate play advocates indicate that training focus should vary between deliberate play and deliberate practice as athletes move towards adulthood. In Côté's stage-based model of athlete development (the Developmental Model of Sport Participation), the early stage of athlete involvement – the *sampling* stage – has a primary focus on deliberate play. As the athlete becomes more mature, and more skillful, there is a shift to a greater integration of deliberate practice in the *specializing* stage. Finally, in the penultimate stage of development prior to expertise – the *investment* years – the athlete has an almost singular focus on deliberate practice.

WHAT THE RESEARCH DOES NOT TELL US

In discussions about the role of training and experience, the roles of innate factors and "talent" inevitably arise. Despite the rhetoric generated in popular scientific discussions about athlete development, studies highlighting the value of deliberate practice actually tell us very little about the role of innate factors. The strong role of training and practice in developing expertise is uncontroversial. The important distinction between scientific camps is whether deliberate practice is *sufficient* to describe the process of expertise development, not whether it is *necessary*.

Let us consider the following example: two young boys find themselves at their first track and field practice. Both are of similar age, coming from similar families with similar financial resources to support their development. Importantly, both enjoyed their track and field experience so much that they decide on the spot to become

18

elite sprinters so they can go to the Olympics to be like their new hero Usain Bolt. Twenty years later, only one of the boys has achieved expert status as a sprinter; the other stopped sprinting before exiting secondary school. An important limitation of the deliberate practice approach is that it typically considers the amount of training at the end point of development without considering the factors that might have moderated or buffered an athlete's ability to train deliberately. Returning to our sprinters, if we looked at only the hours of deliberate practice, even if it was throughout their development instead of only at the end point, we might see differences in the amount and type of training each boy did, concluding that deliberate practice explains the differences in achievement. However, this conclusion might not necessarily be correct; consider, for instance, results from the HERITAGE Family Study (conducted by Claude Bouchard and his colleagues), a multi-site study conducted in the United States that examined the varying influences of genetic factors on predictors of health and disease risk. Families participating in the study were healthy, but untrained, including both biological parents and at least three biological children. In addition to a range of physical and health related tests, participants completed a 20-week standardized aerobic training program. By examining patterns of results between and among families, results from the HERITAGE study conclusively show that several variables related to physical performance (such as VO2max, maximal aerobic capacity) are genetically constrained, but, more importantly, the HERITAGE data shows that an individual's response to a training stimulus is influenced by their genetic makeup. This program of research, as well as many other studies from independent labs around the world, clearly shows that large amounts of the variability in cardiorespiratory function between different people can be attributed to the presence or absence of specific genes and, logically, the level of attainment in activities in which these factors are important (e.g., marathon running) will be higher if a person has an advantageous genetic makeup (i.e., genotype).

Researchers are now identifying individual genes responsible for performance-related outcomes. For example, the *COL5A1* gene on chromosome 9 is responsible for producing the protein for collagen, type 5, alpha 1, which encodes for a specific collagen protein relevant to flexibility of ligaments and tendons and appears to affect an individual's predisposition to tendon and ligament injury. By affecting injury risk, this gene is likely to affect the amount and intensity of training individuals in certain sports can perform throughout their development. These results, and those from HERITAGE, suggest that the ability to accumulate thousands of hours of high-quality deliberate practice is built on a foundation of beneficial genetic raw material.

Despite the evidence noted above, it is easy to be swayed by the deliberate practice approach; however, apart from a small evidence base examining the acquisition of very specific cognitive skills (e.g., Ericsson and Chase's study of memory skill), the research on the development of expertise has been exclusively retrospective (i.e., tracking athlete development backwards from the end points of their development). This type of design, although invaluable for providing information about how training changes throughout development and/or the role of specific influences (e.g., peers, coaches, parents) on expertise development, does not allow us to determine conclusively whether practice is the sole influence on athlete development. This can come only from randomized control group studies that track athletes longitudinally over the course of their development. Ultimately, innate potential may not be an insurmountable obstacle to the acquisition of expertise (although this is unlikely) but, at the very least, based on the existing evidence it is premature to make this conclusion.

THEORY INTO PRACTICE

Regardless of whether or not the notion of talent is valid, few would argue against the conclusion that training is the predominant factor in explaining achievement. No one gets to the top without an extensive period of training. Although this is a simple message, there is a common recurring problem for practitioners. How do we connect and integrate the theoretical "big picture" (i.e., what to do) with the applied activities and training on the ground (i.e., how to do it)? In the following section, we try to describe how coaches, trainers, and athletes can integrate the core concepts of deliberate play and deliberate practice within day-to-day play or training activities.

To summarize the progressive journey toward expertise, Figure 2.1 illustrates the general relationship between training and performance over time, indicating rapid increases in performance at the onset of training, and decreased improvements with additional training. It also summarizes the proposed changing nature of training activity over time. For instance, most athletes, at least in sports with later ages of peak performance (compared with gymnastics, for example), progress from activities focusing on deliberate play to those focusing on deliberate practice. Relatedly, the structure of training also changes during this time from having a flexible or open-ended structure, to a highly structured environment with very little room for flexibility (e.g., compare a child's first unstructured experiences with a soccer ball and the structure of adult professional training). In addition, the training-related changes and adaptations that occur shift from very general adaptations in the physical and cognitive systems (e.g., gross changes in cardiovascular and cognitive function) to highly specific adaptations in these systems (e.g., physical – changes in capillary density only in muscles associated with the task; cognitive – being able to utilize highly precise advanced visual cues from one's opponent). With these developmental changes in mind, we can now consider ways of determining whether particular types of activity or specific training are optimal relative to the age/stage of an individual's development. This begins with a discussion of training emphasis across stages of development.

The starting point: intrinsic motivation

Although a thorough discussion of athlete motivation is beyond the scope of this chapter, it is worth spending a bit of time discussing intrinsic motivation. Given that a long-term devotion to training and practice, in whatever forms it takes, is clearly a necessity for the development of expertise, perhaps the most important element is the need to keep athletes intrinsically motivated throughout the developmental process. Generally speaking, intrinsic motivation refers to motivation that is driven by an inherent interest, satisfaction or enjoyment in the task being performed and is demonstrated by athletes who (a) focus on mastery of the task (as opposed to satisfying ego-related needs through defeating opponents), (b) feel a high degree of autonomy and self-determination in their actions (i.e., they do not feel "controlled" by others), and (c) are not primarily motivated by external factors (e.g., trophies, medals, etc.). The development of this quality is somewhat elusive, although enjoyment clearly plays a role, but it is clear that no one becomes an expert without a high degree of intrinsic motivation. An important element for the coach to consider, in addition to the enjoyment issue noted above, is setting a level of difficulty that is sufficient to challenge the athlete to improve through practice. A moderately challenging task can encourage athletes to practice (e.g., "I know I can do it if I train harder"), thereby developing perceptions of competency, which increase intrinsic motivation, whereas tasks that are too difficult may result in athletes dismissing the challenge as impossible (e.g., "there's no way I'll ever be able to do that"). Developing the appropriate "challenge point" is a key task for the progressive coach. Ultimately, intrinsic motivation is the currency of skill acquisition, and athletes who have high levels of this quality are more likely to persevere through the inevitable difficulties that are experienced on their way to greatness.

Focus on deliberate play in the sampling years

With only a few exceptions (e.g., early-specialization sports such as gymnastics), deliberate play (at the ages of 6–12) in a range of non-sport specific activities appears to provide a foundation for long-term sporting involvement. Advocates of deliberate play believe that involvement in playful, flexible activities at young ages provides a stimulus for the development of intrinsic motivation as well as fundamental motor and cognitive skills through experiential and discovery-based learning. During this phase of development, coaches should ensure that skill development occurs in flexible and adaptive environments that promote a high degree of enjoyment in their athletes.

Integrating deliberate play and practice for the specializing years

The specializing years (generally early to mid-adolescence) are a time when athletes reduce their sport involvement to focus on one or two sports (e.g., rugby and cricket). Beneficial activities at this stage are characterized by a balance of both deliberate play (i.e., high activity/interaction and enjoyment) and deliberate practice (i.e., high concentration, physical effort and relevance to skill acquisition). It is important to note that this guideline is most relevant for athletes looking to progress into the investment years and may not be as important for athletes aspiring to recreational forms of involvement. As a coach, trainer, or parent, consider the overall pattern of activities your athletes participate in and try to provide a balance of both deliberate play and deliberate practice.

Focus on deliberate practice in the investment years and beyond

The investment years (i.e., late adolescence onwards) are strongly associated with a focus on deliberate practice. There are challenges when identifying a general form of deliberate practice, particularly the assumption that, once identified, the nature and structure of that activity remains fixed. On the contrary, by definition, deliberate practice represents the optimum type of training for a particular point of skill development. Once athletes have moved beyond this point, the type of training that constitutes deliberate practice also changes. An important task for every coach is considering how training activity should be manipulated according to the specific task or technical skill required for the athlete's current level of development. More specifically, in order to prevent developmental plateaus, coaches need to understand the factors constraining development at that point in the athlete's career. Once these are identified, training can be modified in order to overcome these constraints.

The stage-based model proposed by Côté and his colleagues provides a good framework for conceptualizing the various types of training and practice athletes experience throughout their careers; however, it is important that coaches, trainers, and athletes are aware that there could be significant variability in athletes' paths to expertise. Some athletes will advance through the sampling and specializing stages more rapidly than others; this does not necessarily mean rapid advancement is an indicator of greater potential or talent. This is not a trivial point; most talent development systems work on a deselection approach whereby athletes who are not selected for the next stage of development are relegated to lower levels of

22

competition. It is extremely difficult for these deselected athletes to re-enter the system later in their development.

Importantly, for all athletes, the coach's approach to training should match the developmental status of the athlete. Integrating too much deliberate practice too soon could be detrimental for athletes who are not far enough advanced in their development for this more intense form of training.

A simple exercise for identifying different forms of practice

Given the stage-based recommendations we have highlighted above, it is important to be able to identify activities that typify the characteristics of deliberate play (i.e., high participant engagement and control, low structure, and inherent enjoyment) and deliberate practice (i.e., high physical and mental effort; high relevance to performance improvement). Table 2.1 provides a framework for identifying different types of practice throughout an athlete's development.

Each type of training/practice can be considered on the different qualities that determine whether it is best described as deliberate play, deliberate practice, or other forms of training (i.e., such as those associated with maintaining existing performance). The various types of training an athlete experiences can be rated on each quality in Table 2.1 using a simple scale such as from 0 (low) to 10 (high); we have provided some soccer-related activities as examples. For each training activity, consider who is involved and the nature and content of the training, and consider the following questions: How directly involved and active are participants in doing the task or skill? Can participants freely engage and interact with each other and/or a parent or instructor? Can participants start and stop activity involvement voluntarily and can they adapt, or have they adapted, the activity/game and its rules? Do they find the activity immediately enjoyable and satisfying (i.e., lots of smiles on faces during the activity)? To what degree does the activity demand physical (e.g., highly intense repeated sprinting) and mental effort (i.e., attentive concentration or problem solving)? Finally, to what degree do you think the activity is likely to lead to an *immediate* improvement in skill or performance?

In interpreting the ratings for each activity, we need to be mindful of the age and stage of development of the participants, as this will influence whether an activity is developmentally appropriate relative to the features of deliberate play and practice. For instance, related to our soccer examples, the first activity, with its high scores on all qualities except for "relevance for immediate improvement" and "mental effort," describes an activity that adheres well to the characteristics of deliberate play. The second suggests an activity that does not reflect the qualities of either deliberate play or deliberate practice, and the third illustrates an activity scoring high on characteristics of deliberate practice.

Table 2.1 Coach guide for determining differences between types of practice

Activity description	On a scale of 1 (low) to 10 (high), what is the level of this in the activity?						
	Active participation	Interaction between participants	Participant control	Inherent enjoyment	Physical effort	Mental effort	Relevance to immediate improvement
Example 1: 6- to 8-year-olds playing backyard adapted game with mini soccer ball	9	9	9	9	9	6	2
Example 2: 11- to 13-year-olds recreational level playing 11-a-side soccer game, under coach supervision	5	5	3	6	8	8	5
Example 3: 18-year-old representative players, rehearsing counter-attack strategy in preparation for an opponent, under coach supervision	5	5	2	3	7	8	9

Based on the needs of participants as they move through development, it will be important to identify, and actively remove or reduce, involvement in activities that are rated consistently low (i.e., 1–3) across feature characteristics at a given stage. Such activities may have little value for participants, even though they may be beneficial at other stages of development. Moreover, activities rated high on one or two characteristics of deliberate play or practice but with one or two characteristics in the mid-range (i.e., 5 or 6), should be reconsidered to determine how the structure of the activity can be adapted to better adhere to the tenets of deliberate play or practice. For example, if deliberate play characteristics are more important for the athlete at this stage of development, then enhancing participant activity time on the task, participant interaction, control, and/or enjoyment will be necessary. Finally, it is important to recognize the subjective nature and variability in scoring and assessing activities. Ratings are likely to vary according to personal perceptions, the activity being observed, and the broader context in which it occurs, as well as the participants within them. If there are multiple coaches and trainers working with a team or group of athletes, it is possible that ratings will be different from one coach to the next. Obtaining ratings from various perspectives (i.e., senior coach, parent, athletes) may help in more reliably identifying training activities deemed appropriate for continued performance progression. Despite these limitations, this simple exercise may be valuable for providing a way to identify and reinforce the most developmentally appropriate training, ensuring optimal training activity for those seeking to continually improve skills and performance.

CONCLUDING REMARKS

As we have noted in the sections above, the general position of books such as those noted in the introduction to this chapter (i.e., that "talent" does not exist or is of minimal importance in athlete development) is not supported by the evidence – at least, the evidence collected to date. A more likely conclusion is that athlete development is the end-result of an enormously complex process of interacting genetic and experiential factors. Regardless of whether or not the theory of deliberate practice stands the test of time and scientific scrutiny, the benefit of these books is that they have brought attention to factors, such as the quality of training, that are actually under the control of the progressive coach and athlete. Athletes cannot do much to change their genetic raw material, but they can improve the delivery of appropriate training at the appropriate time. Although simple in principle, in reality this will require careful attention to how an athlete's day-to-day training links to long-term skill acquisition. Furthermore, successful long-term athlete development will require careful connections between coaches at all levels of competition, across the stages of athlete development (see Chapter 6).

My experience of coaching rugby for the last 25 years or so has meant that I have seen many generations of players emerge. In my opinion, I think the current generation of players is generally not as skilled as previous generations. Obviously there are many reasons for this situation, including the amount of competition from other sports to secure the best talent. However, I think the lack of "deliberate play," as the authors put it, is a key factor. Similarly, I think specializing too early is also limiting the skill development of our younger generation in team sports.

Thinking back to my own playing days, it was not uncommon for me and many others to play an organized cricket match where I would have my bat in the morning, then take off to play in a rugby trial game, and then come back to the field for my cricket team in the afternoon. As a result, I was always thinking about the sports I was involved in. Whether I was aware of it or not, I was probably transferring things I learned from one sport to the other. When coaching, I can clearly pick out those players who have played a variety of sports growing up relative to those who have predominantly specialized in rugby. A key difference is that those who have played lots of sports are usually more tactically astute.

How much play and practice?

I think it is critical that it is play before practice and not the other way around. As detailed in the chapter, if you play a sport for a period of time you start to develop a motivation to want to play it better, which then directs you down the path of more specific practice. This passion for self-improvement is not forced on you from the coach but something developed by the player out of their experiences. This process makes sense to me, rather than starting out with specific practice and perhaps never really developing a passion for the game.

It is logical to me that there should be a progression from play to practice. Primary school children should be exposed to more play and less formal practice. Then, as they get to secondary school at around 12–13 years of age, a format of two specific practice sessions and two play sessions could occur. Finally, as they hit 15–16 years of age, they would then be training and playing competitive games regularly. The play element would still exist outside the formal training and competition times because of the internal motivation the players have developed to want to get better at their sport.

In Australia, the summer–winter program of sports provides an excellent framework to play a number of sports and strike a good balance between play and practice. For me, as I mentioned before, it was cricket and rugby. Summer meant playing cricket. Usually there would be lots of deliberate play after school with others in the neighborhood, and then there would be club or school training to attend and a game to play on the weekend. This would continue for four or five months. Then winter would arrive and rugby would commence; we would play touch footy in school physical education and at every lunch break. In addition to the deliberate play we would attend club training and again play a weekend game. Looking back, I think the fact that the seasons resulted in switching from one sport to another meant I never got bored with the one sport and was always happy to play and practice as much as possible.

One of the interesting facets of being an internationally experienced coach is the opportunity to compare and contrast different countries' cultures and systems. Relative to the Australian system, Japanese players start playing rugby anywhere from 4 to 16 years of age, and practice is never usually shorter than three hours every day and is mostly drill-based. For instance, the current half-back for our national team spent three years in secondary school training four hours every day. The first hour and a half involved a running pass drill in lines of four, and then another hour and a half of positional "units" practice. This was followed by one hour of contact fitness. The same menu was repeated every day. The players only think about how they can survive the session and not get berated by the coach. There is zero deliberate practice. This process then continues for another four years at university, during which time the players, not surprisingly, lose their love of rugby and do not improve their skill level. The proof is in the pudding. No Japanese player has ever played at the highest level of professional rugby in Europe or the southern hemisphere. Interestingly, in baseball and soccer, Japan produce world-class players.

The modern era

Back in Australia, from what I am told, currently many school children do not play any sports during recess or lunch breaks. On occasion, even if the children want to play sport, the schools – for policy (insurance) reasons – ban games such as touch rugby or British Bulldogs (a physical tag game). Similarly, as the students get older and need to be exposed to more competitive play, the school calendar for organized competition is very brief. School rugby teams may play seven matches in a school season. Hence they train, train, train, with only a little competition and deliberate play. Incidentally, much of this training is based around winning the inter-school competition, meaning players are locked into playing positions and roles based on their current playing status (mainly decided by their physical stature). Although they may win the school "A-grade" competition, this approach stifles their overall skill development, producing players with a limited set of skills.

Providing enough competitive play as players get to 16 years of age or older can still be a problem. We need to have our players contextualize what it is they are learning in training into a game format. Unfortunately, players typically train more than they play. I see the benefits of playing more competitive games in other sports. For instance, Australian cricketers travel to England for the Australian winter to compete in the county cricket competitions. While the competitions may not be as testing as the Australian equivalent, the sheer volume of competitive play allows the players to get valuable repetition in a game context. When I relate this Australian perspective to my Japanese experience there are some commonalities and differences, as you would expect. Having first coached in Japan in 1996, and now again since 2010, I see many changes in the rugby here. Players are fitter and faster but no more skillful. It reminds me of the old 10,000 hours of practice story; everyone drives more than 10,000 hours but few of us become better drivers – because there is a lack of deliberate practice.

Creativity is another area where I have seen a decline in modern-day players. I attribute the lack of deliberate play as one of the reasons for this decline. Play fosters inquisitiveness to learn and develop new skills. For instance, "how can I bend this pass around that tree?" or "how can I dodge my mate from next door when playing one-on-one rugby in a narrow backyard?" A lack of creativity appears in all sorts of situations at the elite level. Rarely do players initiate their own warm-up with a ball. They have to be told by coaching staff to get under way. In past generations players would arrive early to simply throw the ball around before the formal training session began. A lack of creativity means we have fewer players with the decision-making skills required to win games of rugby.

In Japan, the lack of deliberate practice, implicit coaching, and games at training produces Japanese players who struggle to make decisions quickly and whose skill level is impaired by the lack of rigorous, well structured training. They tend to play by rote learning, playing what they think they should play rather than what the situation requires. Although the above snapshot of Japanese rugby seems all doom and gloom there is an upside. I was able to take my club team (Suntory) from having won one championship in nine years to winning three trophies in two years essentially by training the players through a game-based approach. Within this was an emphasis on implicit coaching and injecting some love! The level of deliberate practice increased enormously as the players got their love back for the game. I have never seen a team improve so quickly. So, through a game-based approach that encouraged learning, formerly "wooden" players came alive.

A message to other coaches

I found this chapter to be particularly relevant to those coaching at the youth development level. At this level we seem to want to specialize our players too early and the information in this chapter provides us with some good evidence not to specialize too soon. Importantly, we may have to create organized practice sessions to simply provide deliberate play opportunities to the players. This sounds illogical but, until the players get back to discovering and playing the game for themselves, we need to make up this shortfall in school and club settings on their behalf.

KEY READING

Baker, J., Cobley, S., and Schorer, J. (eds.) (2012) *Talent Identification and Development in Sport: International Perspectives*. New York: Routledge.

Baker, J. and Côté, J. (2006) 'Shifting training requirements during athlete development: the relationship among deliberate practice, deliberate play and other sport involvement in the acquisition of sport expertise', in Hackfort, D. and Tenenbaum, G. (eds.) *Essential processes for attaining peak performance*. Germany: Meyer and Meyer, pp. 93–110.

Baker, J., Côté, J., and Abernethy, B. (2003) 'Learning from the experts: Practice activities of expert decision-makers in sport', *Research Quarterly for Exercise and Sport*, 74: 342–347.

Baker, J. and Davids, K. (2007) 'Nature, nurture and sports performance' (Special Issue), *International Journal of Sport Psychology*, 38: 1–143.

Côté, J., Baker, J., and Abernethy, B. (2007) 'Practice and play in the development of sport expertise', in Tenenbaum, G. and Eklund, R.C. (eds.) *Handbook of Sport Psychology*. Hoboken, NJ: John Wiley & Sons, pp. 184–202.

Deakin, J. and Cobley, S. (2003) 'A search for deliberate practice in figure skating and volleyball', in Starkes, J. and Ericsson, K.A. (eds.) *Expert Performance in Sport: Advances in Research on Sport Expertise*. Champaign, IL: Human Kinetics, pp. 115–136.

Ericsson, K.A. (1996) *The Road to Excellence: The Acquisition of Expert Performance in the Arts and Sciences, Sports and Games*. Mahwah, NJ: Erlbaum.

Ericsson, K.A., Krampe, R.T., and Tesch-Römer, C. (1993) 'The role of deliberate practice in the acquisition of expert performance', *Psychological Review*, 100: 363–406.

Greco, P., Memmert, D., and Morales, J.C.P. (2010) 'The effect of deliberate play on tactical performance in basketball', *Perceptual and Motor Skills*, 110: 849–856.

Starkes, J.L. (2000) 'The road to expertise: Is practice the only determinant?', *International Journal of Sport Psychology*, 31: 431–451.

CHAPTER 3

HOW GOOD ARE WE AT PREDICTING ATHLETES' FUTURES?

JÖRG SCHORER AND MARIJE T. ELFERINK-GEMSER

In medieval times, common people as well as lords and kings believed that augurs and seers were able to tell us the future through the use of numerology, palm reading or crystal balls. Although these practices have been discounted, predicting the future is still widely used in many domains, perhaps none so widely as sport. Predicting an athlete's future performance is largely based on the idea of a talent formula, hypothetically grounded in pure scientific evidence and consisting of a number of predictors. Although this approach has increased our knowledge of what might distinguish highly talented athletes from their less skilled counterparts, our knowledge regarding how to predict future success in sport is rather limited.

Two examples from North American basketball nicely illustrate our limits in this area. During his sophomore year, Michael Jordan tried out for the varsity team of the Emsley A. Laney High School in Wilmington, but at 5 foot 11 inches (180 cm) was considered too small to play at this level and was directed to the junior varsity team. He went on to win six National Basketball Association (NBA) championships with the Chicago Bulls, five Most Valuable Player awards during the season and six during the play-offs, and is considered by many to be one of the greatest basketball players in the history of the game. Conversely, one could reasonably propose that predicting performance in the NBA from the sophomore year of high school is difficult; however, a more recent example shows that predicting performance from one year to the next is also complex. Prior to the 2011–2012 season, Jeremy Lin seemed to have no hopeful future in the NBA as a playmaker. He came from a college not recognized for its basketball brilliance (Harvard) and seemed destined to spend his career with the New York Knicks in a supportive role. However, thanks to the right confluence of circumstances – most would say it was because his coach had no other options – he played and performed beyond anyone's expectations (except his own perhaps). As a result, "Linsanity" started and he became a star. For the Knicks, he additionally became a bargain; because most general managers did not believe he had the potential to make an impact on the NBA, he was not even chosen in the NBA draft.

WHAT DOES THE RESEARCH TELL US?

Are these outstanding cases rare or are those responsible for identifying "talent" in sports really so poor at predicting future success in their domain? Do sport scientists have better approaches to this problem? This latter question is what we critically examine in this chapter. First, we try to define what talent is. Second, we focus on the process of talent development. Then we present a list of potential predictors identified in talent research followed by some discussion of the time frames over which these predictors have been evaluated to get an idea about how long we might confidently use them. Finally, we highlight some of the problems we have identified in our talent selection systems. These research topics are followed by recommendations or ideas for the practitioners that might help improve our skill at predicting future success in sports.

Talent definitions

An important first step in understanding the strengths and limitations of current understanding of talent identification and development is having a clear definition of what talent is. Whereas some researchers dismiss the idea of talent (see Chapter 2), and most teachers and coaches say they can see talent once it emerges, the definition of a "talent" is more complex. According to *Webster's English Dictionary*, "talent" is any innate or special aptitude. The *New Penguin Thesaurus* sees talent as "gift, endowment, faculty, flair, aptitude, feel, knack, turn, bent, gorte, genius, aptness, ability, capacity, skill, and/or strength." In most sports, athletes are considered talented if they perform better than most of their peers during training and competition and have the potential to reach the elite level. In line with this, a leading researcher in the field of giftedness and talent, Françoys Gagné (2004) defines talent as the "outstanding mastery of systematically developed abilities (or skills) and knowledge in at least one field of human activity to a degree that places an individual among the top 10 percent of age peers who are or have been active in that field or fields." If a more statistical line of reasoning is administered for these outliers then their performance should be two to three standard deviations away from average performers, which is within the top 5 percent.

Usual practice in sport is that the best 12-year-olds, for example, are put together in a youth selection team for U13 players (i.e., under 13 years of age). It is important to acknowledge, however, that there is no guarantee that the best 12-year-old will be the best athlete at later ages. One important feature of talent development is that the best predictors of initial task performance are usually not the same as the best determinants of final task performance; that is, what distinguishes a person early in their training is not what distinguishes experts from mere mortals. Importantly, to reach the elite level, a talented athlete also needs the potential to develop. Therefore, in sports science, the "identification of talent" typically refers to the process of recognizing current participants with the potential to become elite players, not just the best players of the moment. It entails predicting performance over various periods of time by measuring physical, physiological, and sociological attributes as well as technical and tactical skills, either alone or in combination. Winfried Joch, a retired talent researcher from Münster, Germany, expanded the largely static talent definition by including a dynamic element. The static component of Joch's definition sees the talented athlete as one who has (1) the disposition to perform well, (2) the motivation to perform well, (3) the social environment that enables them to perform well, and (4) current results that are outstanding to others in their respective age group. However, in his talent definition, he extends the definition by highlighting the changes an athlete is able to fulfill over a certain amount of time. This dynamic component reflects athletes who (1) develop actively, (2) are in an active pedagogical accompanied change process, and (3) are trained intentionally for later peak performance. All of these components have to come together to reflect a "talent," someone who is already good but has the potential to become better. This definition illustrates nicely the importance of the developmental factor in identifying and developing sport talents.

TALENT DEVELOPMENT

One way to shed some light on this paradigm is to track the development of young athletes over time. Many factors influence this development, making it a complex process to follow. The development process can be divided into several stages. In the first stage, the performers are untrained and the individuals who differ from the norm in a positive way are "gifted" with natural abilities to perform better than their age peers. In Gagné's *Differentiated Model of Giftedness and Talent*, "giftedness" refers to the possession and use of untrained and spontaneously expressed natural abilities in at least one domain to a degree that places an individual at least among the top 10 percent of age peers. In sport science, the discovery of potential performers who are currently not involved in a sport is known as "detection." In the second stage, the performers start to participate in sports and develop skills while training. The term "talent" appears in a second stage of development and is used for those individuals who differ from their age peers in development of their abilities. According to Gagné, there is no direct bilateral relationship between gift domains and talent fields. Depending on the field of activity, a natural ability can express itself in many different ways. For example, intelligence can be modeled into the scientific reasoning of a physician but also into the game analysis of a chess player or the strategic planning of an elite soccer player. Yet some occupational fields are associated more directly with specific ability domains. For instance, it is intuitively logical that sport skills are built on the foundations of motor abilities. In the last stage, elite players can be distinguished because they have fully developed their abilities to an outstanding level, which places them among the best in the world.

RECENT APPROACHES TO TALENT SELECTION

In cases where the investments in time are long, such as in the road to expertise in sports, it is important to commit facilities and resources effectively. A rule of the thumb is that at least 10 years or 10,000 hours of deliberate practice is needed to achieve expertise in any domain (see Chapter 2). With a good system of talent identification, money and time can be devoted to those talented athletes who are most likely to be successful, thereby reducing the failure or attrition rate. There are several approaches to identifying potential talent predictors. The first looks at the natural abilities of a person as an indicator of future success, similar to the way Boris Becker and Steffi Graf were identified and developed. Their talent selection was based on performance on tests of general abilities such as speed or coordination. The second approach was inspired by expertise research (as described throughout this book) and compares experts to near-experts and novices to identify skills that differentiate between performance levels. These skills can then be tested during talent selections in the hope that they will differentiate between talented and less-talented athletes in phase two of the developmental process. The third approach focuses on this second phase, during which talented athletes are invited in selection teams to further develop their skills towards expertise. Comparisons are then made within the group of selected athletes to identify those with the potential to ultimately reach the top.

Not surprisingly, in sport the underlying components of expertise have been found to be not only physical in nature but also to include sport-specific technical and tactical aspects, as well as motivation. Talented athletes possess multi-dimensional performance characteristics that enable them to perform well in their sport and, as mentioned earlier, they constantly need to develop and improve on these characteristics over time. These qualities can be divided into anthropometric, physiological, technical, tactical, and psychological skills. Depending on the sport, anthropometric characteristics such as height and weight are important for an athlete's performance. For example, if you are tall, you have an advantage in basketball, whereas the opposite is true for gymnastics.

The same holds for the other categories of performance characteristics, including physiological characteristics such as anaerobic (e.g., sprint) and aerobic endurance capacities, technical (e.g., dribbling, passing) and tactical skills, as well as psychological qualities (e.g., being goal oriented and self-regulated). Our research at the University of Groningen has shown that players' technical and tactical skills, and the interplay between those skills, are highly relevant and related to performance in elite soccer and field hockey. Tactical skills are not just about knowing what the right action in a certain situation is (i.e., "declarative knowledge"); even more important is performing that right action at the right moment (i.e., "positioning and deciding"). Other research groups have shown that significant proportions of variance in expert performance can be predicted by visual/perceptual skills and sport-specific cognitive skills using tasks that involve shot prediction, decision accuracy, tactical solutions, and recall of game information.

To determine the relationship between multi-dimensional performance characteristics and the performance level in talented youth field hockey players, a longitudinal study with talented Dutch youth players was carried out measuring anthropometric, physiological, technical, tactical, and psychological characteristics. All talented players were part of a prestigious national talent development program of a field hockey club and were playing at the highest level for their age category in the Netherlands. As part of this program, they received extra training sessions from highly qualified trainers and had the opportunity to compete with and against highly skilled peers. Elite players were also selected by the Royal Dutch Field Hockey Association (KNHB) to represent their district on several occasions. When compared with those of the same age at a regional level, who had experience in field hockey but were not identified as "talented," the talented players scored better on all performance characteristics. When a comparison was made within a group of talented players, elite players outscored sub-elite players on certain aspects of performance characteristics only. In some performance characteristics, such as their sprinting abilities, elites were already better than sub-elites by the age of 12 and remained better, whereas in other characteristics, such as their interval endurance capacity, elites had a faster development.

Results also showed that the elite youth players scored better than the sub-elite youth players on technical (dribble performance in a peak and repeated shuttle run), tactical (general tactics; tactics for possession and non-possession of the ball), and psychological variables (motivation). The most discriminating variables were tactics for possession of the ball, motivation and performance in a slalom dribble. In addition, age discriminated between both performance groups, indicating that the elite youth players were younger than the sub-elite players. This suggests that the better players needed less time to improve their performance characteristics.

This finding was confirmed through longitudinal analysis, which followed these field hockey players for three years. Again, elite players scored better than sub-elite players on technical and tactical variables. Female elite youth players also scored better on interval endurance capacity, motivation, and confidence. Future elite players seemed to excel in tactical skills by the age of 14. Further, they stood out in specific technical skills and over time developed these, together with endurance capacity, to a greater level than sub-elite youth players. During adolescence, both

34

male and female elite youth players had a more promising development pattern for interval endurance capacity than sub-elite youth players. Elite players also had a lower percentage of body fat, participated more in additional training, and scored higher on motivation than sub-elite players. Similar results were found for talented soccer players.

The results above are in line with studies showing that successful athletes get more from their practice sessions when habitually performing similar amounts of practice and, as a consequence, are better able to improve their performance. A possible explanation is that talented soccer players score higher on aspects of self-regulation of learning, especially on reflection and effort, than non-elite youth soccer players. This means that they may be more aware of their strong and weak points and more willing to exert effort in training and during games. As a consequence, they improve themselves to a greater extent. Aspects of self-regulation of learning are not sport-specific; instead these are domain-general qualities and as such can be applied to any domain in which a person wants to get the best out of themself. A line of research supporting this idea comes from Chris Visscher and Laura Jonker from the University of Groningen, which has repeatedly shown that talented athletes are not only very good in their sport but high achievers in school as well. One of the proposed mechanisms underpinning these effects is their high level of self-regulation of learning. To sum up, apart from more sport-specific performance characteristics, research has shown that elite youth athletes distinguish themselves from their less successful counterparts by domain-general performance characteristics, such as their self-regulation of learning. One has to keep in mind, however, that all results of the above-described studies are based on comparisons between groups of players (that is, between elite and sub-elite), whereas within each group a variety of developmental pathways can be observed. This makes it a challenge to apply the results from scientific studies to individual athletes; however, we attempt to provide some practical advice in the next section.

THEORY INTO PRACTICE

From a practical point of view, the main flaw in our recent analyses is that we look mostly at statistics based on the average values of a group of athletes, while the main aim of an elite development system is to look for *the* exceptional athlete. In talent selection systems, sum scores of varying tests or observations are often used to make decisions regarding who should get into, or continue in, the talent development system. While these are generally good strategies, they might result in the loss of athletes who have an exceptional skill in one of the areas but not in others. Current trends in elite sport show that many exceptional athletes have something special about them that differentiates them from the sub-elite in their sport. It might be the special touch of John McEnroe, the technical skills of Lionel Messi, or the anticipation of Jan-Ove Waldner. Our current knowledge of statistical analyses does not really allow us to look for those truly exceptional performers. Therefore, we recommend coaches look out for those exceptional skills that could identify a particularly special athlete.

These problems become even more significant once we look at how good and how repeatable those mean analyses are. A recent study by Joe Baker and his colleagues at York University, Toronto, nicely shows that even short-term predictions in professional sports are relatively poor. They investigated the relationship between career performance (as measured by games played) and draft rounds of players enrolled into the National Football League, National Hockey League, National Basketball League, and Major League Baseball. Although they found some expected trends, such as a high number of games played by athletes from the early draft rounds, the overall amount of variance accounted for was less than 17 percent, which can be considered relatively low. This would suggest that traditional approaches to drafting talent in professional sport are fundamentally flawed, perhaps highlighting why the success story recently depicted in the movie *Moneyball* (based on Michael Lewis's book) is so intriguing.

Since the typical timeline between draft and professional debut is a couple of years, the Baker study examined only short-term prediction; if we look at long-term prediction the findings are even more scarce. A recent study by our research team investigated the validity of predictions from national and regional coaches for female handball players. The study compared coaching decisions made during a talent selection camp in 2001 with where players ultimately ended up in 2011. The national and regional coaches had an accuracy rate of between 75 and 80 percent and, although this seems to be a pretty good prediction, it was not appreciably different from a random choice prediction in which all players were classified as "non-talented." The more interesting element of this study came later when short clips of six to eight minutes from each of the 10 games played at the 2001 talent selection camp were shown to current handball players and non-players, who were then asked whom they would consider as "talented." Their predictions were almost as good as those made by the national coaches. Considering that the coaches actually had the chance to influence the later performance of the athletes because they could have chosen them for talent development systems, these results again highlight how difficult accurate predictions are.

Pick your poison: potential errors in talent predictions

After identifying problems with current approaches to talent identification and prediction from a theoretical point of view, evidence-based approaches to talent selection and development should still be part of a balanced athlete development system. The main step within this system should be to determine what kinds of errors are acceptable and which ones should be avoided. In talent selection, there are four possible outcomes:

1 deselect an athlete who will not make it to a top level (correct classification);
2 deselect an athlete who will make it to the top level (type II error);
3 select an athlete who will not make it (type I error);
4 select an athlete who will make it to the top level (correct classification).

The first and fourth outcomes are, of course, desirable, but, from the studies described above, we know this is difficult to achieve. So the main question is: which kind of error is the most tolerable? At first glance, it would seem that case 3 is the most acceptable, because all athletes would be developed. However, this is very expensive, the best coaching would not be available for the best athletes, and, given the high amount of training necessary to become an expert, many kids would devote their time and effort to trying to become someone they could not become. After more consideration, case 2 might be a better option but, again, this may lead to those with high potential not being developed, resulting in the under-utilization of available talent – a costly outcome, particularly if the pool of potential high achievers is not very large. A final element we cannot currently answer is: what is the criterion for measuring success? Although 100 percent accuracy is obviously unattainable, coaches, trainers, and administrators should have a clear expectation regarding what is a reasonable level of acceptable accuracy.

One potential solution is to run talent selection camps every year – or at least as often as possible – but, although this may be optimal, it is also expensive. For all but the most popular professional sports, funding is limited – for many, extremely limited. National talent selections are costly, and sport governing bodies have to decide how much of their money they want to spend on *talent selection* and how much on *talent development*. Because it is normally favorable to spend as much money as possible on talent development, other coaches who see the athletes more often could be utilized to help with talent selection. United States Gymnastics, for example, administers a coach development program during national talent selection to educate coaches on the latest training skills. This program could be used to educate coaches on how to scout talent in their regions, which could improve both the efficiency and effectiveness of regional talent into a national talent development program.

Individual talent profiles as current best practice

One way to apply the results of scientific studies to individual athletes is to make use of reference values for multiple performance tests from several domains (such as physiological, technical, tactical, and psychological) and develop individual profiles based on multiple measurement occasions. In Groningen, we divide talented field hockey and soccer players' scores into three groups, based on quartiles on each performance test. Field hockey and soccer are played at a high level in the Netherlands and the level of performance is recognized internationally.

- Good: they belong to the best 25 percent of talented players in their age category.
- Average: they score 26–75 percent.
- Insufficient: they are in the last quartile (76 percent and higher); that is, belonging to the "least-good" talented athletes on that particular test at that measurement occasion.

In addition, we look at a player's development within a season and over years of development. For example, Table 3.1 presents hypothetical scores of two field hockey players tested at the end of the season. Compared with same-age talented field hockey players, a player scored poorly on tests for sprinting and interval endurance capacity, average on technique tests, and well on tactical as well as

Table 3.1 An U16 field hockey player's hypothetical talent profile at the end of a competitive season

	Best 25%	26–75%	Lowest 25%	Development
Physiological characteristics			x	
Sprint			x	DOWN
Interval endurance capacity			x	
Technical skills		x		
Dribbling	x			UP
Passing			x	
Tactical skills	x			
Declarative knowledge	x			EQUAL
Positioning and deciding	x			
Psychological skills	x			
Goal orientation	x			EQUAL
Self-regulation of learning	x			

Note: In the last column, a player's development is expressed, with EQUAL referring to a position in the same quartile, UP to a position in a higher quartile, and DOWN to a position in a lower quartile compared with the same player's talent profile at the start of the season.

Jörg Schorer and Marije T. Elferink-Gemser

psychological skills. At the start of the season, he scored in the lowest 25 per-cent on the physiological characteristics and during the season he stayed in this performance quartile (in Table 3.1 depicted with EQUAL in the column for devel-opment). On technical skill tests, at the start of the season he scored in the fourth quartile, however, compared with his talented peers, his performance improved to the second quartile at the end of the season, especially on a test for dribbling (in Table 3.1 depicted with UP). His position in the first quartile on tactical and psy-chological skills stayed similar throughout the season. With this talent profile, it is possible to rapidly see a player's performance characteristics and his development over a season.

Each player's profile is discussed among the trainers, coaches, and staff of the club. They decide the relative importance of a player's performance *and* development on each characteristic. For example, player A and player B both play in the same U16 field hockey team; however, only one of them can stay for next year's season because of limited space in the selected team. Both players have a talent profile with one "insufficient," one "average" and two "good" performance characteristics. Player A scored poorly on the physiological characteristics, average on the techni-cal skills, but good on tactical and psychological skills. He developed himself over the season in technical skills, improving from insufficient to average. In contrast, player B scored good on physiological characteristics, as well as technical skills, but poorly on tactical skills and average on psychological skills. Over the season, he continued to be among the best in sprinting, endurance, dribbling, and passing. Nevertheless, he kept making errors and did not seem to understand the game. His goal orientation and self-regulation of learning dropped during the season.

If the club feels it is more capable of improving player A's level of performance by helping him increase his sprinting and interval endurance capacity (taking into account his high motivation and self-regulation of learning) than of improving player B's tactical skills, it can use this information to decide that player B should leave the selection team. On the other hand, based on the same information, it can decide to choose player B if the club is confident about teaching him how to perform the right action at the right moment. The club may, in addition, consider consulting a sport psychologist to work on his psychological skills. In conclusion, this information can help trainers, coaches, and staff make more well-balanced decisions about talent selection, but is also highly relevant for talent identifica-tion and development. For coaches working with talented athletes, we recommend making similar talent profiles based on your own tests. Remember, it is important to consider not only the level of performance at one moment in time but also the development of each player within and across seasons.

Be aware, though, that reference values are not static. As a consequence, they have to be updated regularly. Our Groningen talent studies showed that the performance of current soccer players from a talent development program of a professional soccer club was much higher on a test for the interval endurance capacity than same-age soccer players from the same talent development program 10 years ago. If we were to apply the reference values of five years ago, over half of the players would have been ranked in the first quartile. Therefore, it is important to work with recent reference values. One way to do so is to use your own team as the reference to which all players are compared.

CONCLUDING REMARKS

Returning to our central question – "how good are we at predicting an athlete's future?" – we must admit that, generally, we are not very good. However, it is difficult to determine how good we might get because the problem we face is an ill-defined one. The practical need to select talented athletes for development pathways, along with limited pools of money, coaches, competitions, and so on, does not help the actors in sport systems. However, at the very least, the measurement of a range of components of an athlete's performance has some pedagogical value to coaches and talents alike, because these provide feedback on the current skills of the athlete. They might improve long-term predictions as well, as they might inform us about how we could have predicted future success. Taken together, we have tried to show the strengths and limits of current approaches to predicting future athletic success. Because talent selection is an ill-defined and dynamic problem it is highly likely there is no perfect solution, but increased research in this area will lead to advancement in understanding; however, this is possible only through solid and long-term cooperation between practitioners and researchers.

COACH'S CORNER
John Keogh
Senior Women's Coach, Rowing Canada, Aviron

Background

I remember rowing in Australia back in the early 1990s when one of the female athletes in our squad at the South Australian Institute of Sport was selected by a talent identification process to train at the Australian Institute of Sport in Canberra. This particular athlete was quite new to rowing and was nothing special in terms of her ability to compete with other athletes during workouts on the lake. However, those running the identification program obviously saw the raw talent and I was pleased for her when she received her gold medal at the 1996 Olympic Games rowing regatta.

40

As a coach, my first exposure to talent identification was in a role at British Rowing as Talent Development Coach with the World Class Start talent identification scheme. My job was to find individuals who possessed what we had identified as key attributes for successful rowers: above-average height, strength, and aerobic capacity. Once they were identified, my job was to coach them to become elite athletes capable of winning Olympic gold medals for Great Britain.

Introduction

My first reaction reading this chapter was one of frustration: another academic piece that spends numerous pages discussing the definition of talent, then remarkably draws upon poor examples to help justify a negative response to the question. Michael Jordan, arguably one of the best players to play in the National Basketball Association, was not selected for the varsity team in his sophomore year at college, but he went on to achieve greatness. Jeremy Lin, lucky to get a start with the New York Knicks, suddenly becomes a star when given the opportunity through injury to team-mates.

In order to answer the question with some accuracy we should be looking at examples of successful identification and development programs from around world, both past and present. Ideally, we should also analyze a wide variety of sports with the aim of identifying the common traits in successful programs. That said, having seen the process of talent identification work as an athlete, and most recently as a coach, I think a better question to pose is: why are some national federations or sporting organizations better than others at predicting athletes' futures?

Definitions

How do I define the success of a talent identification and development program? I use – and I would guess that most coaches worldwide do so also – podium performance by which to measure success, or, simply put, medals won at world championships and Olympic Games.

The British Rowing World Class Start (WCS) talent identification scheme is seen by many in rowing circles as one of the more successful identification programs in recent memory. Currently, the senior team includes approximately 12 WCS alumni, who form 25 percent of the team. WCS athletes have won approximately 40 medals at under-23 and senior world championships, and Olympic Games, since the inception of the scheme in 2002.

Overview

- Number of development centers around the United Kingdom: 9.
- Number of full time coaches: approximately 15.
- Number of high-school aged students surveyed to pre-select for testing: 120,000.
- Number selected to undergo the testing protocol: approximately 24,000.

- Number of athletes selected onto the scheme since 2002: approximately 250.

- Number of World Class Start athletes selected to represent Great Britain at the 2012 Olympics: 12.

- Theoretical number of people you need to survey to find one Olympic athlete: 10,000.

- Theoretical number of people you need to test to find one Olympic athlete: 2,000.

Testing regions

The WCS scheme had up to nine dedicated centers spread around the United Kingdom. The location of these centers was strategic: first, they needed to be located in a rowing club for obvious reasons; second, they needed to be surrounded by a large number of schools and school-aged children so that coaches had access to a large population from which to test and identify talent. The outcome of having many centers around the country was that selected athletes could continue to live at home, attend the same school, and attend training sessions without travelling too far in any one direction. The nine centers also provided athletes the flexibility to transfer to other centers as they continued their education.

Coaching structure

Each of the nine centers had a dedicated talent development coach responsible for identifying and developing talent. Typically, these coaches were young and eager to prove themselves within British Rowing. All the coaches underwent a long induction process to ensure compliance with testing and identification protocols. The current success of the program is, in my opinion, directly related to the impact of these coaches on the athletes under their direction. The coaches at this level must possess a strong technical aptitude, an ability to develop a performance culture within the training center, and, most importantly, an ability to excite and challenge athletes in the daily training environment. The structure also included key positions of "Performance Development Coaches." They were responsible for overseeing the continual progression of both coach and athlete across three centers. They reported directly to the manager of the program.

Testing protocol

This part of the program, or of any identification process, is absolutely crucial. Failure to identify the correct athletes will most likely result in the program failing to produce athletes capable of winning Olympic medals. The first step is to identify key performance factors in your sport. In rowing, we test for height and arm span (long levers affect length of stroke), strength (ability to apply force on the blade), and aerobic capacity. The next step is to validate the tests. National team athletes are tested to establish a base line for data comparison. Ensure the tests are quick to perform so large numbers can be tested in a short period. The tests should not be skill specific, such as on a rowing machine, so that you know you are testing for raw talent. This process does work, as we found students with no training history who had similar leg strength to a multiple Olympic champion rower with 15 years of training. That, by my definition, is talent.

Development

The coach–athlete ratio was set at one coach for every six to eight athletes. This allowed the coach the time to focus on teaching new athletes correct skills from day one. The scheme was unashamedly a high-performance program and the athletes trained at a relatively high level for their experience. Of course the volume increased year-on-year as they progressed and developed.

Regular testing camps were held throughout the year and every athlete on the program had a responsibility to attend. Each athlete would complete a series of land- and water-based assessments and their results were ranked against each other and against national targets. Athletes progressed to more demanding tests once they had achieved a certain performance standard. Also, at the camps, athletes participated in a structured education program in areas such as nutrition, recovery strategies, and sports psychology.

A key to ongoing development is how the coach engineers the training environment. It is this competitive environment, with such things as results ranked against world best times, that drives performance and change. It is my experience that this performance-focused daily training environment ignites the fuse of the exceptional talent.

Conclusions

What is apparent to me is that the specialized coaching structure, a proven and validated identification process of selecting talent, and having a performance-oriented daily training environment are the keys to identifying and developing "rough diamonds" into successful athletes. A flaw In any one part of the process or structure will most likely result in disappointing outcomes. The real concern is that these flaws only appear after years of heading down a certain pathway of talent identification and development. In other words, early mistakes will not be fully realized until years of hard work have passed. So, ensure that your program has self-motivated, well-trained coaches, test until you find suitable athletes who meet the selection criteria, and, most importantly, take the time to carefully develop the athletes into world-class performers. Avoid the lure of taking shortcuts with the process and your chances of correctly predicting an athlete's future will improve.

KEY READING

Abbot, A. and Collins, D. (2004) 'Eliminating the dichotomy between theory and practice in talent identification and development: considering the role of psychology', *Journal of Sport Sciences*, 22: 395–408.

Baker, J., Cobley, S., and Schorer, J. (eds.) (2012) *Talent Identification and Development in Sport: International Perspectives*. New York: Routledge.

Bloom, B. (1985) *Developing Talent in Young People*. New York: Ballantine Books.

Elferink-Gemser, M.T., Jordet, G., Coelho-E-Silva, M.J., and Visscher, C. (2011) 'The marvels of elite sports: how to get there?', *British Journal of Sports Medicine*, 45: 683–684.

Ericsson, K.A., Charness, N., Feltovich, P.J., and Hoffman, R.R. (eds.) (2006) *The Cambridge Handbook of Expertise and Expert Performance*. New York: Cambridge University Press.

Fisher, R. and Bailey, R. (2005) *Talent Identification and Development: The Search for Sporting Excellence*. Berlin: International Council of Sport Science and Physical Education (ICSSPE).

Roescher, C.R., Elferink-Gemser, M.T., Huijgen, B.C.H., and Visscher, C. (2009) 'Soccer endurance development in professionals', *International Journal of Sports Medicine*, 31: 174–179.

Schorer, J., Rienhoff, R., Fischer, L., and Baker, J. (under review) 'Talent selection from a decision making perspective – Are simple heuristics the best predictors of athlete potential?'

Starkes, J.L. and Ericsson, K.A. (2003) *Expert Performance in Sports: Advances in Research on Sport Expertise*. Champaign, IL: Human Kinetics.

Jörg Schorer and Marije T. Elferink-Gemser

CHAPTER 4

FUNCTIONAL SPORT EXPERTISE SYSTEMS

JASON GULBIN AND JUANITA WEISSENSTEINER

Talent can emerge from the most unlikely of places and seemingly from innumerable developmental circumstances. For example, you might expect that Australia's stocks of elite swimmers might come from only a handful of key developmental centers, but instead there are more than 50 different pools at any one time incubating elite swimmers. World and Olympic 100-meter hurdles champion Sally Pearson linked up with her current athletics coach when she was 12 years old and together they hatched their plans for success with a partnership that flourishes to this very day. Then there are the athletes successfully switching over to completely new sports relatively late in their careers (i.e., *talent transfer*), and, in the specific case of Australian sportswoman Ellyse Perry, even competing at senior international level in two sports – cricket and football – simultaneously. Professional sporting teams with their big budgets can seemingly import success onto their pitches, courts, and diamonds of the world, whereas local home-grown environments, such as those of the Rift Valley in Kenya or the Växjö Athletics Club in a remote Swedish forest, continue to consistently produce some of the best athletic talent in the world.

Given the incredible array of developmental scenarios leading to expertise, it might appear to be a bit of a stretch to think that it is possible to develop a system that captures this phenomenon. In truth, systemizing expertise by predicting and manufacturing outcomes associated with individual or team brilliance is incredibly challenging. There will always be exceptions to any rule and the potent effects of positive and negative chance events on expertise development can never be timetabled. However, the goal of a system should be to increase the probability of an expertise outcome rather than bank on its certainty. Athletes, coaches, and elite sport agencies may have little control over the final medal outcome, yet they do have tremendous control over the planning and the process which can lead to the increased likelihood of an expertise outcome. Just as a coach or an athlete will emphasize the technique or the process to achieve a particular result, we propose that there is a parallel technique and process at the system level as well.

This chapter presents a holistic approach for increasing the probability of expertise attainment. It explores the dynamic interrelationships that influence development at the individual, sport, and system levels, and proposes a new framework and practical applications to optimize its utility.

WHAT DOES THE RESEARCH TELL US ABOUT PATHWAYS TO EXPERTISE?

In this section, we will first set the scene by reminding ourselves of the complexity and challenge of expertise development. Second, we will examine the popular influential models within the athlete development literature and critique their relative contribution to our collective understanding of this process. Third, we will provide recommendations for an applied, evidence-based, multi-dimensional, and longitudinal framework that can improve our understanding of the nuances of development, with the primary intention of effectively guiding and assisting sports and their system partners – collectively termed the "stakeholders."

Realistic pathways

Understanding, negotiating, and maximizing athlete development is a complex challenge for those working at the sporting front line. For example, it is expected that coaches, in addition to fostering and refining skill acquisition, can correctly interpret and negotiate biological and cognitive maturation and its impact on development and performance, monitor physiological training loads, be sensitive to athlete over-reaching, improve tactical decision making, oversee the timing and negotiation of key developmental transitions (e.g., junior to senior competition levels), and all the while keep their young charges motivated, stimulated, empowered, and committed to achieving sporting excellence.

Added to this, coaches attempting to identify new cohorts of talent have to contend with more prominent deficiencies in the movement literacy of the talent feeding into the high-performance pathway. Increasing economic and socio-contextual constraints are resulting in declining sports participation rates and alternative interests and lifestyle choices. The quantity and quality of Physical Education is disappearing, along with large family backyards, and the precarious connectivity between the participation and elite ends of the developmental spectrum continues to create additional pressures on what is an already vulnerable developmental journey.

Although the pathway to expertise is testing, it is also incredibly diverse. A recent investigation by Gulbin and colleagues examined the developmental trajectories of

46

256 senior Australian elite athletes (including 51 Olympians) from across 27 sports. Results illustrated the incredible variability in pathway progression with a number of complex ascending and descending developmental trajectories described. Even the order and timing of transition between junior elite and senior elite competition levels was extremely diverse. In some instances, athletes regressed one, two, and even three major competition levels in order to ultimately achieve an elite senior status. The common perception that the development pathway from novice to expert follows a relatively predictable and linear ascent was not supported. Furthermore, this study was able to provide evidence that athlete development may even adopt a particular pathway "signature" depending on sport type. For example, athletes in non-*cgs sports* [i.e., those measured in units other than centimeters (c), grams (g), and seconds (s), such as soccer, water polo, hockey, and volleyball], experienced a higher incidence of concurrent junior and senior competition investment (50 percent) in the same calendar year, compared with athletes in *cgs sports* (19 percent) (e.g., canoeing, cycling, rowing, and swimming).

Theoretical pathways

There exists an ever-widening gap between theory and practice due to limitations, inconsistency, and contradictory messages emanating from the athlete developmental literature. It is unsurprising that stakeholders possess and articulate a healthy skepticism regarding the meaningfulness and utility of some of the extant academic research. It is also more than understandable why there can be a tendency to gravitate towards more popular digestible literature such as Daniel Coyle's *Talent Code* and Malcolm Gladwell's *Outliers*, both of which, incidentally, fail to present a balanced perspective regarding the dynamic and multi-dimensional nature of athlete development and sporting expertise. Is it any wonder sporting stakeholders are confused and pathway practitioners remain piqued at the chaos in the brickyard?

A case in point exists between the starkly contrasting approaches to expertise supported by one philosophy of specializing in a sport as early as possible, and the other of diversifying in sports as early as possible and specializing much later. According to Anders Ericsson's construct of "deliberate practice," a monotonic relationship between practice and performance exists where a specific investment of 10 years or 10,000 hours of effortful, not inherently enjoyable, task-specific practice leads to expertise. In line with this thinking, it is proposed that expertise cannot be fast-tracked and early specialization in a single sport is central to expertise. If an athlete commits to a 10-year investment to practice it is assumed through this conviction that they will become an expert. However, the evidence from athlete-centric research to support this theory is far from convincing, with many other investigations showing that expertise can be achieved with far less quantitative investment than 10 years or 10,000 hours.

Contrary to this early specialization approach, Jean Côté's concept of "deliberate play" – a major component of the Developmental Model of Sport Participation (DMSP) – advocates for an early and diversified sporting investment resulting in much later specialization. In addition to reducing athlete dropout and the incidence of repetitive sporting injury, it is thought that this contrasting approach leads to the acquisition of a well-rounded, extensive, and therefore adaptable repertoire of sporting skills from which an athlete can draw and invest in their main sport. However, the DMSP model provides a simplistic and generic depiction of developmental trajectory and it does not address the totality of development. Now, what to do as a parent? Enact the popularized messages based on Anders's theory of single sport specialization or spread the sporting joy more broadly and sign up to Côté's philosophy of engaging in diversified movement experiences and specialize later?

Both of the deliberate practice and deliberate play models feature in Table 4.1 as examples of influential, challenging, yet ultimately imperfect models of expertise development. Three others in their class have also been identified: Istvan Balyi's *Long-Term Athlete Development* (LTAD) model, Françoys Gagné's *Differentiated Model of Giftedness and Talent* (DMGT), and Kristoffer Henriksen's complementary models of *Athletic Talent Development Environment* (ATDE) and *Environmental Success Factors* (ESF).

In consideration of the other models, Gagné's DMGT is essentially multi-dimensional in that it acknowledges the contribution and interaction of intrapersonal, developmental, environmental, and chance factors. It has broad utility for many other domains of expertise; however, its breadth of coverage relative to the sporting environment is limited to what we would describe as the pre-elite and elite levels. For example, the model eloquently characterizes the development of the top 10 percent, yet the formative experiences in leading to this benchmark are not well represented. This is an important feature of the sporting landscape which departs from Gagné's original gifted and talented education-focused model.

Insight offered by Henriksen's complementary models of ATDE and ESF is limited to understanding the features, dynamics, and interrelationships at play within the high-performance environment, specifically the interaction between pre-elite and elite levels. Utilizing a holistic and ecological perspective incorporating a detailed case study approach, Henriksen and colleagues focused on the key environmental features of successful talent development environments specific to distinct cohorts within the sport of sailing (i.e., Danish National 49er sailing team), athletics (i.e., Swedish athletics club IFK Växjö), and canoeing (i.e., Norway's Wang School of Elite Sports kayak team). These included influential others (i.e., family, coaches, managers, peers, experts) and organizations (i.e., school, clubs, the sports federation, educational system, and media). Although this series of in-depth investigations reveals the environmental and supportive influences on athlete development within a small number of sports, the intrapersonal attributes (such as tactical, technical, and psychological skill) of the athlete cohorts remain unknown.

Balyi's LTAD model provides a chronologically prescriptive and generic "one size fits all" model of athlete development which is predicated on maturational and physiological benchmarks. The LTAD model spans the entire athlete pathway from an *Active start* (0–6 years) and *FUNdamental* level (females 6–8 years; males 6–9 years) to *Active for life*, incorporating recreational sporting pursuits and life after sport (retirement and retention). LTAD provides guidelines for the sport practitioner specific to training and competition loads associated with the developmental levels of *Learning to train* (females 8–11 years; males 9–12 years), *Training to train* (females 8–11 years; males 9–12 years), *Training to compete* (females 15–21 years; males 16–*c.*23 years), and *Training to win* (females 18+ years; males 19+ years). Although this model has been widely adopted by national sporting organizations within Canada and the United Kingdom, it has also been widely criticized for its over-prescription and focus on physicality and conditioning, to the detriment of other recognized components of development and performance such as tactical and technical skill.

Although these influential models in Table 4.1 offer helpful insights for sport, they are still essentially sub-set models in their contribution to the understanding of athlete development. Essentially, what is being presented is a segmented view of development. If you like, vanilla ice-cream is being extracted and served from what is categorically rainbow-flavored ice-cream. As a result, it is difficult for the coach, parent, manager, and organization to decipher and translate the vanilla teaser into the full rainbow-flavored experience. Table 4.1 reinforces that these leading models:

- are not always multi-dimensional in their examination of the athletic profile required for exceptional performance, but instead can be uni-dimensional in their focus – examining a factor, attribute, or characteristic in isolation;
- are only applicable to a limited span of the athlete development pathway;
- do not consider the dynamics and interaction of athletic attributes with environmental factors across all levels of the athlete development pathway and associated facilitators of athlete development;
- do not consider the characteristics and requirements of developmental transition, both normative and non-normative in nature;
- are essentially descriptive (do not incorporate a control group within their research design);
- incorporate small and sport-specific samples of participants.

Table 4.1 Popular and influential models related to the development of expertise

Model/construct	Main tenets/core constructs	Discipline origins
Deliberate Practice (Ericsson, Krampe, and Tesch-Römer, 1993)	Expertise is the end product of an extensive amount of deliberate practice: 10,000 hours of goal-oriented, effortful practice that is neither inherently enjoyable nor intrinsically motivating. A monotonic relationship is inferred whereby differences in practice investment equates to differing levels of performance	Psychology
Developmental Model of Sports Participation (DMSP) (Côté, Baker, and Abernethy, 2007)	Recent iteration of model presents three distinct developmental trajectories, i.e., (i) *Sports Sampling* (6–12 years) leading to *recreational* sports participation; (ii) *Sports Sampling* (6–12 years) and *Sports Specialization* (13–15 years) leading to *elite performance*; (iii) *Early Specialization* (6+ years) leading to *elite performance*	Social/ developmental psychology and pedagogy
Long-Term Athlete Development (LTAD) (Balyi et al., 2006)	Recent iteration of model features seven stages, five of which are specific to the athlete development pathway. Advocates the use of measures of physicality to guide practitioners regarding appropriate volumes and ratios of training and competition for each level	Exercise physiology and anatomy
Differentiated Model of Giftedness and Talent (DMGT) (Gagné, 2003)	Details the transformation of "gifts" into "talent" and is inclusive of both innate and developed sporting traits and characteristics. Features three integrated sub-components: activities, investment, and progress, which are influenced by environmental and interpersonal catalysts and chance factors	Psychology and education
Athletic Talent Development Environment model (ATDE) (Henriksen, Stambulova, and Roessler, 2010)	The ATDE provides a framework for examining the dynamics of the micro/macro athletic environment. Complemented by Environmental Success Factors (ESF), i.e., human, material and financial preconditions, everyday activities, organizational culture, and athletic achievement	Ecological psychology

50

Original methodology	Longitudinal coverage of athlete development	Cross-sectional coverage of athlete development	Overview
Qualitative and quantitative case studies (musicians)	Non-elite to elite	Athlete factors only (task-specific practice)	Uni-dimensional examining the factor of practice in isolation from other athlete factors and environmental factors. Conflicting findings in the contemporary sport literature, with some findings not substantiating the construct
Review of the literature; retrospective qualitative data (interviews); retrospective quantitative data specific to play and practice investment	Non-elite to elite	Athlete factors and environmental factors (developmental investment in deliberate play and deliberate practice; coaching and family)	Presents a generic and simplistic depiction of the athlete's developmental pathway featuring broad stages bounded by chronological age ranges. Does not acknowledge the inherent variability of development and its trajectory within and between sports. Based on Canadian and Australian athletes from a relatively small number of select sports
Literature review, observations and anecdotal evidence	Non-elite to elite (and beyond to retirement)	Athlete factors only (morphological and physiological components)	"One model fits all" philosophy which is overly prescriptive. Limited empirical evidence to support and questionable application in the field due to its physiology/conditioning centricity
Review of literature and empirical observations	Limited to pre-elite to elite	Athlete factors and environmental factors (intrapersonal, developmental, and environmental characteristics and chance factors)	Applicability of full model still to be verified fully within a sporting context. Relative contribution of select components to elite performance (i.e., psychological attributes, coaching, chance, etc.) is supported. Applicability restricted to pre-elite to elite spans of athlete development pathway
Review of literature and qualitative data (case studies incorporating interviews, participant observation, and document analyses)	Limited to pre-elite to elite	Environmental factors only (influential others, e.g., coaches, peers, team mates, experts, family; organizations, e.g., clubs, governing sport bodies, media, education, etc.; and cultural setting)	Framework tested within the sports of sailing, athletics, and canoeing but restricted to specific Scandinavian cohorts. Does not incorporate athlete factors and the relative impact of environmental factors and context on these attributes. Applicability restricted to pre-elite to elite spans of athlete development pathway

Advancing the conceptualization of development

As a result of the inherent limitations within the existing literature, knowledge gaps continue to exist, serving only to constrain our collective understanding of athlete development. For instance, we are limited in our understanding of:

- the biopsychosocial requirements at each developmental level across the full span of the athlete development pathway;
- what aligned support is needed for optimal talent development across the entire athlete pathway;
- the facilitators and barriers underpinning successful transition from one developmental level to another;
- the intrinsic and extrinsic factors that need to be considered and negotiated when recruiting and developing sporting talent;
- the characteristics and attributes of world-class performers and the requirements of sustained performance excellence on the world stage.

The athlete development process has been reconceptualized in Figure 4.1 taking into account the current gaps in knowledge and the formative work of our most influential but imperfect models. Figure 4.1, entitled "3D-AD," shows a three-dimensional representation of athlete development and highlights the leading factors (athlete, environmental, system, and chance) modulating this outcome. The 3D-AD model recognizes the combined interaction of these factors, which permeate throughout the entire developmental sequence of the non-elite, pre-elite, and elite phases. In brief, "non-elite" refers to a formative or recreational level of sport participation (e.g., early sporting experiences, local club, or school competition); "pre-elite" refers to those with the potential to become elite, as identified by the relevant sporting benchmark; "elite" refers to those athletes competing internationally at a senior national level of representation. The bottom of Figure 4.1 presents a cross-sectional depiction of the 3D-AD model and connotes the temporal variability in the model's key factors. The extent of this variation will depend upon the sport and the individual.

Featured within the model are seven broad athlete-related factors which have been the focus of much research activity and, within each, it is implicit that sub-factors provide further differentiation and specialization. These include genetics, physiological capacity (e.g., speed, endurance, power, strength), morphology (e.g., anthropometric and biological maturation), psychological attributes (e.g., self-regulation, mental toughness, coping abilities, confidence, self-belief, motivation), sport-specific skills (incorporating perceptual, cognitive, and motor components), practice and competition investment, and socio-developmental background (e.g., family, place of residence, investment in other sports). Despite

52

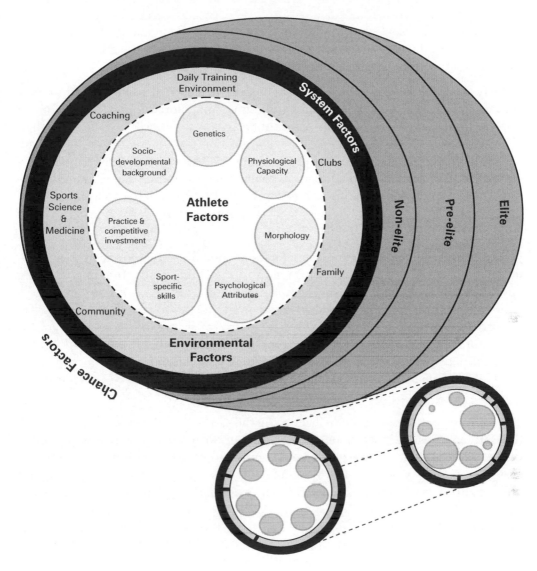

Figure 4.1 The 3D-AD conceptual model of expertise development demonstrating the interplay of the athlete, environmental, system, and chance factors over the full developmental cycle. The bottom schematic presents a cross-sectional depiction of the 3D-AD model and its elements. Note the capacity for changes in their relative weighting and importance over the developmental cycle.

the limitations of the two-dimensional representation of the model, these athlete factors flow completely through the developmental phases with one underlying proviso. The athlete factors do not have an equal impact on development, but are capable of contracting and expanding throughout the developmental phases. For example, the cross-sectional graphics at the bottom of the model represent conceptual "slices" of the athlete factors at different time points and the arbitrary change in their relative weighting or importance to performance.

By way of example, the relative contribution of perceptual, cognitive, and motor skill components are optimally coupled in elite team sport athletes. Similarly, the relative importance of psychological attributes to performance – such as self-belief, self-regulation, mental toughness, and coping ability – increases as an athlete traverses further along the high-performance pathway. Therefore, the relative contribution of each skill component to development – and ultimately to elite performance – will vary depending on the developmental level of the sport participant (i.e., where they are on the developmental continuum) and on the specific sport and sub-discipline they participate in.

Just as the athlete factors extend through development, so too do the environmental factors, which include family, community, coaching, clubs, the daily training environment, and sports science/sports medicine guidance and support. In a similar vein, these co-factors of development are not static contributions but also concertina over the developmental time course. For example, the relative contribution of sporting involvement at a school or formative club level would diminish as an athlete progressed further up the pathway to an elite status. In short, the three-dimensional development cores would show great variability between sports and among the individuals within them.

The athlete and environmental factors in the 3D-AD model generally represent the daily or constant operational components of development. However, there are two more important factors which impact on the optimization of the daily factors: system and chance factors. The system factors represent the strategic, policy, and philosophical decision making by the national sports system, which can greatly affect the degree of targeted investment into the operational elements. For example, in Australia the sports of ice hockey and table tennis receive minimal developmental support because of their lack of popularity, yet for Canadians and Chinese respectively such a system decision would be unfathomable. Similarly, the system decisions will also affect the degree of clinical, research, and sports science support provided to the daily training environment of athletes.

Encapsulating the entire development milieu are the broader chance factors which are essentially beyond the control of the athlete or stakeholder. Chance is a key catalyst in Gagné's DMGT, which translates to all of the positive and negative chance events that might influence development. Chance events may include being born to a particular set of parents, the "luck" of living close to a fantastic coach, or the "bad luck" of sustaining terrible injuries in an accident. Likewise, De Bosscher and co-researchers have also reinforced the notion that macro-level factors – such as geo-political ones – will also shape development. That is, the

54

international elements of geography (water, mountains, population, etc.), politics, and culture (think opportunities for Saudi Arabian women or how a nation values sport) directly impact on the other influential factors. These macro-level factors are also represented by the generic chance factor description, yet share the same unmodifiable qualities.

Beyond concept to application

The 3D-AD "beehive" model brings together a more holistic and multi-dimensional perspective on development. It considers the inherent gaps in the existing literature and the subsequent limit to our current understanding. It is a key reminder and reinforcer to future researchers that we need to be careful that sub-set models are not popularized to such a level that it generates a "cause and effect mentality" in the community (see Chapter 2). It is necessary for researchers to admit and declare that sub-set investigations are not developmental magic bullets and perhaps future publications might come with a "*caveat emptor*" warning: "user beware – it comes with limits!"

Having now presented what we think is an improved conceptual model of development, it is equally salient that we recognize the limitations of our own work. Although we encourage others to "behoove the beehive," a conceptual model such as this is limited in its "user-friendliness" or in its ability to be interpreted and sensibly actioned by sport and its stakeholders. To assist sport and its stakeholders to improve their approaches to expertise development, we have developed a framework that helps with the actual practice of finding and developing champions at the coalface. It is not that coaches or administrators cannot handle the concepts or the theories (although there are some who cannot), but high-performance environments are relentless in their demands and are highly pressurized and time-poor. There can be a limit to the stakeholder's sphere of influence, and then there are the realities of insufficient resourcing and the prioritization of first "getting" the talent ahead of developing it. Competition season runs ever more quickly into pre-season, and the downtime needed to think critically and systematically is compromised. It is completely understandable why the path of least resistance is a well-trodden one. It is simply a survival mechanism.

The application of our thinking around an applied framework is discussed in the next section. Informing such a framework is accrued inductive and deductive evidence whereby observation and experience "in the field" is complemented by accumulated empirical evidence. We believe that such a coordinated and holistic "doing" framework offers great unifying potential for the sport practitioners, stakeholders, and academics serving to address and reduce the current gap between theory and practice.

TRANSLATING THEORY INTO PRACTICE

This section attempts to translate theory into practice by providing a practical method to assist sporting stakeholders construct a more functional development system. Gulbin and his sport practitioner colleagues at the Australian Institute of Sport have recently published their logic behind the need for a more integrated athlete and sport developmental framework. In essence, their FTEM framework is designed to resonate with those at the sporting coalface by aiming to provide a more realistic industry-based view of the development pathway while devising the application strategies to enhance the framework's utility.

FTEM architecture

It is not within the scope of this chapter to re-examine all of the details and nuances of the FTEM framework, so we recommend that you read the original work by Gulbin and his team. For now, the illustration of the FTEM framework is represented in Figure 4.2 and provides a summary of the key architectural elements including:

- the integration of the three key outcomes of sport participation (i.e., an "active lifestyle," "sport participation," and "sport excellence"), with sport excellence our focus here;
- the four broad elements which represent the FTEM acronym: Foundations (F1, F2, and F3); Talent (T1, T2, T3, and T4); Elite (E1 and E2); Mastery (M);
- the incorporation of a "mastery" benchmark as the recalibrated end point of the high-performance pathway, clearly defined as representing T1 through to M;
- the overall connectedness of the talent supply chain, and its points of differentiation;
- a non-prescriptive framework allowing broad user flexibility and adaptability;
- a semi-linear design, permitting all possible movement variations up, down, and across the FTEM framework, including concurrent sports participation at multiple levels.

FTEM elements

Once again it is worth reinforcing that the original research paper should be reviewed in order to better understand the elements of the framework. However, for the purposes of this chapter, the following condensed summary and key phrases defining the respective elements are provided:

56

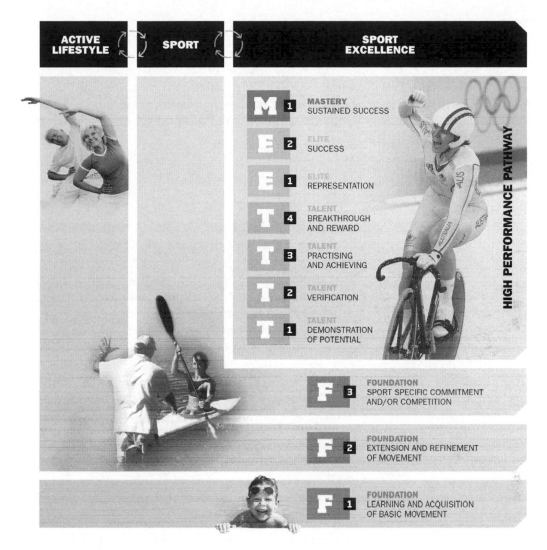

The FTEM framework diagram contains the following labels:

ACTIVE LIFESTYLE · SPORT · SPORT EXCELLENCE

HIGH PERFORMANCE PATHWAY

M 1 MASTERY — SUSTAINED SUCCESS
E 2 ELITE — SUCCESS
E 1 ELITE — REPRESENTATION
T 4 TALENT — BREAKTHROUGH AND REWARD
T 3 TALENT — PRACTISING AND ACHIEVING
T 2 TALENT — VERIFICATION
T 1 TALENT — DEMONSTRATION OF POTENTIAL
F 3 FOUNDATION — SPORT SPECIFIC COMMITMENT AND/OR COMPETITION
F 2 FOUNDATION — EXTENSION AND REFINEMENT OF MOVEMENT
F 1 FOUNDATION — LEARNING AND ACQUISITION OF BASIC MOVEMENT

Figure 4.2 The FTEM framework to assist in the planning, review, and development of expertise systems. Image courtesy of the Australian Sports Commission: http://www.ausport.gov.au

- F1 (*Basic Movement Foundations – BEGIN*). The focus here is on the beginning of very basic movement foundations, such as throwing, kicking, jumping, skipping, and so on.
- F2 (*Extension and Refinement of Movements – EXTEND*). This phase extends and exposes the participant to greater movement challenges and usually involves more professional levels of instruction.

- F3 (*Sport-specific Competition or Commitment – COMPETE*). Movements are now undertaken within the rules and conventions of sport. It manifests as formal competition or self-competition in the instance of personal best pursuits.
- T1 (*Demonstration of Potential – EXPRESS*). Gifted movers emerge at this level and are identified as having the potential for high-performance sport. Entering the high-performance pathway would involve out-performing approximately 90 percent of one's peers.
- T2 (*Talent Confirmation and Verification – CONFIRM*). "Coach's eye" and *in situ* challenges specific to an athlete's self-management, "coachability," and "train-ability" are crucial here to confirm whether initial expressions of potential can be sustained.
- T3 (*Practicing to Achieve – COMMIT*). Athletes are committed to achieving higher levels of sport performance and they practice and compete intensively to reach their goals.
- T4 (*Breakthrough and Reward – ACHIEVE*). Athletes reach a significant break-through performance and are rewarded for their efforts, such as selection in a national age team, or earning a valued sporting scholarship.
- E1 (*Senior National Representation – PERFORM*). Athletes are selected onto the senior national team and compete internationally.
- E2 (*Podium Success at E1 – WIN*). Athletes win medals at peak international competitions.
- M (*Sustained Success at E2 – DOMINATE*). Athletes achieve sustained success at E2 by repeating their wins over multiple high-performance cycles (for more than four years).

Applying FTEM

The FTEM pathway framework is couched in terms that are associated with the progression of athlete skill or performance development. Although it makes sense to focus on the end-user, it would be erroneous to conclude that FTEM is simply an analogue of athlete training volume, intensity, or some other performance sub-component. Therefore it is important to first unpack FTEM's overall intent.

Greatly influencing the development of the FTEM framework are the observations and experiences gleaned from over two decades of applied programs and initiatives incubated within the Australian Institute of Sport (AIS). These could be distilled into a unifying theme called "deliberate programming." This term was coined by Bullock and colleagues, who demonstrated that they were able to identify and then fast-track a novice skeleton athlete into the Olympic Games within a 14-month time frame. It was not deliberate practice in isolation that was responsible for this achievement, but rather the deliberate intent to program specific experiences

58

which would enable rapid development to occur – a hallmark of the AIS. Thus, the strategic and combined layering of sports science and sports medicine, excellent coaching, early and aggressive competition immersion, close program and individual case-management, challenging and enjoyable daily training environments, upward pressure through competitive cohort immersion, and novel qualification and selection strategies collectively typify the multi-dimensional aspect of performance progression central to the FTEM philosophy.

In a broader sense, deliberate programming is the sport-specific version of more classical business-planning methods. Thus, getting the most out of the FTEM framework involves four key approaches. The first step is to establish the *ideal* pathway for a given sport through collective discussions and available evidence (i.e., where would you like to be?). The second step is to undertake a *gap analysis* to assess where the sport currently sits relative to the ideal (i.e., where are we at?). Third, appropriate *actions or interventions* to reduce these gaps should be devised, with the aim of the fourth and final step being to *monitor or review* the progress towards the ideal.

Establishing the ideal

This process begins by asking three simple but deceptively challenging questions repeated for each of the 10 FTEM elements. These self-reflection questions can be applied to the specific sport of interest or to the broader overall sport system. These critical three key questions are:

Q1. What is needed for an athlete to be here?
   At the heart of this first question is the understanding and cataloguing of the biological, psychological, and social elements peculiar to the FTEM level. Collectively, these biopsychosocial aspects equate with the athlete and environmental factors highlighted in Figure 4.1. This type of questioning could be summarized as being *horizontal*, that is, concerned only about each respective FTEM level on its own merit. To illustrate this concept further, early foundational movement experiences are contingent upon modest biological requirements (e.g., little more than healthy functional bodies), but expressing talent at T1 might be contingent upon quite specific biological attributes in some sports (e.g., speed, height, power, strength, endurance). Similarly, non-high-performance club coaches at F3 are likely to need more pedagogical qualities to optimize broad learning outcomes whereas, in contrast, coaches at E1 need far more detailed technical and tactical knowledge. Applying this sequential logic for all elements will generate a clear understanding of what developmental catalysts need to be in place.

Q2. What is needed for an athlete to move?

This second question is focused on facilitating the transition from one FTEM level to a higher one. The philosophy is to plan proactively for sequentially higher levels of sport engagement, rather than passively waiting for it to happen. Therefore, one is encouraged to think *vertically* and to examine transitionary facilitators. Again by way of example, sport participants at T3, who are committed to achieving a high-performance outcome, will be able to achieve a key benchmark performance at T4 (e.g., college or government scholarship, U18 national team selection) only if they are able to meet selection requirements in key selection processes or competitions. Therefore, pre-planning considerations need to be addressed well in advance in order for this important transition to occur. At a lower level of the FTEM pathway, transitioning from F1 to F2 may potentially require a shift in parental "coaching" to a more professional level of movement delivery and feedback (e.g., teachers, specialists). Similarly, the identification of future talents (T1) requires a clear process to be implemented by the sport to facilitate the targeting and recognition of gifted movers at F3 and for the athlete to ensure known markers of potential in their sport are being developed at F3 to achieve the T1 transition.

Q3. How does this level interact with the other levels?

The third line of questioning might be viewed as being *diagonal*, that is, reflecting on how one FTEM level influences any other. These interrelationships may not be well understood and a command of the talent supply chain throughout the FTEM framework will be enhanced with this deeper understanding of the co-factors of development. For example, how important are each of the "Foundation" components (F1, F2, and F3) to achieving elite performances in sport (i.e., E1, E2 and M)? Are athletes who make the senior national team (E1), yet fail to achieve medal success (E2 and M), thwarted in their endeavors because of earlier pathway experiences? Could it be that sustained international sporting success requires creativity, innovation, reinvention, and adaptability – elements potentially fostered at lower levels of the FTEM pathway? Perhaps first-contact club coaches at F3 remain critical in developing confidence or passion for progression and continuation through subsequent FTEM Levels. What impact can a great coaching eye or that of a "super scout" at T2 have on international selection (E1)?

Gap analysis and intervention

The concept here is relatively straightforward. Devise an evaluation tool using a series of probing questions to objectively assess current sport performance against each of the FTEM elements. However, the proviso to this step is that the objective criterion measures reflect the drivers or facilitators of development and are established by that respective sport. That is, the stakeholder "fits out" the framework by loading their specific variables of interest. Therefore, a matrix approach of the development drivers (rows) multiplied by each of the 10 FTEM elements (columns) would provide the ideal gap analysis tool by ensuring that any analysis is deeply layered and methodically addressed. Typical drivers might include themes such as coaching, sports science, research, competition, management, communication, and education. However, other key variables of interest will be highly sport dependent. For example, veterinary care may be a critical driver in the sport of equestrianism; infrastructure becomes vital in the sports of diving and shooting; equipment and technology are key drivers in sports such as sailing and alpine skiing. The bottom line is that the sport should build and refine their driver models. Once the matrix is completed, each driver-by-FTEM level can be evaluated and then the appropriate or prioritized intervention actioned and its impact subsequently measured.

The achievement of a sport (and ultimately its individual or team of athletes) must take into account the broader environment in which it operates. As represented in the 3D-AD model in Figure 4.1, development does not occur in a vacuum and is affected by chance factors, but also by system factors. The influence of the national sports system or the strategic investment and policy decisions have the potential to galvanize the sum of the parts. Therefore, improving the probability of expertise requires optimization of the sport, but also the broader system which has the capacity to support or, regrettably, to hinder.

The FTEM framework can also be utilized to review the performance of the broader national and system elements. In keeping with the wider strategic business-planning principles, the ideal system environment can be evaluated and reviewed against an objective gap analysis process. Necessarily, the questions associated with a gap analysis of a system will be thematically broad rather than narrow and sport specific. Importantly, however, both approaches will go some way to enhancing the probability of a sport expertise outcome.

The suggested approach would be to independently review each of the sports using a standardized review process – or, if you prefer, a common overall pathway health-check. The review would assess each sport's overall FTEM pathway, as well as each of the FTEM sub-components. Weighted scores or other indices of pathway performance can then be calculated. The key to understanding and evaluating the pathway functionality of the system (or nation) is to aggregate the data from the standardized tool to assess common gaps and establish prioritized areas of action.

The aggregation of these system data provides opportunities for governments or elite sport agencies to establish intervention strategies which support sports collectively. For example, if it were identified that there was a shortfall in resources

Table 4.2 An example of an FTEM framework gap analysis and representative intervention solutions at both the sport and system levels

	Identified gap	Sport-level intervention example	System-level intervention example
F1	Limited information, guidelines, and opportunities in relation to parents/carers, etc., encouraging and facilitating early movement experiences	Consideration to develop and market early age-appropriate movement experiences through existing club infrastructure. A commercial enterprise that would offer the community a product that would be generic and appropriate for multiple sports	Development of intra-governmental alliance between Sport, Health, and Education to build a unifying strategy targeting the assistance of parents and child care centers to promote basic movement exploration with pre-school children, supported by a national awareness campaign
F2	Quantity of professional Physical Education instruction in primary schools is very low	Sports to consider offering coaches, athletes or other delivery specialists (e.g., human movement graduates) to help schools with creating challenging, stimulating and enjoyable state of the art movement environments	Lobby Health and Education sectors to improve the numbers of teacher-training places offered at university and to promote the importance of increased movement specialists employed within primary schools
F3	The participant retention rates for those sampling the sport/club for the first time are low	Ensure that individuals who have a role in first contact with children, parents, or older participants possess a skill set that is commensurate with the demographic	Aim to increase more broadly the quantity and quality of coaches within the sporting system. Develop incentives to encourage volunteers to take up coaching or mentoring roles in sport
T1	The quality of emerging talent suitable for high-performance sport is low	Develop strategies and networks to more systematically identify, recognize, and develop the pool of gifted movers within and outside of the sport at the F3 level	Implement national talent identification strategies across multiple ages and sports to aid in a broader awareness of an athlete's potential for high-performance sport in a current or alternative sport
T2	Coaches are selecting talent for teams who subsequently drop out or under-achieve at higher levels	Review coach education throughout the organization to ensure that there is alignment in talent selection diagnostics for the long term (E1) and that relevant biopsychosocial factors are incorporated into their decision making	Elite sport agencies to conduct education and training on behalf of sports and provide education, resources, and appropriate tools to assist them with talent diagnostics

	Challenge		
T3	Highly talented athletes receive little support or direction during their development	Appoint the equivalent of an FTEM athlete pathway manager who is responsible for the overall integrated functioning of the talent supply chain. Gifted movers at F3 who are talent identified and verified at T1 and T2 are case-managed and supported throughout	Establish deeper systems of athlete support using a variety of available resources and agencies. This may include private providers, regional sports academies, specialist sports schools, universities, notable clubs, etc.
T4	Poor conversion rates for the transition of the junior/U23 elite into the senior elite levels of competition	Improve planning and coordination of transition strategies. Ensure athletes are equipped for senior demands in a technical and tactical sense, but also from a self-regulatory and coping perspective	Improve the vertical integration of pre-elite and elite athletes beginning with clearer sport planning expectations and the provision of quarantined resources to support transition through training camps and international competitions
E1	Difficulties converting near success (e.g., fourth or fifth place, finals) into medal success	Post-competition/tour reviews and feedback from athletes, coaches, and managers. Assuming athletes and coaches are suitable, consider whether sports science and medicine provision before and during the tour/competition is adequate	Better planning, coordination, and allocation of system service providers to national sporting organizations and teams
E2	Athlete success brings greater resourcing challenges usually at the expense of other pathway levels and activities	Develop a means-tested "pay-back" scheme whereby any successful athlete who has been the recipient of support understands that a degree of "philanthropy" is required in return	Relieve the financial burden on sport through medal incentive programs or other direct athlete payment schemes using the combined resources of government, Olympic Committee, and sponsors
M	Poor developmental understanding of the life-cycle of the Mastery athlete	Ensure a minimum retrospective assessment of Mastery athletes is conducted with a view to capturing prospective data as athletes progress and transition through the FTEM pathway	Research to be conducted with Mastery athletes from multiple sports to develop a much clearer picture of the biopsychosocial profile and transition requirements throughout FTEM. Goal is to maximize investment by producing more Mastery athletes

supporting the education and training of coaches and athletes in the key development support areas such as strength and conditioning, recovery, nutrition, or sport psychology, then the most efficient response might be to coordinate tools, resources, or alternative servicing models without the duplication of an individual sport's time, effort, and financial resources.

Table 4.2 is an abbreviated example of how the FTEM framework allows for a differentiated gap analysis, and how a bespoke intervention can be applied at the sport and system levels. It should be clear from Table 4.2 that the sport intervention selected is appreciably buttressed by the identification of a system solution as well. In concert, both approaches are necessary to reduce the identified gaps in the athlete and sport developmental pathways.

CONCLUDING REMARKS

The fascination with elite athletes and their developmental stories has clearly not waned, with bookstores full of the biographies and autobiographies of our Mastery-level athletes. It has been two decades since Ericsson's paper advocating that 10,000 hours of practice leads to expertise was first published, yet we have failed to expand upon what is now clearly a superficial account of expertise. With the recent wave of popular books related to athlete development, there may now be a greater pool of unfulfilled researchers, coaches, athletes, and administrators, who have been inspired to look to, and demand more from, the expertise "experts." There is a tremendous opportunity to harness the exponential intellect and activities of the expertise community and to collaborate on more realistic and representative models of development that will ensure that we can move much further in the next 20 years.

Future research efforts should begin with a reinforced and consistent terminology or language of development and the adoption of a model which is more realistic and penetrative and sets a more agreeable tone. With a commitment to longitudinal, prospective research designs featuring a higher level of variable control, we look forward to reducing the gaps in our knowledge about the developmental experience of champions. These longitudinal projects need not be tedious and laborious. Wonderful controlled environments are readily accessible in talent transfer programs, where performance outcomes can be achieved relatively quickly. A "within-squad" setting allows for training environments and other resources to be standardized and, for more uncommon sports, lifetime training can be quantified from day one (see Bullock *et al.*). These improved levels of environmental control will also allow us to obtain a better understanding of the athlete factors.

Finally, let us remind ourselves that it is crucial to engage with those at the coalface to establish a more practical and authentic system of expertise development. This action research approach, encompassing the real life observations and experiences of practitioners living out the models, may very well encourage longer-term commitment to athlete development when there are significant resourcing and employment pressures to deliver in the most immediate high-performance cycle.

COACH'S CORNER

Tricia Heberle
High Performance Director, Hockey Australia

I always try to be open in my thinking and look for alternatives to existing understanding and knowledge, so I was excited to be shown the FTEM and to be able to talk with Jason Gulbin and his team as they presented a variation on my previous experiences of the more traditional Balyi LTAD framework. Although the Balyi framework is easy to understand and provides a long-term view of development, I felt that the FTEM framework was a much more complete model of development that provided a more realistic and flexible fit within our sport.

Initially, Hockey Australia (HA) has used FTEM as a catalyst for challenging our current thinking, for creating discussion and debate, and to assist us in our research in respect of how we develop and then introduce a "whole of sport" Athlete Development Model (ADM). Ultimately, once we have completed our scoping and investigations of what we need to do, I can see the FTEM model being utilized as a foundation for the establishment of our "customized" HA ADM. This remains somewhat in the future but having the model as a starting point, and being able to make use of experts, has allowed us to build more understanding, to create discussion and debate, and to define some of the tasks we need to carry out before we can shape our own framework.

With the exception of a small number of high-profile professional sports, I believe that for many national sporting organizations it remains a challenge to attract, retain, and develop participants. Therefore, for hockey, it is imperative that we are able to provide a sport with all the associated training/competition activities and environments that provide people of all ages and from different backgrounds an activity that they want to be involved in for life. This presents us with great challenges in being able to support people participating in hockey through whatever agenda they may have, be they beginners, social members, veterans, or the elite. Having a strong foundation of understanding for how we run and structure our sport, and what we want to achieve for the betterment of all involved, is critical to hockey remaining contemporary, culturally significant, and a sport of popular choice. We are hopeful that the introduction of an ADM will allow us to lead our sport in a positive manner and to make better decisions around some of the most critical areas, including financial investment, staff skill set, policies/rules/structures specific to junior development, appropriate and effective competition structures, coach education, talent identification, integrated pre-elite and elite development systems, and so on.

We are looking forward to having dialogue and sharing experiences with other sports, using the FTEM framework and language. There is a great opportunity for HA to tap into the insights and experiences of other sports who share similar challenges. We are particularly interested in seeing what range of interventions are being applied and how these may also shape and inform our own practices.

Adam Sachs
High Performance Manager, Gymnastics Australia

My initial reaction to the FTEM model was very positive, primarily because it aligned so well with the structure and pathways in gymnastics but also because it gave a bit more substance (i.e., filled in some gaps) to the LTAD model that we have all been working with for some time. All of the people in gymnastics who have been exposed to FTEM have also responded positively because it fits so nicely with our sport's "levels-based" programs and competitions. The amount of research evidence that sits behind the FTEM model has provided us with the confidence that we should sign up to it, whereas LTAD just left some lingering doubts because the background evidence seemed lacking.

Although gymnastics is one sport, it comprises six or seven disciplines which all have their own unique programs and cultures. In addition, not all of these gymsports are resourced the same way and so, over time, they have developed at different rates and sometimes in different directions from one another. This has led to a massive duplication of effort – lots of "reinventing the wheel" – which in turn has led to Gymnastics Australia (GA) struggling to deliver effective services and support across its gymsports (i.e., business services, events, coach and official education, club development, etc.), particularly as resources become more limited.

In the coming months, GA will be working closely with each of its gymsports to review their current four-year plans and commence preparation of the plans that will guide their development (and GA's support for the same) over the next four years. GA will undertake a gap analysis using the FTEM model as a common framework across gymsports as they progress through this review/planning process. It is anticipated that the FTEM model will help people within each of our gymsports to review their current pathways, programs, and events more comprehensively because they can identify all of the different levels and how they interrelate. It is also expected that, by creating a common language across gymsports, GA can encourage better sharing of information at all levels of, and across, the organization.

Australia's sporting system is incredibly complicated and often disjointed and the delivery of national objectives is often undermined by a lack of integration and alignment

66

(i.e., vertically and horizontally) within the system. I believe that our national sporting system could benefit from, and is ready for, a common framework and language to describe our pathways and how their constituent elements fit together to create a successful and sustainable whole. FTEM can provide this framework, although I would like to see more specific recommendations coming out of the FTEM model (i.e., the "how") which would help our sport with its future pathway planning.

KEY READING

Bailey, R., Collins, D., Ford, P., MacNamara, A., Toms, M., and Pearce, G. (2010) *Participant Development in Sport: An Academic Literature Review*. Commissioned report for Sports Coach UK. Leeds: Sports Coach UK.

Balyi, I., Cardinal, C., Higgs, C., Norris, S., and Way, R. (2006) 'Long-Term Athlete Development – Resource Paper V2', www.canadiansportforlife.ca/sites/default/files/resources/CS4L%20 Resource%20Paper.pdf

Bullock, N., Gulbin, J.P., Martin, D.T., Ross, A., Holland, T., and Marino, F.E. (2009) 'Talent identification and deliberate programming in skeleton: ice novice to winter Olympian in 14 months', *Journal of Sports Sciences*, 27: 397–404.

Côté, J., Baker, J. and Abernethy, B. (2007) 'Practice and play in the development of sport expertise', in Tenenbaum, G. and Eklund, R.C. (eds.) *Handbook of Sport Psychology*. Hoboken, NJ: John Wiley & Sons, pp. 184–202.

De Bosscher, V., De Knop, P., Van Bottenburg, M., and Shibli, S. (2006) 'A conceptual framework for analysing sports policy factors leading to international sporting success', *European Sport Management Quarterly*, 6: 185–215.

Ericsson, K.A., Krampe, R.T., and Tesch-Römer, C. (1993) 'The role of deliberate practice in the acquisition of expert performance', *Psychological Review*, 100: 363–406.

Gagné, F. (2003) 'Transforming Gifts into Talents: The DMGT as a Developmental Theory', in Colangelo, N. and Davis, G.A. (eds.) *Handbook of Gifted Education*. Boston, MA: Allyn and Bacon, pp. 60–74.

Gulbin, J.P., Weissensteiner, J.R., Oldenziel, K.E., and Gagné, F. (2012) 'Patterns of performance development in elite athletes', *European Journal of Sport Sciences*. DOI: 10.1080/17461391.2012.756542

Gulbin, J.P., Croser, M.J., Morley, E.J., and Weissensteiner, J.R. (in press) 'An integrated framework for the optimization of sport and athlete development', *Journal of Sports Sciences*.

Henriksen, K., Stambulova, N., and Roessler, K.K. (2010) 'Holistic approach to athletic talent development environments: a successful sailing milieu', *Psychology of Sport and Exercise*, 11: 212–222.

PART II

EXPERT OFFICIALS AND COACHES

CHAPTER 5

THE SPORT OFFICIAL IN RESEARCH AND PRACTICE

HENNING PLESSNER AND CLARE MACMAHON

> In the name of all the judges and officials, I promise that we shall officiate in these Olympic Games with complete impartiality, respecting and abiding by the rules which govern them in the true spirit of sportsmanship.
>
> (Officials' Olympic Oath since 1972)

Without a doubt, judges, referees, and umpires are an essential component of sport competitions, such as in the Olympic Games. They are responsible for evaluating athlete performances and for enforcing rules. They often have a direct impact on the outcome of a competition, and their decisions can be the center of media attention and public debates, or, at the worst of times, fan, athlete, and coach abuse. Although a great deal of the information in this book can be applied to the official, there are unique aspects of the official's role. Despite this, the bulk of sports science research has not addressed the sport official directly. Whereas a number of early studies focused on stress and the impact of crowd behaviors, recent work acknowledging this role follows the trends in athlete research by (a) assessing the demands of officials, (b) examining characteristics of decisions and the influence of different features on decision making, and (c) tracing the training of elite performers.

In this chapter, we will talk about the research in these three areas. We will show that for some officials physical demands are often a priority which is reflected in their training. We will also show that the research approach to officiating decisions differs from that used for athletes, where officiating decision making often follows a socially driven thinking process. Although factors that influence decisions are sometimes framed as biases, we will show how they are due to the difficulty of the task and simple human nature, and often take place on an unconscious level. Finally, because there is still a great deal of research to be done with officials, we will often ask the questions that remain to be answered. Although there are a variety of different types of sport officials, from the basketball referee to the judge in dressage, the research we will review deals mostly with judges (e.g., gymnastics), referees (e.g., soccer, rugby), and umpires (e.g., baseball).

CLASSIFICATION OF OFFICIALS

In order to address a group as complex as that of the official, we must acknowledge the variety of demands faced by different *types* of officials. These demands will dictate the relative importance of different research questions, findings, and thus training. To this end, we have identified four dimensions which we feel are the key sources of variation between types of officials. These dimensions are: knowledge and rule application, contextual judgment, personality and management, and physical fitness. Of course, we acknowledge that all officials need knowledge and rule application and that physical fitness will always be an asset; however, the volume and complexity of knowledge varies from sport to sport and some officials must remain stationary whereas others must do a great deal of running and sprinting.

As an extension of this differentiation, Figure 5.1 proposes some general *categories* of officials. These categories are based on two major collapsed dimensions: the amount of interaction with athletes on the playing/competition surface and the number of athletes or cues that are being monitored. In interaction with athletes, personality and management become important. In some cases, physical fitness is also highlighted. Examples are the soccer referee and the cricket or baseball umpire. With fewer athletes to monitor, the wrestling mat official and the boxing referee are also examples of this category, labeled as *interactors.* Interactor officials have an impact on the pace of the competition at a micro level, ensuring that the rules and laws are enforced. They are also instrumental in ensuring the safety of the athletes. Most open-sport officials fall under this category.

With little to no interaction with athletes, the gymnastics judge is an example of a *monitor*, who does not determine the pace of the competition (except the head judge who signals the start of a performance and sometimes deals with protests), but observes and assesses the quality of performance in relation to a points system. While monitors most often assess one performer at a time, albeit with the potential for a great number of cues to consider, synchronized swimming judges are an example of monitors who evaluate a relatively larger number of athletes at once. For this type of official, perceptual-cognitive skills become increasingly emphasized. As we will see, the overwhelming demands to process high-speed action may also lead to some characteristic errors.

Finally, we have identified *reactors* as the types of officials who are responsible for only one or two cues and do not largely interact with athletes. An example here is the tennis line judge. The assistant referee in soccer may also straddle the reactor

72

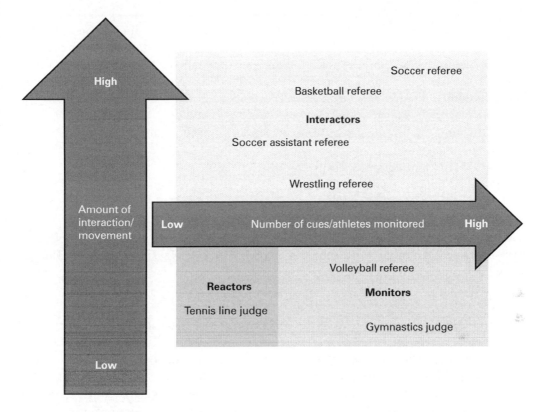

Figure 5.1 Classification of sport officials based on movement, interaction, and perceptual demands.

and interactor categories. Similarly to *monitors*, perceptual-cognitive demands are often highlighted for this group.

Figure 5.1 has illustrated our proposed categories by placing some examples of specific officials approximately along the two dimensions. Clearly, the exact placement of officials in categories can be a matter of discussion; there is not necessarily always an exact spot. Moreover, such a discussion helps us to consider the different demands of different types of officials. This consideration is relevant for training, research, and performance evaluation.

THE DEMANDS AND CHALLENGES OF OFFICIATING

Considering the dimensions we noted in our classifications, there is no doubt that officiating is a demanding role. When we consider examples of some of the best referees and officials, it is obvious that there is a need for a basic level of fitness and a deep knowledge of the rules. However, high-performance officials also display skills that speak to additional demands. The best officials seem to possess *intangible* personal judgment and the ability to manage contests without dominating them. Taken from work in rugby union which identified "cornerstones of performance," the following demands will be addressed in five sections:

1 knowledge and application of the laws or rules of the sport;
2 game management;
3 personality and communication;
4 physical demands and positioning;
5 developing skill and expertise.

This discussion will help us understand the often substantial challenges officials face. In a second step, we will then discuss solutions or ways that these challenges have been addressed or continue to be addressed.

(1) Knowledge and application of the laws or rules of the sport

In many sports, officials make a substantial number of decisions throughout a game or contest. In one study, researchers watched all of the games from the EURO 2000 soccer tournament and counted the number of observable decisions (e.g., when the referee made a signal). The results showed that during the course of a game, the match referee made an average of 137 decisions. With an estimated 60 or so unobservable decisions, such as deciding *not* to blow the whistle, this put the average number of decisions up to around three or four *per minute* during a game.

What makes these decisions even harder is that there is often intentional deception – from the gymnast or skater who tries to cover up a fault, to the catcher in baseball who frames a pitch to get a strike call, or the soccer player who uses a little bit of acting to draw a penalty. Although dealing with athletes and coaches can make or break an official, one of the most demanding aspects of the role is that officials must evaluate intentionally deceptive fast-paced action under time pressure, with very little information. As a result, officials need to gain as much information as possible. In many sports, to get the key information and to deal with deception, officials become aware of typical tactics and practices and counter them by using key cues. As we will see when we discuss physical demands, the need for the best information is why positioning and mechanics are so important and why much of this knowledge is based on personal experiences both as officials and former competitors or coaches.

Even with the best positioning and the best experience and knowledge, there are many situations where task demands overwhelm resources and information is missing. Because of this, officials sometimes fill in the blanks with knowledge derived from general memory structures (e.g., stereotypes), which may lead to systematic error. In addition, there is some evidence that officials' judgments may also be biased by specific memories of athletes' prior performances. For example, such influences have been studied in an impressive series of experiments by Diane M. Ste-Marie and her colleagues. They investigated how the memory of prior encounters with an athlete's performance could influence actual performance judgments. In these experiments, judges first watched a series of gymnasts perform a simple element and decided whether the performance was perfect or flawed. The judges' task was the same in the second phase that followed, except that some of the gymnasts were shown during the second phase with an identical performance as in the first phase (e.g., almost perfect performance both times), and others were shown with the opposite performance (e.g., first perfect and then flawed). It was found that judgments on the second phase were influenced by the performances from the first phase. For example, a perfect performance in the second phase was less likely to be judged as such by the judges if they had seen this athlete with a flawed performance in the first phase. The robustness of these findings led the authors to the conclusion that judges inevitably rely on retrieval of prior episodes from memory. In principle, the only way to avoid these biases would be to prevent judges from seeing the gymnasts perform before a competition. However, given the limited number of top athletes and the limited number of top officials in most sports, this may be an unrealistic proposal. One may also argue that the observed memory effect is a by-product of a functional mechanism that in most situations in fact supports the judgment process and helps officials to detect true performance differences between athletes.

In other judgments, the input or perception is not the problem. It is interpreting the action. This interpretation may be based on factors that are not immediately performance relevant, but are used by officials to help them fill in the gaps of missing information. In figure skating and gymnastics, for example, coaches create an order for their athletes to compete, putting the better skaters or gymnasts at the end. This creates an expectation for the quality of the performance based on this order. Several studies have shown this effect: when the same gymnastics routine or skating program is seen later in the order, it is scored significantly better than when that exact same routine or program was seen as one of the first performances.

These expectations are created not only in the often-criticized *judged* sports. For example, baseball umpires can be influenced by a pitcher's reputation as being either "controlled" or "wild" (no control over his pitches). In several studies, athletes' and teams' reputations, as well as many other sources of expectancies such as stereotypes, have been found to influence judgments of sport performance. Although these influences are mostly treated as unwelcome, again, it should be noted that expectancies which mirror true differences can also improve accuracy in complex judgment tasks.

Another way that officials fill in missing information is to use comparisons. For example, the judgment of an athlete's performance is frequently based on the comparison with other athletes or with prior judgments of other athletes' performances. In principle, comparisons can be very helpful in order to achieve fair judgments that mirror true differences in performance. However, research also suggests that such comparisons can lead to biased judgments. In an experiment by Lysann Damisch and colleagues, experienced gymnastics judges had to evaluate two routines on vault in a sequence. The two athletes were introduced to the judges as belonging either to the same national team or to different teams. Although the second routine was the same in all conditions, half of the judges first saw a better routine whereas the other half first saw a worse routine. It turned out the second gymnast's score was assimilated toward the standard when both gymnasts were introduced as belonging to the same team. The opposite effect occurred when the judges believed the gymnasts belonged to different teams. In other words, when the gymnasts were believed to be from the same team the two routines were scored similarly, but when they were believed to be from different teams the scores were less similar or in contrast.

(2) Game management

The research that we have presented so far refers primarily to officials' goals of accurately applying the rules of the sport or the "enforcement of the laws of the game." However, most sport game referees are also motivated by the goal of game management (i.e., to ensure the flow of the game, to be/appear unbiased, consistent, and impartial, as the Olympic Oath suggests). Accordingly, some authors suggest that the official's task is not only to make accurate decisions but to make so-called "adequate decisions." Accurate decisions are correct according to the laws of the game, whereas adequate decisions take the specifics of the respective game (the context) into account. This concept of game management has recently received some attention in an impressive series of studies by Christian Unkelbach, Daniel Memmert, and colleagues, on so-called "calibration processes." These authors propose that, in general, judges avoid extreme categories in the beginning of a judgment series because extreme judgments reduce their degree of freedom for following judgments. For example, if a gymnastics judge awards a score of 9.80 points for the brilliant execution of the first routine in a competition, she would have little room to reward an even better execution within the following athletes. Only when judges have calibrated an internal scale (i.e., they have developed a feeling for the range of performances that they can expect on the day) are they able to use extreme judgments. The necessity of calibration processes has been nicely demonstrated in a study of yellow cards in soccer. It showed that, among others, referees' foul-decision behavior in the first half of games is different from their behavior in the second half. Specifically, they award fewer yellow cards earlier in games. This effect remains even when alternative explanations have been controlled for (e.g., fewer fouls actually occurring at the beginning). According to the authors, referees need to "get a feel for the game," and avoid yellow card decisions in the beginning because it could lead to a flood of yellow (and red) cards if they like to be consistent throughout the game.

Rule application and game management have been compared in the literature as the tools of a craftsman and an artist respectively. Referring to our categories of officials, monitors should put the greatest emphasis on the craftsmanship aspect of their task (rule application), whereas interactors must also focus (at least sometimes) on the artistic aspects (game management). However, it is not always clear which aspect is more important for certain tasks of officiating.

(3) Communication and personality

It is a common assumption that becoming an official may be more attractive to a certain type of person. Consequently, some research has addressed the question of whether officials differ in personality from the "average person" or if a certain personality profile is advantageous for top level refereeing. By and large, only little evidence has been found so far that, for example, soccer referees score higher on personality traits such as extraversion or conscientiousness. However, as with athletes, differences may be more important on the social-psychological level; for example, on communication skills.

Naturally, a key component of effective game management (see above), particularly in gaining acceptance for decisions, is communication. Many officials need to interact with athletes and coaches in order to officiate. Still others not only interact with both athletes and coaches, but they also interact with each other or operate in officiating teams.

Officials learn the appropriate hand signals to communicate calls; however, many sports require skill in dealing with players and coaches before as well as after decisions. In most sports, referees and umpires will tell you that one of the most important things is to show *confidence*. Many sports also emphasize spectator appeal and maintaining *flow*, discouraging officials from calling unnecessary stoppages (which is also an aspect of game management). This often leads to informal interactions and *preventive refereeing*, where an official may instruct a player to prevent him from committing a foul or offense (e.g., "number 3, get onside!").

Although it is difficult to study or assess things like personality and management skills, a review of psychological and performance demands describes the adaptation of a conflict management style grid in rugby referees. An example of conflict is given when a player addresses the referee by saying, "come on, ref, he's offside; that's ridiculous!" The cooperation and assertiveness used in response combine for five different conflict management styles as shown in Figure 5.2. As the authors of this work point out, there is no research yet that can be used to guide referees for *when* to use which style. Researchers also acknowledge that the details of communication are often unplanned, with personal style an influential factor. Different styles can also be equally effective and hence an awareness of the different options or styles available is a starting point for the individual referee to begin to experiment with.

In more specific terms, a study of rugby and soccer officials, by Mikel Mellick and his colleagues, identified seven areas of behavior that are key in recognizing both effective and ineffective communication (see Table 5.1). Underpinning these behaviors is engaging the offending player in order to communicate, appearing confident in the decision, and promoting the decision as fair by the laws of the game and from how the official viewed the action. In particular, a lack of confidence in communicating a decision may lead to argument and aggression.

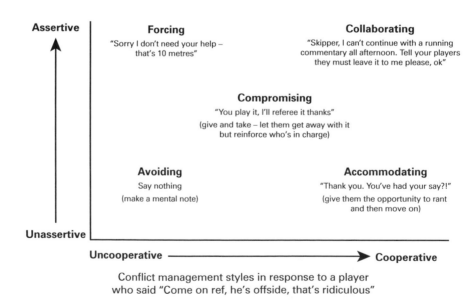

Conflict management styles in response to a player
who said "Come on ref, he's offside, that's ridiculous"

Figure 5.2 Thomas and Klimann's (1974) Conflict Management Style Grid adapted for Refereeing. (From Mascarenhas, O'Hare, and Plessner, 2006.)

Table 5.1 Examples of descriptors of skillful and unskillful referee communication

	Skillful communication	Unskillful communication
Whistle	Loud, sharp, denotes offense type	Delayed, insufficient to control players
Gaze	Eye contact with offender, incident zone in view	No eye contact with offender, incident zone not kept in view
Posture, movement	Strong, firm stationary position, looks calm, close proximity to incident	Head down, backs away from incident when making decision, skipping action, rushing in, touching player
Hand/arm signals	Prompt, clear, obvious, 3–4 seconds arm extension, illustrates offense and direction of call, uncomplicated, definitive, obvious to players, crowd	Messy, weak, unclear, confusing, too short, too early, hurried, no signal indicating offense, no direction of call, incorrect signal, sloppy, too much gesticulating
Verbal explanation	Explanation to team captain, offending player and others involved, verbal reasoning for decision, explanation of how to avoid repeat offense, concise	No verbal explanation, no explanation to necessary players
Control style, composure	Manages, controls interpersonal space, isolates and identifies offender, controls restart, immediate, non-aggressive, calm, deliberate, positive, definite	Allows players to control the situation, allows ball to be kicked away, offender not isolated, no appointment of blame to player, no presence, too calm/relaxed, confrontational, loss of composure
Time management	Takes time	Reactions too slow, not enough time taken to explain decision, too long to get to incident

Adapted from Mellick, Fleming, Bull, and Laugharne (2005).

One of the seven major categories of behaviors described in the study led by Mikel Mellick is verbal explanation, which is used to communicate, explain, and even provide the reasoning around the offense being called. However, what is notable in the other major categories is the variety of ways that officials communicate, with an emphasis on non-verbal means. The authors make the point that many elite officials will encounter athletes who are not native speakers in their language, which places even greater importance on non-verbal communication. Whistle use, as an example of a non-verbal category of behaviors, can be used to indicate the type of offense, with a long, loud whistle for a dangerous penalty. Similarly, hand and arm signals are unarguably a key skill for soccer and rugby referees, with the fast pace of games. Clear, timely signals reduce confusion and allow players to react quickly. The communication of non-calls is also often essential in order to signal ongoing control over the game.

Two other categories of communication behaviors include time management, which can include slowing down a game when needed without interrupting the flow of the game, and control style and composure, which encompasses controlling the space when placing the ball for a penalty or pulling an offender aside when calling a penalty. From our point of view, although these behaviors encompass communication, they are also major tools for game management as our previous discussion shows. That communication tools are game management tools is seen with most of the categories identified by Mellick and colleagues, for example, using verbal communication to provide the reasoning behind a call or to help players avoid penalties. This is particularly the case with the category of time and control style.

The last two categories of communication behaviors identified are gaze and posture and movement. Behaviors described in these categories include those used to portray confidence, such as making eye contact with an offender, looking calm, and standing firm. However, other behaviors under these categories make clear links to the physical demands in soccer and rugby as interactor-officiating sports; for example, using gaze in order to keep the incident in view and using movement to place oneself in close proximity to incidents. It is thus clear that communication is an excellent link between game management, which we discussed in the previous section, and physical demands and positioning, to which we turn in the next section.

As mentioned, beyond communicating to coaches and athletes, which was the focus of Mikel Mellick and colleagues' work, it is also important to consider that the majority of officials do not work alone. Of the average 137 observable decisions during Euro 2000 games, 64 percent were made in communication with the assistant referee. Teamwork and communication are especially highlighted in sports such as Canadian football (gridiron), where a crew of seven officials must coordinate throughout the game, or in the three-referee system in basketball – or the two-referee system in rugby league – where communicating well helps increase the consistency of calls. In these cases, the role and responsibilities of each official are specialized and well defined, arguably more so than the roles of athletes in many team sports.

There are times when officials are asked to interpret actions, with many rules based on the intentions of a player. The ability to read and interpret emotions, both in rule application and in dealing with confrontation, and even to predict reactions, is a sub-component of what some psychologists have identified as "empathic ability" or as "emotional intelligence." For example, it is crucial for a good referee to sense when players are becoming too heated. The stringency of calls may then be adjusted, and captains spoken to in order to avoid a brawl or unnecessary and dangerous fouls. Although, as we say, this has always seemed to be an intangible skill, researchers can use questionnaires to produce data and examine emotional intelligence in officials. Although the questionnaires have their limitations, we might expect that more successful referees and umpires show greater emotional intelligence, but that the same is not true for sports where the officials do not have as much interpretation and interaction with the athletes (e.g., gymnastics, skating). This is all speculation at the moment as this work remains to be done. As one of the best known and most respected soccer referees, Pierluigi Collina, has said:

> If you have good relations with all the players in a match, including the coaches, it's possible to have a better match – the players can do their job, and the referee can control the match better. If the players trust and accept a referee and his decisions, I feel that it makes for a better game of football.

However, it should be noted that this philosophy is not shared by all officials in all sports and even many soccer referees would insist that it is better for them to be as blind as possible towards the participants of a game. This also highlights the differences we pointed out before, whereby some officials may be more focused on accurate rule application (e.g., in gymnastics) and some on game management (e.g., in basketball).

(4) Physical demands and positioning

Research that quantifies the demands of sport officials has been the most comprehensive when addressing the *interacting* official who must move about the playing field and interact with the athletes. A soccer or rugby referee must keep pace with up to 30 players moving about a field that is up to 110 meters long and up to 75 meters wide. At any moment, a kick can move the action 50, 60 or 70 meters away. Heart rate monitors were placed on referees and assistant referees during the final games of the EURO 2000 soccer championships and the data collected showed that match referee heart rates throughout the game were between 80 and 90 percent of their maximum. These physical work rates are as high as, if not higher, than those of the players. What is more, the average age of a 2007 study sample of FIFA and UEFA soccer referees was 41, whereas the players being refereed were in their mid to late twenties. This highlights how hard referees must work to keep pace with players and the action they are evaluating.

As mentioned, officials are often asked to make important judgments with partial information. It seems like a straightforward judgment to decide whether a rugby player has touched the ball down to score a try. It is made much more difficult, however, from a distance with opposition players obscuring the view. In a key study in soccer, Raôul Oudejans and colleagues showed how the positioning of the assistant referee could lead to perceptual errors in judging offside. In soccer, a player is in an offside position if he or she is nearer to the opponents' goal line than both the ball and the second-last defender at the moment the ball is played by a team member. In order to judge offside, assistant referees are instructed to position themselves in line with the second-last defender. The Dutch researchers found that the high percentage of errors in offside decisions in soccer mainly reflected the viewing position of the assistant referee (see Figure 5.3). Although they should have been standing in line with the second-last defender, on average they were positioned too far behind. By considering the retinal images of referees (i.e., the projection of the scene being viewed onto the eye's retina), the researchers predicted a specific relation of frequencies in different types of errors (wrongly indicating offside as opposed to not indicating an actual offside) depending on the area of attack (near or far from the assistant referee and inside or outside the defender). In an analysis of 200 videotaped matches, this prediction was confirmed, thus demonstrating that assistant referees' decisions directly reflected the situations as projected onto their retinas. Similar results were obtained from studies in sports where officials have fixed viewing positions, for example, in gymnastics. The main message from these studies is that even experienced officials are influenced in a predictable way by basic perceptual illusions as they are determined, for example, by their imperfect viewing positions.

In many sports, officials, athletes, and spectators alike hold the view that having experience as an athlete in that sport is useful, if not essential, for proficient officiating. For example, it has frequently been claimed that certain incidents on a soccer

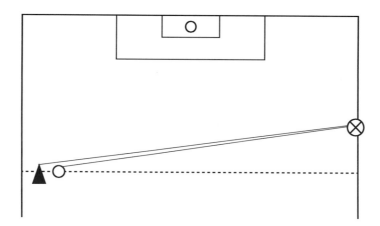

Figure 5.3 Optical errors in judging offside positions. Positions of defenders are indicated by circles and attackers by triangles. The offside line (in line with the second-last defender) is indicated by a dotted line. The typical position of the AR just ahead of the offside line is marked by a circle with a cross. From this position, the attacker furthest away (who is actually onside) appears to be ahead of the second-last defender and the AR is likely to commit a flag error. (From Mascarenhas, O'Hare, and Plessner, 2006.)

pitch can be accurately assessed only by a referee who has past playing experience. In recent years, this assumption has gained some theoretical support through the so-called "embodiment perspective." It emphasizes the significance of the mind's connections to the physical world. Consequently, perceptual and motor systems are considered to be highly relevant for the understanding of central cognitive processes such as judgment and decision making. For example, prior motor experiences with certain movements have been found to facilitate the recognition of these movements when performed by other people. Thus, it appears to be quite plausible to assume a positive relationship between prior specific sport experiences and officials' performances. In some sports, prior success as an athlete is even an official requirement for becoming an official on a higher level. However, the systematic investigation of officials' decision making from the viewpoint of an embodiment perspective has begun only recently. For example, Alexandra Pizzera and Markus Raab examined the relationship between previous motor and visual experience and officiating performance in a sample of 370 sport officials from soccer, handball, ice hockey, and trampoline. They found that officiating performance is related to motor, visual, and officiating experience to differing degrees in the analyzed sports. They suggest that, depending on the sport, officials should either specialize early in officiating, or gather visuomotor experience as an athlete or spectator first and then switch roles to become a sport official. Thus, their main finding is that gathering prior experience as an athlete is not automatically of an advantage for an official in all sports.

(5) Developing skill and expertise

There continues to be a great deal of focus on training within sport expertise studies. The most influential research is the theory of deliberate practice, which proposes that to become an expert in a field one needs to engage in a large volume of practice (up to 10 years or 10,000 hours). This practice must also be highly effortful and relevant to improvement with opportunities for feedback and correction. We will leave the detail on this theory and on training research to Baker and Cobley (Chapter 2) and simply present and make comments on the research findings with respect to officials.

In a study of 26 elite soccer referees from FIFA, UEFA, and the English Premier League, the referees were asked to report the time they had spent in different training activities for their first year of formal refereeing, in 1998, and in 2003. For example, they were asked how much time they had spent per week in on-field activities such as speed and agility training, high-intensity runs, and recovery runs; off-field activities such as strength training, flexibility, and video training; and match or match-related activities such as refereeing league or exhibition games.

These three years were chosen to get a picture of practice changes over time, as well as the impact of structured training programs which were put in place in 1998 and remained in place in 2003.

The results of the study showed that elite officials were unique to athletes from a training perspective. These elite performers were not simply retired players or coaches. Supporting the suggestions that Alexandra Pizzera and Markus Raab made with regard to training for certain sports, these soccer referees had specialized relatively early as referees and spent many years training. For example, the 14 FIFA referees in the group had started formal refereeing at an average age of 18 and it took a little over 16 years on average for each of them to reach the FIFA list. All of the referees reported doing very little weekly training in their first year but gradually increased both the amount and also the different types of training activities. For example, the referees typically reported that in their first year they would do an hour a week of high-intensity running and perhaps 30 minutes of low-intensity running. They would also engage in other training such as bicycling for fitness. Over the years, they maintained their focus on high-intensity running, with an average of one and a half hours per week, but also increased the amount of time spent in other activities such as speed endurance and agility training, recovery runs, video training, and technical skills. At the same time, the other training dropped off, showing their specialization in activities that mimicked the physical demands of on-field performance.

One of the basic ideas around the theory of deliberate practice is that the most useful practice provides an opportunity for learning through feedback. The provision and reception of feedback is a tricky issue in learning to officiate. Even delayed feedback from assessors is often in short supply for referees, especially as they are making their way up the ranks and acquiring skill. Probably as a result of this, the referees in the study discussed above reported that refereeing league games is the most relevant activity for improving performance, even ranked ahead of refereeing exhibition games, which are less formal, may have less pressure, and often are not assessed.

The essential nature of experience is highlighted in a study of rugby union referees that identified the concept of "deliberate experience" as an alternative way to develop refereeing expertise. A number of rugby referees observed and interviewed by researchers felt that traditional training alone was not sufficient to reach expert levels of performance. One ex-international official stated that:

> To be a good international standard referee, you have to referee international games. It's the same for the guys who want to move up to Zurich [a

Henning Plessner and Clare MacMahon

higher level of competition]. The games are totally different and you are constantly learning.

Later in this chapter we will discuss training methods that seek to fill the gap between traditional training and on-field experience. So far, however, it is not clear if these methods are successful in this goal.

The study of rugby union referees also acknowledged that experience in other roles contributed to referee proficiency in a transfer of skills. The researchers reported that referees felt experience gained from playing helped them to know how a player thought. However, as we reported with the current research from an embodiment perspective, this may not always be the case and may differ between sports. Echoing our earlier statements related to the demands of officiating, the referees also felt that personality, confidence, and assertiveness contributed to refereeing and that these were often developed in one's occupation but transferred onto the field.

The fact that skills such as management and assertiveness are developed over time and transferred from other roles, combined with the need for deliberate experience through actual game refereeing, may explain why it took the referees in the soccer study 16 years to reach the FIFA list – a lengthier time than expected by the theory of deliberate practice. On the one hand, sport bodies must acknowledge that development in officials is arguably more complex than that of athletes, with the need for (a) the development of officiating skills, (b) the development of a positive reputation, and (c) the negotiation of the politics of promotion. This lengthy skill acquisition and promotion process has an impact on the age at which many officials are at their peak. Some officials may thus simultaneously encounter the beginning of age-related declines and a need for increased recovery from bouts of demanding officiating. However, we know very little specifically on whether these declines have an impact on performance. For example, although an older official may have less physical capability such as running speed, the experience of knowing where to be and how to anticipate the play may compensate so that there is no loss in performance.

On the other hand, it may be that officials can shorten the length of time it takes to become a top performer by increasing or refining their training methods. It seems certain that some sport officials will benefit from an increase in deliberate experience in the form of refereed games. There are limits, however, and it may be unrealistic to expect that a novice official will have access to a large number of games for training purposes. In the next section, new video-based training programs, as well as other training programs, will be reviewed. These programs may help to accelerate the way to top expertise.

RESEARCH INTO PRACTICE: ADDRESSING THE CHALLENGES

In this section, we will again address the five "cornerstones of performance," as adapted from work in rugby union. However, the focus is now mainly on practical issues, that is, how can officials improve their performance and address each of these cornerstones?

(1) Knowledge and application of the laws

The most basic requirement in officiating, on which licensing and accreditation is often based, is knowledge of the rules and laws of the sport. Arguably more so than athletes or coaches, officials are required to have a strong foundation of declarative knowledge, which is often defined as rule-book knowledge. The implementation of the rules is referred to as procedural ("how to") knowledge. For both learning of the rules and learning of rule application, most sports provide materials in the form of commentaries and accompanying videos that help the novice official to become familiar with the specific rule system beyond the mere study of the written rules. These materials are important because laws are typically written with the main purpose of being exact and not of being user-friendly. In addition, in some sports, learning the rules is already the greatest challenge for the future official. For example, the Code of Points in gymnastics is rather complex and comprises, among other things, a detailed list of hundreds of value parts that need to be recognized in a competition. Accordingly, research has pointed to the fact that in such sports the main difference between novices and experienced judges is their knowledge structure. This research argues that experienced judges have specific knowledge that helps them to process performances faster and more efficiently. They know what information is relevant, what to expect, and what the typical interrelations are among variables. Again, it seems that this kind of knowledge is not attained as an automatic consequence of mere experience in a sport – for example, as an athlete – but is acquired through specific, structured, and effortful training. Apart from video materials that can be helpful in order to learn both the rules and how to implement them, officials are also advised to frequently observe and discuss athletes' performances either in training sessions or competitions.

As has been discussed in prior sections, quite a few biases have been identified in officials' judgment and decision making that stem from different processes of information integration. A first step in order to prevent theses biases is to make officials familiar with them. However, it should be noted that some of these processes work in a rather automatic fashion and are, therefore, difficult to control even if judges are aware of them. In addition, processes such as comparisons can be helpful guides in an uncertain environment. That is, if judges for some reason are not able to apply the rules in the supposed way, the use of direct comparisons

86

will bring them much closer to the *true* value of a performance rather than simply guessing. Therefore, some general advice in order to prevent biases on this step of information processing is the training of accurate rule application that leaves no room for interpretation.

Feedback training, possibly using video, has been suggested by many authors as a measure to improve accuracy in categorization tasks such as recognizing an offensive pattern in soccer. For example, Geoffrey Schweizer and colleagues developed a video-based online training tool for improving soccer referees' decisions. It is based on the assumption that referees' decision making in contact situations mainly relies on intuitive processing. For improving intuitive decisions, feedback on the correctness of decisions is essential. From this theoretical perspective, one can even go so far as to state that explanations are not required. Referees who take part in the training watch videos, make decisions, and receive immediate feedback. The researchers found evidence of the training's effectiveness even in a study with expert referees. Thus, immediate feedback on the correctness of decisions seems to be sufficient for increasing decision accuracy. Other researchers found similar results with video-based training programs focused on offside decisions in soccer. Together, these studies suggest quite some potential for tailor-made video training as a complement to traditional training forms (see also Chapter 12).

(2) Game management

From the viewpoint of game management, that is, adequate instead of accurate decision making, video-based training tools raise some of the most interesting and hardest questions when dealing with officiating: How do we decide on the *correct* call? How do we appropriately evaluate performance by officials? In many sports, a video replay of the action does not provide the same point of view that the on-field or on-court official had at the time. Nor can an isolated clip of action provide the context that an official might use to influence decision making. In many areas, the "biases" used in judgment and decision making can be considered as adaptive and helpful. These factors are what probably contributes to the difficulty in creating sensitive tools to assess and train referee skill. For example, in creating a research tool or test where an expert panel, which may be composed of coaches, ex-officials, and administrators, cannot agree on the correct decision for a clip of action, we decide that it would not make a good testing item and exclude it. However, this may result in a pool of clips which are *too easy* and do not discriminate between more and less skilled officials, or even between officials and players. It also eliminates the type of plays that prompt criticism and second-guessing of an official's decision – the *key* decisions. In the "real world" of the referee and referee assessors, key decisions need to be evaluated.

From both a research and an officiating evaluation perspective, there needs to be an acknowledgement that there are, in fact, *ambiguous* actions for which the call may change depending on the context. However, little is known about how contextual judgment and decision making could be incorporated into the abovementioned training tools.

From a practical point of view, it appears to be helpful for officials to prepare for each game and/or athlete they encounter next. This could even prevent the calibration effects we discussed earlier. Knowing the demands and typical decisions at different levels of play may also help to create a smoother transition for developing officials. For instance, a typical rookie error for Canadian Football League officials is to call a player offside believing they could not have been *that fast*. This is an example of how officials need to adapt to the physical capabilities of players at a higher level of competition. They may also encounter different tactics, requiring adapted positioning, and an increased frequency of higher-order skills such as a drop kick during open play in rugby. They may no longer be expected to let some calls go and must now adapt to a new set of unwritten rules. These may all be captured through analysis of key decisions and typical errors and contrasted across levels of officiating. However, it will be difficult to keep the balance between careful game preparation and the creation of (inadequate) expectancies about athletes' performances.

(3) Personality and communication

Most sports develop a specific language of communicating assessments and decisions. The acquisition of this language is a natural part of officials' basic training. For example, Figure 5.4 presents typical arm signals of handball referees. In addition, the officials' training could also include the teaching of effective versus ineffective communication styles, such as the examples given in Table 5.1. It may be helpful to work together with professional communication programs and trainers on these issues. This may be most important for the non-verbal communication of interactors. As has been said before, good officiating could be considered as engaging the offending player in order to communicate, appearing confident in the decision, and promoting the decision as fair by the laws of the game and from how the official viewed the action. In particular, a lack of confidence in communicating a decision may lead to argument and aggression.

88

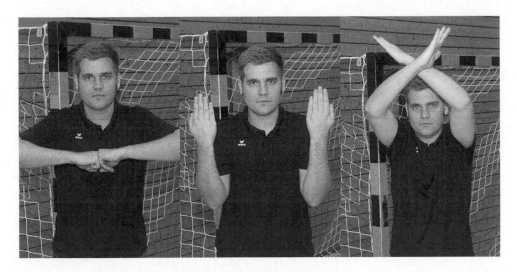

Figure 5.4 Typical arm signals of handball referees.

(4) Physical demands and positioning

With regard to officials' physical fitness, which is mainly of concern for interactors, there are excellent training guides available, at least for professional sports such as soccer. Of course, most educational programs for interactors also include the training of correct positioning. In addition, there is some evidence that at least some of the perceptual illusions due to inappropriate positioning (which we discussed earlier) can also be overcome using feedback training. In a training study by Gernot Jendrusch and colleagues (2002), electronic devices were installed on a tennis court to objectively assess the point where the ball hit the court. In a training group, line judges received accurate feedback about their decisions during several sessions a week. Their decision making improved markedly in comparison with a control group that did not receive training. What is most interesting about this study is that, according to all kinds of physical measures, there was no improvement in the perceptual abilities of the training group's line judges. Rather, they learned what to look at to make decisions. That is, they used relatively valid perceptual cues to assess the point at which the ball hit the court; for example, the shape of the flying curve. The message from this work is that creating learning environments that help officials to use multiple valid cues should be an important aspect of developing decision training. In addition, it should be noted that we can figure out the best viewing position for an official by analyzing the details of their perceptual demands. For example, a study in baseball found that repositioning the home plate umpire as suggested in visual perception research literature improved the accuracy of ball-strike judgments.

(5) Developing skill and expertise

As suggested throughout the chapter, the demands and skills vary a great deal between different types of officials, from the smaller differences between the referee and assistant referee to the bigger differences between a gymnastics judge and a rugby referee (see Figure 5.1). This limits our ability to provide concrete guidelines for all officials. Nonetheless, the general points below should be considered by researchers, sport bodies, and individual officials themselves. We have already addressed some basic training for officials, which is why we move directly on to issues that may be of additional relevance as they acquire skill and resources become more available. First, however, we briefly discuss the problem of evaluating officials' performance.

The acknowledgment of ambiguity and "fuzziness" of many decisions that we addressed in relation to the aspect of game management will also benefit assessors who are concerned with evaluating the performance of an official. Evaluators need to be mindful and sensitive to the fact that they may be assessing an official's decision based on less (e.g., absence of context), more (e.g., slow motion), or different (e.g., angle of view) information than the official had at the time of making a call or decision. In addition, once officials are made aware of potential biases and factors that have been found to influence decisions, evaluators may look to see if an official has fallen into a judgment trap.

Although it is understandable that assessors may look to create evaluation systems that are objective and quantitative measures of performance, great detail and statistics do not always translate into a great evaluation system. The research which presented the five cornerstones of referee performance for rugby union advises evaluators to avoid diminishing the task into a skeleton of itself. Evaluators should consider the characteristics and skills of several of the sport's top performers, what skills or qualities are not captured in a "ticks and checks" evaluation system, and where there are different but equally successful *styles* of refereeing. An appropriate evaluation should provide the opportunity to cater to an individual so that it is *meaningful* and provides *specific feedback* on which an official may take action and seek further training and refinement. For example, a referee may be told to reconsider positioning for a specific type of play. This section will also provide some advice on aspects to consider in evaluating officiating performance.

Officials are often left out in the cold in terms of a research basis for their training. They are left to rely on what we know about training for the athletes in their sport. For some skills this is not entirely inappropriate. For example, the fitness and physical training of the soccer official should be somewhat similar to that of the soccer athlete; however, we should strive to obtain a clear understanding of the specific demands of the official, keeping in mind that some of these are additional and/ or different to those of the athlete. Again, it is also worth mentioning that these demands may differ depending on the level of play that is officiated and the gender of the athletes. Demands may be assessed by watching a selection of videotape performances and coding the action using a number of categories:

- movement patterns (e.g., forward, sideways, backwards; sprinting, jogging, walking);
- communication (e.g., length and number of communications with other officials, athletes, coaches);
- number and type of decisions.

Once the demands are understood, these can be used to identify key decisions, typical areas of difficulty, and even sources of error. This can be based on noting the source of arguments with coaches and players, discussion with other officials, and even the impact of a decision. For example, a penalty decision has a major impact if it leads to point scoring. The information-processing approach is helpful to identify the stage at which errors have occurred. Thus, for example, positioning may be a large source of perceptual difficulty which leads to error in a particular decision. Once again, key decisions may differ by level of play and undoubtedly for different types of decision-making systems (e.g., a panel of judges versus an on-field referee). This type of analysis can provide information on common practices, types of systems, and their influences on decision making; for example, the use of a panel of judges responsible for providing a global mark for an athlete as opposed to split responsibilities (e.g., technical and artistic assessments as in gymnastics).

The next obvious step is to use the information gained from an assessment of demands and errors to guide training. In physically demanding officiating, training should build an aerobic base and mimic the on-field demands. With regard to decisions, officials can now become sensitized to which key decisions require additional focus in video tools, the law book, and positioning. While training should acknowledge that high volumes of deliberate practice in relevant activities are associated with improving skills, we also encourage officials to increase and maximize their deliberate experience, and do as much *actual officiating* as they can. The influence of context and realistic scenarios must be emphasized.

As we have discussed in previous sections of this chapter, officials face demands that are not necessarily observable or captured by ticks and marks. These skills and their relative importance to the overall proficiency of an official should be communicated to create an assessment, training, and promotion system that is as transparent as possible. For example, the cornerstones of success for rugby referees that we have repeatedly referred to provide specific areas for assessment and skill development. When evaluations are concrete but meaningful, assessors can direct officials to the tools for improvement. Moreover, as we mentioned above, *teams of* officials can be evaluated where appropriate to assess the impact of consistently training and performing together.

CONCLUDING REMARKS

We have shown that officiating is a diverse role within sport: there are many different *types* of officials with different demands. Research has focused on describing these demands, tracing the training of the top performers, and understanding the characteristics of decision making. The official is both similar to and different from the athlete in many respects. These characteristics and demands should be understood in order to provide focused training, assessment, and improvement. It should also be noted that demands may change based on the level of play being officiated. In addition, age-related declines may need to be considered at present, but perhaps avoided in the future, if we are able to shortcut the path to proficiency in officiating by improved training.

There is still a great deal to do in understanding the demands, training, and skills specific to sport officials. Although we have provided some general practical guidelines, just as important are the potential research areas we have highlighted. Although many officials are accustomed to shunning the spotlight, and in fact strive to be somewhat invisible, understanding and improving their skills is an area where it would do them well to raise their voices and draw some attention. Finally, optimal training of officials that is based on scientific insights will also help them to fulfill their Olympic Oath.

COACH'S CORNER

Ralf Brand
12-year first league basketball referee

What first came to mind when I read this chapter was: well done, Clare and Henning! This is quite a comprehensive picture of what we are doing. However, I then began thinking about what we are doing *where*. Now, after some time, I have come to the following conclusion: this chapter most thoroughly describes the state of refereeing research. Still, I feel that there are some gaps to be closed over the next few years until we, as researchers, have reached a level from which we can not only describe (and, from time to time, explain) what happens on the court, but actually inform practitioners on what they have to do instead of, or in addition to, the things they are already doing.

Undoubtedly, it is very important to know why, for example, certain decisional biases occur. It is interesting to see that researchers have found evidence of calibration processes during the beginning of matches. Every experienced referee who has ever had a referee supervisor giving him feedback after a match (and, believe me, all of them have) knows that this is a crucial problem referees have to solve at the beginning of every match. They just would not call it calibration. Knowing that biases or other psychological phenomena exist, or explaining the reasons why they occur, does not make you a better referee. Rather, what is interesting in practical terms is how referee boards create the conditions for the best referee performances possible.

What I think is the next evolutionary step for referee researchers is to develop some kind of a "big picture" of sport game officiating. And if we want to paint it appropriately it is crucial to talk with referee experts not only from the academic but also from the very applied side. So far, to draw this picture, blank spots have to be filled in, separate picture parts have to be related to each other, and some words about what this big picture means (what it can and what it cannot achieve) have to be written. Let me give you some examples of what I mean.

Blank spots that have to be filled in

Referees will always have to communicate their decisions. Not predominantly by using words, though. They literally have to "stand" behind their decisions even if they themselves may doubt them. Particularly at the highest level of refereeing it is all about presenting calls and selling them by using the appropriate body language. The coaches, the players, the audience, they all have to find trust in the referee's expertise, neutrality, and willingness and ability to avoid mistakes. Referees need to convey a sense of trustworthiness, even after situations in which they might have been wrong, as the game must go on. I have not read much about this core aspect of modern refereeing so far in the academic literature.

Connected with this, researchers should also think about the following: my impression is that there is an implicit assumption that blowing into the whistle is a kind of commentary on what has happened an instant before. This is only half of what really happens (or of what should happen), because the other part of the story is that players and coaches should understand through a referee's actions how comparable situations will be judged in the subsequent development of the game and thereby get to know how they should play on. Referees are not only "reactors." Excellent referees are able to give direction (e.g., by preventively de-escalating plays between some hot-blooded opponents). And all of this happens, not least by physically "representing" their duties.

Separate picture parts have to be related

Though not depicted in this chapter, there is literature on how referees should cope with the stressful situations that arise during matches. As you might suspect after reading my paragraph above, it is very important that the public (players and coaches foremost) do not notice this, so referees have to control their body language very carefully. However, as a game goes on, physical and psychological exhaustion on the part of the referee will begin to play a role. Controlling oneself becomes difficult under circumstances of physical as well as mental fatigue. I have not read one study yet in which the interaction of physical demands with cognitive (e.g., exact decision making) and emotional skills (e.g., controlling one's facial expressions) has been investigated. Another example is that very seldom have I read about the effect that a certain referee's behavior (e.g., setting a more generous foul/no-foul standard with regard to incidental physical contact between opponents) has on the subsequent development of the game.

What does the picture mean (and what does it *not* mean)?

Knowing that calibration processes occur, for example, does not automatically inform practitioners about what to do. Thus, an important question for practitioners would be whether there are recommendations on *how* one should calibrate. To put it formally, technical rules (knowing what one has to do to make things happen) cannot directly be derived from prescriptive rules (if "a" then "b"), but must be empirically tested separately: if you do "x" then "y" will result.

We have to be very accurate in what we write with respect to what we have done in the laboratory (incidentally, quite a few studies) and what has actually been tested in intervention studies (considerably fewer studies). Reporting that we know a lot about some basic mechanisms might stimulate applied research. However, neglecting to analyze and then clearly report what we formally were able to achieve with our experiments might hinder further development of applied research with our knowledge of basic psychological processes. The worst part of neglecting to analyze and report what we are able to achieve through experiments is discouraging practitioners from reading our texts and, as a result, from gaining any value from this work.

KEY READING

Damisch, L., Mussweiler, T., and Plessner, H. (2006) 'Olympic medals as fruits of comparison? Assimilation and contrast in sequential judgments', *Journal of Experimental Psychology: Applied*, 12: 166–178.

MacMahon, C., Helsen, W.F., Starkes, J.L., Cuypers, K. and Weston, M. (2007) 'Decision-making skills and deliberate practice in elite association football referees', *Journal of Sport Sciences*, 25: 65–78.

Mascarenhas, D.R.D., Collins, D., and Mortimer, P. (2005) 'Elite refereeing performance: Developing a model for sport science support', *The Sport Psychologist*, 19: 364–379.

Mellick M.C., Fleming, S., Bull, P., and Laugharne, E.J. (2005) 'Identifying best practice for referee decision communication in association and rugby union football', *Football Studies*, 8: 42–57.

Oudejans, R.R.D., Verheijen, R., Bakker, F.C., Gerrits, J.C., Steinbrückner, M. and Beek, P.J. (2000) 'Errors in judging "offside" in football', *Nature*, 404: 33.

Pizzera, A. and Raab, M. (2012) 'Perceptual judgments of sports officials are influenced by their motor and visual experience', *Journal of Applied Sport Psychology*, 24: 59–72.

Henning Plessner and Clare MacMahon

Plessner, H. and Haar, T. (2006) 'Sports performance judgments from a social cognition perspective', *Psychology of Sport and Exercise*, 7: 555–575.

Ste-Marie, D.M. (2003) 'Expertise in sport judges and referees: Circumventing information-processing limitations', in Starkes, J.L. and Ericsson, K.A. (eds.) *Expert Performance in Sport: Advances in Research on Sport Expertise*. Champaign IL: Human Kinetics, pp. 169–189.

Schweizer, G., Plessner, H., Kahlert, D., and Brand, R. (2011) 'A video-based training method for improving soccer referees' intuitive decision-making skills', *Journal of Applied Sport Psychology*, 23: 429–442.

Unkelbach, C. and Memmert, D. (2008) 'Game-management, context-effects and calibration: the case of yellow cards in soccer', *Journal of Sport & Exercise Psychology*, 30: 95–109.

CHAPTER 6

DEVELOPING THE EXPERT PERFORMANCE COACH

JEAN CÔTÉ, KARL ERICKSON, AND PAT DUFFY

The term "coaching" is used in many different contexts to describe various roles that individuals take to nurture someone else's development and performance. Coaches enable people to perform to the best of their abilities in different domains of life such as business, personal development, career, finance, health, and sport. In the sport arena, coaches have the broad responsibility to mentor and teach the physical, mental, technical, tactical, and social skills that empower athletes to participate and perform. In 2007, the European Coaching Council defined sport coaching as "the guided improvement of sport participants and teams in a single sport and at identifiable stages of the athlete/sportsperson pathway." This definition of sport coaching suggests that there are several coaching contexts in sport that require different types of coaching knowledge and behaviors.

Jean Côté and his colleagues proposed a typology of four different coaching contexts in sport based on athletes' level of competitiveness and age:

1 participation coaches for children;
2 participation coaches for adolescents;
3 performance coaches for young adolescents;
4 performance coaches for older adolescents and adults.

According to this typology, each of these four categories requires coaches to have different types of knowledge in order to meet the specific needs of the participants. This chapter focuses on "performance coaches" (3 and 4 above), those who work with aspiring and elite athletes to nurture their talent and maximize their level of performance respectively.

Before discussing the development of expert performance coaches, we need to define what expert coaches are and the role they have in the development of aspiring and elite athletes. Biographies of professional coaches and stories of their interactions with athletes are sources of information often used to describe the development and behaviors of successful performance coaches; however, these stories are not always reflective of all the developmental activities necessary to become an expert coach and the knowledge and behaviors used by coaches to develop aspiring and elite athletes. This chapter will use the most current research findings to focus, first, on defining expertise in coaching and, second, on defining the developmental activities necessary to become an expert coach.

WHAT DOES THE RESEARCH TELL US?

Defining coaching expertise in a performance environment

It is well known that the development of talent in sport lies in the constructive relationships between athletes and coaches. Coaches support, supervise, and facilitate the healthy development and performance excellence of athletes in sport. In this context, coaching expertise is defined by the highly variable roles that coaches assume and reflects the constant personal exchanges and interactions that coaches and athletes have in a performance environment.

Jean Côté and Wade Gilbert proposed an integrative definition of coaching effectiveness and expertise that focuses on the integration of coaches' knowledge, athletes' outcomes, and the different contexts in which coaches typically work. The definition, based on a thorough review of coaching, teaching, athlete development, and positive psychology research is:

> The consistent application of integrated professional, interpersonal, and intrapersonal knowledge to improve athletes' competence, confidence, connection, and character in specific coaching contexts.

This definition is comprised of three components: coach knowledge, athlete outcomes, and coaching contexts. Coach knowledge extends beyond the commonly examined area of professional knowledge (sport-specific knowledge) to include both interpersonal (interaction and connection with others) and intrapersonal (openness to continued learning and self-reflection) forms of knowledge. Coaching contexts refer to the varied sport settings in which coaching can take place in terms of competitive levels (performance or participation) and major life periods (childhood, adolescence, and adulthood). The final component of the integrative definition is athlete outcomes, which are defined as the "4Cs" (i.e., competence, confidence, connection, and character). While the nature of the knowledge required by coaches in different sporting contexts is highly variable, the "4Cs" remains a stable indicator of athlete outcomes.

According to this definition of coaching expertise, the ultimate role of a performance coach is to develop their athletes' competence, confidence, connection, and character so that they are ready to advance to the next stage of their development and/or compete at their highest level of performance on a consistent basis. Sport competence in elite athletes is the most obvious and recognizable outcome that results from expert coaching. For example, the development of athletes' sport competence can be broken down into general dimensions – such as the teaching of technical skills, mental skills, tactical skills, and physical skills – in such a way that they can be reproduced in competitive situations where decision making and positive responses to pressure are of the essence. A second goal of performance coaches is to instill the belief and confidence in their athletes that they possess the capability to be successful and compete in the sport they practiced, while the third is to develop their athletes' connection with others because elite sport is a social venue that requires interactions with a broad range of individuals for optimal performance. Performance coaches need to foster a climate in which their athletes engage in meaningful and positive relationships with their team-mates, peers, and others involved in their sport environment and their life. Finally, it is important for coaches involved in nurturing talent in athletes to promote the development of character so that athletes make appropriate and ethical decisions regarding their training and their overall involvement in sport.

The "4Cs" provides a concise yet comprehensive framework to measure performance (competence) and psycho-social outcomes (confidence, connection, and character) in long-term talent development programs for athletes. Together, these four constructs represent a holistic approach to talent development that incorporates traditional goals of sport programs (e.g., skill development and performance) with an added emphasis on positive psycho-social development.

According to the definition of coaching effectiveness and expertise described above, coaches working with athletes at different stages of their development will require a mix of professional, interpersonal, and intrapersonal knowledge tailored to the specific context in order to develop athletes' competence, confidence, connection, and character. For example, preparing a 16-year-old long-distance runner for a national championship will require different coaching expertise from preparing a 28-year-old long-distance runner for the Olympic Games.

Coaches' professional knowledge includes understanding of the sports sciences (psychology, physiology, biomechanics, etc.), sport-specific demands and techniques, and the pedagogical knowledge used to teach sport skills. The professional knowledge that coaches need to be effective in specific situations could be referred to as the "science" of coaching. On the other hand, interpersonal knowledge involves the understanding that coaching is essentially about the relationships developed with athletes and that these relationships are based primarily on social interactions (coach to athlete, athlete to coach, *and* coach to other stakeholders involved in supporting the performance of the athlete). Interpersonal knowledge in a sport-coaching context might best be framed as a combination of emotional intelligence – the ability to understand and connect with others (players, other coaches, media, administrators, officials, etc.) – and transformational leadership – the ability to help and inspire others to grow as individuals and transcend their current abilities to reach higher levels of functioning. The interpersonal and social skills involved in leading individuals to higher levels of performance can be referred to as the "art" of coaching. Lastly, the third type of knowledge – intrapersonal knowledge – is most aligned with the concepts of self-awareness and reflection. It has been shown repeatedly that effective coaches have a keen sense of self-awareness, are aware of their strengths and limitations, and are prepared to act on insights gained. The development of this awareness occurs through constant reflection about current and past actions.

The developmental activities that lead to coaching expertise

The professional, interpersonal, and intrapersonal knowledge needed to coach at a high level of performance is acquired through a variety of structured and unstructured experiences and training strategies over the course of many years. Although formal classroom learning is an important activity of coaches' development, other less-structured sources also play major roles, including experience as an athlete, learning from a mentor, observation and interaction with other coaches, and hands-on learning such as being an assistant coach. There have been several research initiatives focusing on how different sources of knowledge afford learning opportunities for developing coaches. According to Penny Werthner and Pierre Trudel's view of coach learning situations, a coach's cognitive structure will change under the influence of three complementary types of learning situations: mediated, unmediated, and internal. In mediated learning situations, the learner is directed to salient information by a more experienced other (e.g., coaching courses, clinics, mentors). Unmediated situations involve the learner deciding what is important or useful and choosing what to learn under their own initiative (e.g., on-the-job experiences, observing other coaches). Finally, internal learning situations involve no presentation of new information but instead consist of deliberate review of existing practices and ideas (e.g., reflection on experience). This framework sheds light on the process of learning; however, it provides little information on the types of activity that appear to be most relevant in the development of expert coaches.

Accordingly, some studies have quantified the specific developmental sport experiences of high-performance coaches and suggested developmental activities that are consistent in most performance coaches' development. For example, having previously played the sport that they now coach at a competitive level and having formal leadership experiences as an athlete are experiences reported by most coaches. With regard to coaching experience, initial coaching positions at a lower but still competitive level and being mentored by a more experienced coach were consistent experiences of these coaches. Finally, formal or informal education such as an undergraduate degree in Physical Education or attending coach education programs and clinics were important regular activities. These developmental experiences contribute to the nurturing of performance coaching expertise by affording coaches mediated (e.g., coaching classes), unmediated (e.g., watching other coaches), and internal (e.g., use of a mentor to reflect on their own coaching) learning situations.

According to retrospective studies of expert high-performance coaches it is possible to suggest a certain amount of time spent in specific developmental activities to become head coaches at the performance level. More specifically, expert performance coaches accumulate 9,000–12,000 hours of experiences in sport during their development, figures which are then often significantly surpassed in the case of coaches with long careers. The 9,000–12,000 hours identified in the research to date may be divided into the following developmental categories:

1 athletic experience, for example, as an above-average athlete in a specific sport, or someone with leadership roles as an athlete involved in different sports (3,000–4,000 hours);
2 coaching experience, for example, as an assistant coach coaching at a lower but still competitive performance level (3,000–4,000 hours);
3 informal and formal education, for example, through mentors, formal education in Physical Education or a related profession, a coaching certification (3,000–4,000 hours).

This developmental profile provides a possible structural framework for informing the development of training programs for performance coaches; however, it is important to shed light on how athletic experience, coaching experience, and informal and formal education may contribute to the development of performance coaches.

Athletic experience

Previous research suggests that extensive and diverse sport experiences as athletes aid coaches' development by providing unmediated learning situations. Being involved in multiple sports or teams as athletes provides future coaches with opportunities to observe the coaching, teaching, and interpersonal practices of several different coaches and, thus, to acquire coaching skills, knowledge, and values. Developmental psychologists have shown, through many years of research, that extra-curricular activities such as sport provide an ideal context for developing a thriving youth that will eventually give back to his/her community. A prominent developmental psychologist, Reed Larson, showed that sport activities provide young people with a context they enjoy and that requires concentration and effort over time. He suggested that these three characteristics of organized activities are critical to the development of initiative and overall positive life skills. This type of context is different from their other time-consuming activities such as school or watching television. For instance, in school, youth may experience concentration without a great deal of enjoyment; conversely, watching television can provide an enjoyable experience but generally lacks effort and concentration.

Sport participation is enjoyable and challenging and contains unmediated learning experiences that can lay the foundation for important knowledge and skills required for coaching. By providing this unique context, sport can help young people develop into physically, socially, psychologically, and emotionally healthy people. This resulting overall positive development (exemplified by the "4Cs") is posited to be the necessary prerequisite for the final "C" of positive youth development: contribution. As thriving youth develop into adults, they often choose to contribute or "give back" to their community, in this case by promoting the positive development of the next generation of youth in sport through coaching. In particular, studies have suggested that leadership experiences in this context (e.g., being a team captain) may be an important link between positive experiences as an athlete and the desire and ability to contribute to other athletes' development as a coach.

The context of sport as a unique developmental experience helps explain its importance in terms of preparing future coaches. Other extra-curricular activities such as music and art could possibly replace sport as a foundational activity to coaching in that they share the critical characteristics (enjoyment, concentration, and effort over time), facilitating positive youth development and thus promoting eventual "contribution"; however, the advantage of sport over non-sport extra-curricular activities resides in the added value of being immersed in a culture that is directly applicable to coaching. An individual who plays sport in a positive environment will develop as a competent, confident, and connected person who possesses character and who will have the desire to contribute back to sport as a coach. It is certainly plausible that the development of competence, confidence, connection, and character occurs through involvement in non-sport extra-curricular activities; however, this pathway is less common in the development of performance coaches. The positive assets and integrated knowledge base that participation in sport provides set the basis for young adults to develop a coaching career and eventually sustain a sporting system in which other young people may thrive. Overall, this section highlights the importance of designing sport programs that provide athletes with diverse experiences and opportunities that can eventually be transferred into coaching skills. Based on past research, we therefore propose that athletic experiences can be seen as an essential early experience of future coaches.

Coaching experience

Coaching experience is also an important element for the development of expert performance coaches. Coaching experience provides coaches with on-the-job learning situations in which they can gain knowledge and reflect on their own coaching practices and behaviors. Wade Gilbert and Pierre Trudel suggest that practical learning situations such as coaching present three different contexts for reflection – reflection-in-action (during games or practices), reflection-on-action (after games or practices), and retrospective reflection-on-action (at the end of the season) – with each context affording slightly different opportunities for coaches to further their knowledge. The mechanism of knowledge gain through coaching experience may in fact be reflection in and on these experiences. By consciously monitoring what behaviors, decisions, or strategies are successful or unsuccessful and why, coaches may discern components of personally effective coaching practices.

Based on their studies of expert coaches, Gilbert and Trudel suggested a process to understand how good coaches translate experience into knowledge and skills. They developed a model of experiential learning based on reflection, comprising a number of different components. In particular, once expert coaches have identified a coaching issue (i.e., something to be changed or altered) within their self-defined role as a coach, they proceed through a loop of sequential components comprising strategy generation (i.e., brainstorming), experimentation (i.e., implementing a strategy), and evaluation (i.e., did it work and why?). Expert coaches often cycle through this loop numerous times for any given issue. Connected cycles through a reflective conversation often result in what coaches sometimes define as insights. These somewhat spontaneous revelations are in fact the result of numerous cycles of reflective conversation that are based on real coaching experiences. Coaching experiences combined with deliberate reflections on these experiences are an important source of expert performance coaches' acquisition of professional, interpersonal, and intrapersonal knowledge.

Formal and informal education

Coaching knowledge can also be gained by way of learning situations provided by formal education or informal learning experiences. In general, formal learning situations such as coaching education classes and clinics have been found in some studies to be of relatively low overall impact on coaching knowledge and effectiveness in comparison with the more informal learning situations where coaches spend most of their time. Despite rating formal education as less important, expert coaches still get involved in several hours of formal training and these types of experiences will no doubt lead to the development of coaches' professional knowledge.

Comprehensive coach education programs that focus primarily on professional knowledge have been developed in many countries around the world. These formal programs have many similarities in content and are typically structured around courses in sports sciences (psychology, physiology, pedagogy, biomechanics, etc.), general coaching theory, sport-specific techniques and tactics, and supervised coaching practice. Similar content is often reported by coaches who have post-secondary Physical Education training. Formal coach education has been found to be important in coaches' development by increasing perceived coaching efficacy, facilitating the social development and growth of athletes, and decreasing the rate of burnout in coaching.

On the other hand, informal education – such as mentorship, observation, and communities of practice – has emerged in the coaching literature as a significant source of knowledge for coaches' development. Mentoring is often cited as being one of the most effective ways of passing on knowledge to a developing coach. Through a mentor, a developing coach can develop his or her own coaching style and philosophy. Observing other coaches has also been reported as a primary source of coaching knowledge. Often referred to as an informal apprenticeship of observation, this observation can occur as an assistant coach or head coach by watching other coaches in action. Finally, as a mid-point between mentoring and the self-directedness of observation, communities of practice have been proposed as a particularly fruitful approach to fostering coach learning. Composed of a group of individuals (often with differing levels of experience) who share a common interest in informal professional development, communities of practice bring coaches together on a regular basis to interact on the "practice" of coaching. Through this sustained interaction and sharing with other coaches in person or through social media, communities of practice can collectively negotiate meaning from each other's coaching experiences in order to learn from one another.

Formal education such as sports science, coaching courses, and coaching clinics and informal educational experiences in the form of mentoring and communities of practice are consistent developmental experiences of expert performance coaches. These types of experiences contribute to coaches' acquisition of professional knowledge, interpersonal, and intrapersonal knowledge and skills.

THEORY INTO PRACTICE

Developmental activities

The integrative definition of coaching expertise we outlined at the beginning of this chapter suggests that expert performance coaches use professional, interpersonal, and intrapersonal knowledge to improve their athletes' competence, confidence, connection, and character. Ultimately, coaching expertise should result in positive changes in all of these athlete outcomes.

Although a major component of coaching expertise resides in one's ability to teach sport-specific skills (professional knowledge), coaching expertise is also about the ability to create and maintain relationships with others (interpersonal knowledge), and the ability to learn from one's own practice (intrapersonal knowledge). Figure 6.1 summarizes the type of activities that have been shown to have an impact on the training of expert performance coaches and ultimately the acquisition of professional, interpersonal, and intrapersonal knowledge. As noted earlier, expert performance coaches typically accumulate 9,000–12,000 hours of experiences in sport during their development, divided between the categories of (1) athletic

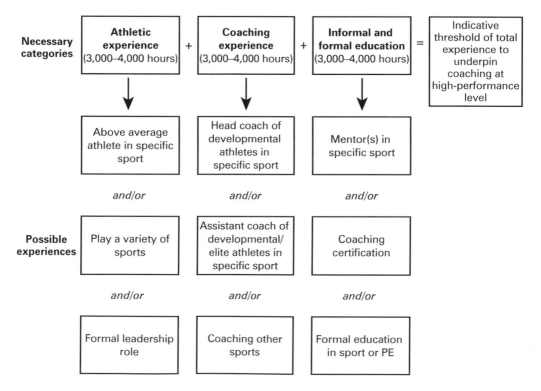

Figure 6.1 Activities and experiences of performance coach development.

experience (3,000–4,000 hours), (2) coaching experience (3,000–4,000 hours), and (3) informal and formal education (3,000–4,000 hours). Within each of these areas, coaches participate in a variety of activities that, added together, contribute to the overall training of an expert coach as illustrated in Figure 6.1.

Assuming that the minimum total number of hours (e.g., 3,000 hours) in an area of activities represents a threshold amount of the total developmental sport experiences required to become a performance head coach, these hours could be experienced in a number of different types of activities (e.g., coaching certification, mentors) that constitute the general area (e.g., formal/informal education). For example, two expert high-performance coaches can both accumulate over 3,000 hours of formal and informal experiences; however, one coach may have a Physical Education degree whereas the other coach may gain most of her formal education at coaching clinics without the benefits of a degree. Thus, variability is expected and has been documented in the specific activities that coaches experience within each of the three general areas of developmental experience shown in Figure 6.1 (athletic experience, coaching experience, and formal/informal education); however, each of the general areas of developmental experience facilitates the development of a unique set of abilities and knowledge necessary to become an expert performance coach.

Figure 6.1 clarifies the type and amount of experiences necessary to become a high-performance coach; however, it does not shed light on the timing of these experiences during the development of a coaching career. The next section will outline a chronological pathway of experiences that can be considered developmental milestones during the emerging career of a performance coach.

Developmental milestones

A performance coach's development is characterized by five stages, each delineated by important milestones (see Figure 6.2). This stage-based model was developed from research on the development of performance coaches in several countries. The first two stages are descriptive of an athletic career in which future coaches develop the positive assets that will set the stage for a future coaching career. These developmental assets (i.e., competence, confidence, connection, and character) could possibly be acquired through other types of extra-curricular activities such as music and art, but youth sport participation is the most common extra-curricular activity of expert performance coaches. Although the athletic experience of a young athlete between the ages of approximately 6 and 19 is difficult to assess in terms of impact on a future coaching career, it is well understood that sport can provide a developmental context that encourages individuals to contribute back to their community. Therefore, a positive youth sport environment serves as the building

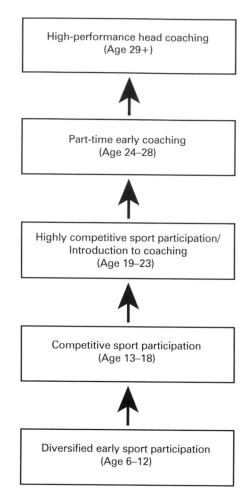

Figure 6.2 Stages of high-performance coach development. (Adapted from Erickson, Côté, and Fraser-Thomas, 2007.)

block of a sporting system that can influence young athletes to become coaches and eventually contribute back to the next generation of athletes.

Figure 6.2 illustrates that the first stage of a successful performance coaching career starts with a *diversified early sport participation* at approximately age six. This stage is characterized by participation in many sport activities, both team and individual in nature, and most often on a recreational basis. The second stage, *competitive sport participation*, occurs at approximately age 13. In this stage, at least one sport is played at a competitive level. For team sport coaches in particular, it is during this stage that most formal leadership opportunities (i.e., being a captain) occur, both in the sport they currently coach and in other team sports.

The third stage, *highly competitive sport participation and introduction to coaching*, occurs at approximately age 19. While the main focus at this stage is still on individuals' own sport participation, often at the elite level, it is during this stage that most coaches first gain coaching experience. Coaches often help with developmental teams after their own competitive season finishes or hold other relatively low-responsibility coaching positions. The fourth stage, *part-time early coaching*, occurs at approximately age 24. As their highly competitive athletic participation ends during this stage, coaches often begin other major activities (e.g., jobs, graduate studies) while coaching part-time. During this stage, most coaching experience occurs as a head coach at a slightly lower competitive level or as an assistant coach at a high-performance level. Coach mentoring usually takes place during this stage. Coaches commonly still participate in sports on a recreational or informal basis at this stage, but the primary focus has shifted from their own participation to coaching others. The fifth and final stage is when a coach obtains a *performance head coaching* position, which occurs at approximately age 29.

The stages of developmental sport experiences for performance sport coaches (Figure 6.2) are an attempt to explain what experiences are needed throughout development to reach a stage of consolidated expertise as a performance-level coach. The definition of the roles associated with such expertise are still under development but, for the purposes of this discussion, a coach taking on a role that involves leading a sustained performance program is deemed to be a "head coach." Within the current international dialogue, head coach roles would appear to equate to senior coach roles. This framework is based on existing data and will clearly need further research from a sport- and country-specific perspective. The initial sport experiences outlined in Figure 6.2 (diversified early sport participation and competitive sport participation) are essentially the same type of contexts that lead to elite performance as an athlete, suggesting a common developmental thread shared by athletes and coaches. Other stages of athletic participation are also roughly equivalent for both athletes' and coaches' development; however, coaches have additional experiential requirements (e.g., leadership for team sport coaches during the competitive sport participation stage and initial coaching experiences for all coaches during the highly competitive sport participation/introduction to coaching stage).

The current model provides an explanation of the transitions from athlete to coach and from initial coaching involvement to high-performance head coaching in terms of the experiences needed to successfully navigate through these transitions. The pursuit of a performance coaching career (e.g., obtaining formal qualifications and engaging in educational coaching experiences) tends to occur during or prior to the final stage of athletic participation, which also coincides with initial coaching experiences. The developmental path of performance coaches presented in Figure 6.2 (and the research on which it is based) also provides support for Simon and

Chase's "10-year rule" (see Chapter 2) regarding the development of expertise in any domain. Specifically, the current model outlines that the difference between average age of initial coaching involvement and average age of obtaining a high performance head coaching position is approximately 10 years.

CONCLUDING REMARKS

The "what," "how much," and "when" analysis presented in this chapter is intended to be directly applicable to structured coach education and development. More specifically, these findings could be used in the development of future coaches by helping to identify and support potentially successful future coaches and to more efficiently educate experientially deficient coaches. For example, formal coaching education might be tailored to meet the specific experiential needs of individual coaches, given their previous experience and current developmental stage. In addition, sport organizations, particularly those with small participation bases who have difficulty developing and retaining performance coaches, might look to identify athletes with the experiential potential to become performance coaches and tailor their sport experiences appropriately.

The more immediate practical implications of each stage of coach development – with their associated activities within the three general experience domains – should also be considered. In the first stage (diversified early sport participation), it seems that future coaches would benefit from exposure to many different sports in a fun-focused environment. A similar conclusion is implicit in the high levels of deliberate play during the sampling years described by emerging models of athlete development, suggesting that such a structure might benefit all athletes, future coach or not. During the second stage (competitive-sport participation), sport environments should be explicitly structured to promote the "4Cs" of athlete development and allow as many athletes as possible to hold leadership roles, as this seems to represent a requisite experience for performance coaching and is generally seen as a life skill that is beneficial in many professional settings. This stage seems critical in developing the desire to contribute back to the sporting community as a coach (the final "C" of positive youth development). Given that the final stage of athletic participation (highly competitive sport participation and introduction to coaching) appears to coincide with the decision to pursue a career in coaching, allowing elite-level athletes opportunities to become involved with coaching experiences tailored to fit their still-demanding athletic schedule might be of utmost importance for the development of future coaches. Finally, in the last stage of development before becoming a performance head coach (part-time early coaching), the most pressing implication seems to be the pairing of these new coaches with a more experienced mentor coach. Although most coaches report gaining access to a mentor coach at this stage through chance meetings or previous connections, there might be benefit to working with a mentor coach from the beginning of one's coaching involvement. Accordingly, providers of coaching education might do well to consider making such pairings a part of their mandate to encourage the development of new coaches who might not have access to a mentor coach on their own, rather than leaving to chance what seems to be a vital experience in the development of professional, interpersonal, and intrapersonal knowledge. The process of supporting the development of more junior coaches should also be more formally identified as part of the responsibility of more experienced coaches, thus making for a stronger on-the-job orientation in the professional development of high-performance coaches.

COACH'S CORNER

Patrick Hunt
Applied Technical Advancement Coach, Australian Institute of Sport

It is great to see the continued emergence of some academic interest in coaching development and expertise. Based on my experiences as a coach and coach mentor I have found that coaches develop their skills in a variety of ways. The list below summarizes most of these.

How do coaches develop?

- playing experience;

- formal coach education courses (Level 0, 1, 2, and 3 coaching diplomas, degrees);

- informal coach development experiences;

- trial and error practice experiences;

- competition experiences;

- program planning and implementation experiences;

- critical evaluation of coaching experiences in both practice sessions and games;

- life experiences.

Obviously all these experiences add up to make you the coach you are. Hence, one problem I see with the scientific need to develop "a model for everything" is that in creating a model it tends to oversimplify the complexity and diversity of experiences that go into the development of coaching expertise. For instance, in the model presented in Figure 6.1 it strikes me that, if coaching development plays out as described, why are there not more high-level ex-players as coaches? Similarly, I always worry when I see numbers of hours tied to a stage of development. This reminds me of the "deliberate practice" approach. Coaches often simplify this theory to the need for them to provide their athletes with 10,000 hours of practice to become elite rather than consider the *quality* of the practice. I hope we do not interpret the model presented in Figure 6.1 in the same manner. However, equally I think the use of the "and/or" approach to recognizing the cumulative and diverse range of experiences that contribute to coach development is an accurate representation. For instance, in my experience, 70 percent of coach development is by way of informal or "on the job" education and the remaining 30 percent is through formal means. However, what contributes to these percentages and the quality of experiences will obviously vary. For instance, although coach education courses are vital, they are only one small part of the coach development process but are often considered all that is needed. I think coach education courses need more content that is focused on the real world of coaching, which I like to term "practically applied coaching."

It might sound like a cliché but the best coaches learn from every experience they have. A significant proportion of coach development time can emerge from the practical experiences that a coach accrues. If coaches can take advantage of this as a learning experience through specific evaluation of their performance, their coaching expertise will continue to develop. A message to the researchers: we need more research that examines what is the best method of evaluating coaching performance. We need a method or system for this evaluation that is non-threatening to the coach and provides practical feedback that a coach can then go away and work on.

Over time I have found the development activities listed below to be particularly beneficial for our coaches:

- less experienced coaches working side-by-side more experienced coaches in development camp settings;
- coach evaluation/feedback sessions;
- international study tours;
- interaction with visiting international coaches;
- coach exchange programs.

All of these experiences involve coaches interacting with other coaches. Informal and formal mentoring opportunities develop from such programs and attendees are exposed to different ways of preparing a player or handling a situation. Mentoring is a hot topic at present in coach development programs. I think there is great potential in mentoring but it needs to be a one-to-one format and structured to achieve specific aims. This will look very different from a more informal approach where a "mentor" coach may be more a critical friend whose opinion is sought typically only in difficult circumstances.

Jean Côté, Karl Erickson, and Pat Duffy

Stages of a basketball coach's development

I have my own version of Figure 6.2. If I were to attach a timeline to someone's coaching life-cycle as it evolves from a first-time beginner coach through to an advanced coach, I would describe the process as follows (see Table 6.1). As you can see, there is a basic progression from the mechanics of coaching – such as developing a good database of drills and strategies – to the more personalized aspects of coaching, which are all about developing effective relationships with players and other staff.

Table 6.1 Stages of a coach's career

Stage of career	Coaching need	Description
Beginning	"Yearning for drills"	Looking for textbook drills
	"Yearning for plays"	Looking for textbook plays
Intermediate	Reinforcing detail	Developing acceptable standards of skill execution at practice
	Game coaching techniques	When to call a time-out, player match-ups, strategic changes
	Coaching on the run	Using succinct coaching terms
	Changing behavior techniques	Using different coaching methods as required
	Anecdotes	Use as another means of getting a message across
Advanced	Detailed information	Imparting necessary but large amounts of information pitched to an individual's skill level
	Implementation information	Does practice transfer to the game?
	"The art of coaching"	Knowing how to change behavior at an individual and group level and integrate
	The "coachable moment"	Recognition of when it occurs
	Personal examples	Use personal coaching and playing experiences

Those coaches that reach the advanced stage of coaching usually find they need to spend more time developing what I refer to as the "non-technical areas of coaching." These include:

- conflict resolution;
- negotiation skills;

- IT user-friendly skills;

- management techniques/planning evaluation;

- group dynamics;

- stress management;

- managing relationships: other coaches, support staff, athletes.

Summary

The development of coaching expertise is a continual process of formal and informal experiences that, if evaluated, can improve one's coaching skills. I do not think coaching expertise can be categorized as something that one reaches after 10 years or 10,000 hours, as most expert coaches continually refer to how much they are still learning.

KEY READING

Côté, J. and Gilbert, W. (2009) 'An integrative definition of coaching effectiveness and expertise', *International Journal of Sports Science and Coaching*, 4: 307–323.

Côté, J., Young, B., Duffy, P., and North, J. (2007) 'Towards a definition of excellence in sport coaching', *International Journal of Coaching Science*, 1: 3–17.

Erickson, K., Côté, J., and Fraser-Thomas, J. (2007) 'The sport experiences, milestones, and educational activities associated with the development of high performance coaches', *The Sport Psychologist*, 21: 302–316.

European Coaching Council (2007) *Review of the EU 5-level structure for the recognition of coaching competence and qualifications*. Köln: European Network of Sports Science, Education and Employment.

Fraser-Thomas, J.L., Côté, J., and Deakin, J. (2005) 'Youth sport programs: An avenue to foster positive youth development', *Physical Education and Sport Pedagogy*, 10: 19–40.

Gilbert, W. and Trudel, P. (2001) 'Learning to coach through experience: Reflection in model youth sport coaches', *Journal of Teaching in Physical Education*, 21: 16–34.

International Council for Coach Education and the Association of Summer Olympic International Federations (in press) 'The International Sport Coaching Framework Version 1.1'. Champaign: Human Kinetics.

Koh, K.T., Mallett, C.J., and Wang, C.K.J. (2011) 'Developmental pathways of Singapore's high-performance basketball coaches', *International Journal of Sport and Exercise Psychology*, 9: 338–353.

Lyle, J. and Cushion, C. (eds.) (2010) *Sports Coaching: Professionalization and Practice*. Oxford: Elsevier.

Werther, P. and Trudel, P. (2006) 'A new theoretical perspective for understanding how coaches learn to coach', *The Sport Psychologist*, 20: 198–212.

PART III

CONTEMPORARY COACHING APPROACHES

CHAPTER 7

OBSERVATION AS AN INSTRUCTIONAL METHOD

NICOLA J. HODGES AND DIANE M. STE-MARIE

INTRODUCTION

Learning through watching others appears to be a pervasive method of skill acqui-sition. The fact that observing someone else perform a skill can positively impact on one's own skill is not debated. What is of interest and debate, however, concerns how learning is achieved through watching others (or oneself), what information is being imparted, and how this depends on the complexity of the action, the skill level, and the goals of the watcher. This information filters down to techniques for imparting knowledge through demonstrations, such as understanding when demonstrations should be given and what they should contain. This, perhaps, becomes even more relevant when we consider that practitioners have more tech-nology available to them than ever before and it is no longer a cumbersome process to provide video models to assist with motor skill acquisition and performance. The mere observation of a model providing a demonstration, however, does not necessarily lead to benefits. Rather, it is important for practitioners to be informed of potential factors that aid or reduce its effectiveness. Our goal in this chapter is to provide an overview of these factors in relation to current research and theory.

DEFINITIONS AND MEASUREMENT

Let us start with some definitions of observational learning. In the literature you will see the terms "observational learning," "observational practice," "imitation," "emulation" and "modeling." In all cases an observer watches a dynamic demon-stration or static image of a "model" performing a skill in order to later re-enact that skill. The model might be a skilled individual, a learner, oneself, a computerized biomechanical display, or an edited video. If the goal is to copy the exact action, technique, or expression, then this might be referred to as "imitation." Probably more common is "emulation," whereby an individual attempts to achieve the same goal(s) as the model. These are both encompassed by the term "modeling," as frequently an observer is trying to use movement-related information to achieve an end goal (e.g., throw a ball a particular distance by adopting the technique of a more skilled individual). "Observational learning" and "observational practice" have been differentiated by the presence or absence of interspersed physical practice respectively. In applied settings it would be rare to watch multiple demonstrations without the chance to physically practice. However, the study of pure observational practice allows researchers to make direct inferences about information that is imparted through watching (uncontaminated by knowledge gained through physically performing). Given the more frequent use of demonstrations interspersed with practice, we will use the term "observational learning" in this chapter to more generally refer to the process of learning through observation.

As with any measure of learning, it is important to consider how demonstrations impact rate of skill acquisition and short-term performance (i.e., how quickly someone gets better) and how well a skill is retained (i.e., how well a skill is remembered across time), as well as what has been learned in terms of generalization to new contexts or similar skills (i.e., transfer). Typically, observational learning benefits are assessed by measurements of accuracy (is a person reducing their error?) or measurements of form (is a person performing more like a model?). In rare cases, visual gaze has been studied to enable inferences about what information is gleaned from a model and how this changes with practice, as well as measures of brain activation to isolate similarities or differences from physical practice or other more covert measures of practice such as imagery – using techniques such as functional magnetic resonance imaging (fMRI), electroencephalography (EEG), and magnetoencephalography (MEG). Although sophisticated equipment is needed to gain accurate information about these features, such as eye trackers, brain-imaging equipment, and motion analysis systems, simple and cost-effective solutions are available in the field to record and analyze movement – such as Dartfish video-editing and analysis (www.dartfish.com) – as well as gain information about where people are looking (e.g., head-mounted web cameras).

How do demonstrations work?

It is likely that a considerable amount of learning from demonstration occurs through the imparting of a strategy or a specific technique that is highly related to task success. For example, to throw a dart accurately, one strategy might be to minimize movements of the shoulder and the elbow. It has been argued that learning through observation is more than just picking up on strategies and this has been supported by research showing that verbal or written instructions are not

Nicola J. Hodges and Diane M. Ste-Marie

always as effective as demonstrations. However, it is possible that demonstrations convey multiple strategies that cannot easily be conveyed through instructions or that demonstrations impart more subtle knowledge than can be imparted explicitly (such as realizing the time of release of an object).

It is thought that demonstrations enable a representation or image of an action that can be used to guide later attempts (much like a perceptual blueprint). There is also evidence that it is difficult to image something that cannot be physically performed, such that this representational mechanism might be limited to skills that are relatively simple or that merely need refining or sequencing (such as perfecting a kick or learning to sequence some dance moves). Indeed, we know that experience modifies the patterns of brain activation seen when observing moves that can or cannot already be performed. There has been evidence to suggest that demonstrations can function to improve learning in a more implicit manner, potentially through a "simulation" process whereby motor-related areas of the brain and possibly muscles are activated (at a reduced level in comparison with actual execution) during observation. Although there is considerable evidence to show that there are cortical brain similarities between physically performing and observing for well-practiced actions, this more implicit type of motor simulation is less likely for novel actions and in the early stages of learning. For the practitioner, this means that the same demonstrations will potentially work differently, depending on the existing skills of the learner. Although there is value in providing demonstrations throughout different stages of skill acquisition, early in the practice of a relatively novel skill, demonstrations might provide more of a strategic value than later when the observer might be able to activate their motor system to covertly practice or simulate what they are seeing. Further research is needed to elucidate what this simulation might involve and when and how it is achieved.

What are demonstrations used for?

In addition to skill-based functions of demonstrations, that is, learning and the acquisition of skill-related information (whether these are perceptual blueprints, strategies, or more implicit information), demonstrations are also believed to provide an important affective role. Albert Bandura, who could easily be considered one of the most influential theorists of observational learning, identified both cognitive and affective processes that could potentially aid performance and learning through observation. A person's perceptions of competency or success at a task (i.e., self-efficacy) were shown to be promoted through vicarious experiences of a given task; that is, observation led to higher levels of self-efficacy. Self-efficacy perceptions are important because they promote persistence and effort, ultimately resulting in improved performance. There is also evidence that watching a model can lead to reductions in fear and anxiety, which might be associated with high task difficulty and chance of injury (e.g., a somersault on a trampoline or a spring-board dive).

The functions of demonstrations have also been explored through an assessment tool called the "Functions of Observational Learning Questionnaire." Through the sampling of a large number of athletes from a variety of sports, demonstrations were reported to broadly serve three functions, with varying frequencies. Not surprisingly, "to learn and improve skill execution (skill function)" was the most common. Less frequently, athletes reported that they used demonstrations "to learn and improve strategies and game plans (strategy function)." Least often, observation was reported to play a "performance function," aiding mental and physiological arousal. In terms of research, most attention has been directed to the skill-function of observation.

How do we use observation effectively?

There are many factors to consider in answering questions about how to use demonstrations as an effective practice or competitive enhancement tool. These factors have been noted by a number of different authors over the past few decades but most recently these factors have been integrated into an applied model for the use of observation (see Figure 7.1). The characteristics of the observer and the task should be given early attention. For observers, factors such as their age and stage of learning (novice or advanced) will influence the success of the observation experience. Task characteristics can include factors such as skill complexity, action goals, and whether the skill to be learned is discrete, serial, or continuous. Discrete skills are those that have a defined beginning and end, such as a cartwheel. When discrete skills are combined together they form serial skills (e.g., cartwheel to back walkover), whereas continuous skills are those that have an arbitrary beginning and end (e.g., running or swimming). Observation effectiveness is dependent on these task characteristics, so they need consideration before embarking on observational practice interventions. The second level of the applied model is based on the reasons why the learner is using observation (i.e., function) and the situational context (e.g., training versus competition). These factors listed above will impact on (a) the type of model to use, (b) the content of the demonstration, and (c) when they should be administered and the structure of the training session (before, after, during, intermixed), as well as (d) how they should be provided (e.g., frequency, speed, control of viewing). We review some of the literature on each of these four modeling characteristics (i.e., who, what, when, and how), but recognize they are limited in scope and encourage readers to expand on this content by perusing some of the selected works recommended at the end of this chapter.

118

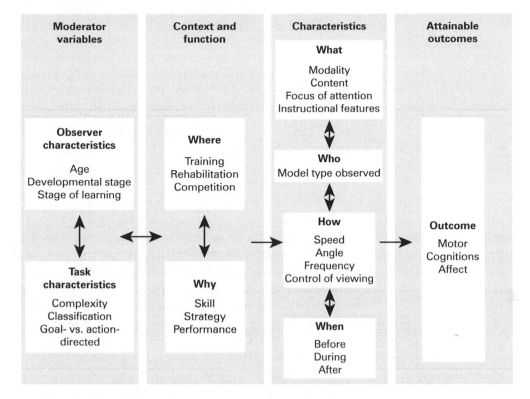

Moderator variables	Context and function	Characteristics	Attainable outcomes

What

Modality
Content
Focus of attention
Instructional features

Observer characteristics

Age
Developmental stage
Stage of learning

Where

Training
Rehabilitation
Competition

Who
Model type observed

How

Speed
Angle
Frequency
Control of viewing

Outcome

Motor
Cognitions
Affect

Task characteristics

Complexity
Classification
Goal- vs. action-directed

Why

Skill
Strategy
Performance

When

Before
During
After

Figure 7.1 The applied model for the use of observation. (Reprinted with permission from Ste-Marie *et al.*, 2012.)

THEORY INTO PRACTICE

Whom should I watch?

There are a variety of model types to choose from, with a basic distinction being the observation of others as opposed to that of the self. When observing others, one can observe a skilled model that is showing "ideal" execution, or an unskilled model showing errors in execution, or even learning models that progress from "incorrect" to "correct" execution. Although a correct model might be referred to as a "mastery" model, some researchers have added verbal statements during the observational learning period to highlight this mastery component and to tap into the skill-based function of observational learning as well as the affective component. For example, a skilled model that also verbalizes self-efficacious statements, such as "I know I can do this skill" and low task difficulty (e.g., "this is an easy task for me") is referred to as a "mastery model." In contrast, a "coping" model is one that progresses from low to high(er) skill, as with learning models, but might also be accompanied by low to high self-efficacy statements and high to low statements concerning task difficulty perceptions.

Viewing others

Skilled models have frequently been shown to provide a skill acquisition benefit and this benefit has been linked to the formation of a strong mental representation of what to do (i.e., a goal template) as well as increased attention from an observer to a model that they perceive to be highly skilled and competent. Researchers initially argued that only a skilled model could be effective for teaching because of the importance of or need for a correct mental representation of the skill. It is now recognized that an unskilled or learning model can assist observers with skill acquisition as long as the performance-dependent feedback provided to the model is also available to the observer. For example, it is not enough to see the action required to perform a throw or kick; rather the observer must also be able to hear any corrections to the movement provided by the coach and see or be told where the ball landed. Augmented feedback, coupled with the observed demonstration, engages the learner in problem-solving processes related to the motor solution and thus also facilitates learning as long as the learner is clear about what he or she is trying to achieve. Moreover, a model that is perceived to be more similar to the observer has sometimes been shown to be more effective for learning, perhaps as a result of greater attention and ease of simulating or copying than that of a highly skilled model. Thus, when a skilled model is not immediately available, practitioners can use others in the group to model the skill, but they must be sure to provide the necessary corrections to skill performance for all to hear.

When comparing mastery and coping models, it is noted that the type of model can influence what is learned through observation. Perhaps not surprisingly, mastery models have been shown to be more effective for enhancing skill execution, but coping models have had more of an effect on observers' perceptions of self-efficacy. Accordingly, practitioners who want to first focus on an athlete's self-perceptions of confidence to do a task could begin with a coping model and then transition into a mastery model as they begin to target more physical aspects of the performance.

Watching oneself

Observation of the self is an alternative way of modeling desired behavior and some research has shown that the self can be a better model than others. There are two basic forms of self-as-a-model interventions. The first is standard video replay, termed self-observation, wherein the learners observe their previous attempt(s) of the skill. In effect, this type of demonstration also functions as feedback as the observer gains access to the visual consequences of their actions, often allowing them to see features of the action which were hidden from them during performance. The second form is self-modeling and involves video editing before viewing.

Self-observation research has yielded somewhat equivocal findings that make it difficult to assess its usefulness for skill acquisition. The varied findings highlight that there are important factors related to the effectiveness of self-observation. One factor concerns the observer's stage of learning. Novice learners need to be guided in terms of the relevant features in the display to which attention should be directed, whereas advanced learners can use self-observation without such direction. Researchers have also shown that novice learners who see their own performances alongside that of an expert (or a correct model), either in a split-screen format or immediately preceding a demonstration, obtain additional benefits from self-observation as compared with only viewing themselves or only viewing a demonstration. Thus, comparative information can enrich the learning experience provided by self-observation. Finally, equivocal findings in research may be related to the lack of information surrounding the frequency of viewings, when videos were used, who controlled when a video was viewed, what instructions accompanied a video, and other such variables that can be manipulated. More research on these issues is needed to further guide practitioners in the use of self-observation. We are unaware of any negative effects associated with self-observation for motor learning and, especially for actions that are difficult to see (i.e., you cannot see what your arm is doing when it goes behind your head during a cricket bowl or tennis serve), making the "unobservable observable" would appear to be a sound principle.

For self-modeling, two techniques have been used to edit the video. The positive self-review technique involves the elimination of poor performances, such that the observer only sees their best performance attempts. The feedforward technique is different in that it entails editing the video to show the individual executing at a performance level that has not yet been attained or in a context in which that task has yet to be executed. In Figure 7.2 we have shown six video stills showing different phases of a gymnastic stunt (i.e., back handspring) assembled from multiple attempts at this action. With reference to skill acquisition, again the research has yielded relatively mixed results. Self-modeling has been shown to enhance certain skills, such as in trampolining and swimming. In studies of gymnastics, figure skating, and volleyball skills, however, athletes who used self-modeling techniques in addition to physical practice were no better than those who used physical practice alone. These discrepant findings may be related to the skill level of the athletes or to the type of self-modeling technique used (positive self-review or feedforward). For the two skills where benefits were noted, the feedforward technique was adopted

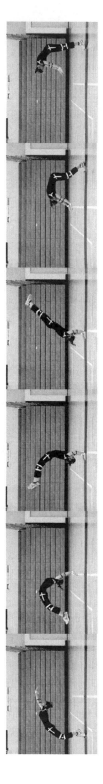

Figure 7.2 An example of a "feedforward" video shown for illustration as six consecutive still frames. In this example the gymnast is performing a handspring which has been assembled from different phases of her best attempts at performing this skill.

with novice learners, whereas, in the studies that failed to show benefits, positive self-review was used with intermediate skilled athletes. Therefore, although further research is needed to isolate the important variable behind self-modeling benefits and potential learner–technique interactions, watching oneself perform a "future" behavior seems to have more power to effect change, particularly during early learning, than positive review of current performance. What is worth considering, however, is that a fair amount of labor and time is needed to construct self-modeling videos than using self-observation, so we question its utility in all skill acquisition settings.

There is also some evidence that self-modeling videos provide an important performance enhancement role. Research with gymnasts showed that higher competitive scores were obtained when the gymnasts watched a feedforward self-modeling video than when they did not watch one. Despite the time needed to create the video, the advantage for the gymnasts was three-tenths of a point: an increase in score that can make the difference between fourth place and first place on the podium. Interviews with the gymnasts revealed the important role of the video for increasing self-efficacy and placing them in an optimal arousal state prior to competition (performance function), as well as inciting other strategic functions (e.g., using imagery).

In summary, when considering who should be observed, the practitioner needs to consider that skilled, unskilled, mastery, and coping models all have a role to play depending on the skill level of the learner and the goal of the observation experience. Self-as-a-model techniques also have merit, with self-observation augmenting the skill-learning experience when consideration is given to the observer's stage of learning and guidance is provided as needed. Feedforward self-modeling appears to be more effective than positive self-review and self-observation for skill learning. Feedforward self-modeling may be of most benefit in the competitive sport performance environment and in the early stages of skill learning.

What should a demonstration contain?

The observer's existing skills (or what might be referred to as "functional task difficulty") and the difficulty of the to-be-learned skill (what has been referred to as "nominal task difficulty") are important considerations when making decisions about what information a demonstration should contain as well as where attention should be directed. Rather than try to comprehensively address all the various information manipulations and measurements of critical information, we highlight below a few cautionary notes about the content of demonstrations. First, a learning context that includes demonstrations conveys multiple goals and thus it is important for the observer and the practitioner to be aware of their main or primary goal throughout practice. It is important to consider whether the primary goal is to copy the action or to achieve an outcome. There is evidence to show that technique is sacrificed at the expense of goal attainment if insufficient emphasis is put on movement form. Children are especially susceptible to this prioritizing of outcome goals at the expense of movement goals. Although outcome attainment might be more rewarding for an individual and allows for creative and self-determined solutions for outcome success, in some skills this sacrifice of movement quality for outcome success could have later repercussions. For example, an inefficient cricket bowling or tennis service action might lead to fatigue or injury during competition. Certain techniques are inherently more variable than others (perhaps because of the number of joints involved). Under conditions which are likely to promote further variability, such as increased competitive pressure, the original more variable technique is likely to be more negatively affected. Therefore, if modeling a desired technique is viewed to be a primary goal of the observational learning process, it may be necessary for the practitioner to de-emphasize outcome attainment by rewarding form-related goals at the expense of outcome attainment.

Related to this issue above and the need to prioritize actions or outcomes during observational learning, there is some debate about whether individuals should be guided to acquire an "ideal" technique and hence focus on form-related goals. For researchers who advocate a constraints-based method of teaching, it is believed that the movement itself or the technique should be viewed as one potential solution to an outcome goal and not a prescription for individuals to copy. If an individual is shown only a technique-oriented demonstration that is not clearly related to the outcome, or if form rather than outcome success is emphasized as the goal, arguably the learner might copy a movement solution that is not optimal for their stage of learning, body size, or strength. However, there is clearly some benefit to be gained from guiding people to find efficient and effective movements. Therefore, the practitioner or learner must consider the relationship between actions and outcomes and find a balance between prescribing what to do and allowing the learner to sculpt a solution that allows them to achieve the task outcome quickly and appropriately based on their existing skills and needs. Awareness of these potentially conflicting goals and needs is important for successful teaching.

Data from visual gaze tracking and occlusion studies (where key areas at specific time points are degraded or removed during observation) suggest that the critical information from a model performing a goal-oriented action pertains to the action end point. This might be the trajectory of an object to be thrown, the foot that is kicking a ball, or the bat or arm that is swinging during a batting or golfing action. If a kicking action is being taught, an observer will typically focus their attention on the foot of the model, although there is suggestive evidence that the focus becomes less distal (away from the body's midline) and more proximal (towards the body's midline) as both physical and observational practice proceeds. Interestingly, people do not even need to see the actions of the model to gain from observational practice. Trajectories of objects (such as a ball or Frisbee® disc) convey information about the throw or kick such that the movement solution can be discovered as a result of trying to "match" an outcome effect. There is considerable evidence to support such an "externally" oriented focus of attention during performance and learning in order to attain maximal skill outcomes. What practitioners must promote, however, is change in performance when observation is serving a skill acquisition function. That is, if one type of demonstration is not leading to a change in the learner's form (and that is the desired goal of the instruction), then a new type of model might be needed and/or a change in instructions and feedback.

For some individuals, change can be brought about by focusing externally and attempting to emulate what they are seeing, whereas others seem to need more prescription (i.e., this is how you do something) in order to bring about a change in an ineffective or immature movement pattern or technique. Cueing has been shown to be an effective technique to help learners pay attention to information within a demonstration that is believed to be critical for success (depending on the observer's needs and current skill level and technique). Although a body-focused cueing technique might be helpful for practice and changing movement form, it is generally agreed that, for optimal performance in competition, attention to the external action effects is more likely to result in skill efficacy and efficiency than attention to body-related components (see Chapter 10). It is worth noting that both a body focus and an outcome focus can be independently encouraged through video, depending on how the video is edited and the goals of the demonstration.

When do I show (and tell)?

Much like physical practice, retention advantages are gained from scheduling of demonstrations in such a way that the observer is maximally engaged in the task. This means actively trying to detect errors, looking and thinking about ways errors are corrected, and watching with the intention to learn and later re-enact (see Chapter 8). For example, if the intention is to learn a number of different skills, such as a forehand Frisbee® disc throw, a backhand throw, and a left-hand throw, then it is more beneficial to show these skills in a mixed or random schedule than it is to repeat the same skill multiple times before demonstrating the next. It also helps to let people choose when to see a demonstration during observational learning. Demonstrations are most effective if they are provided early in practice, rather than just interspersed during practice or only provided later in practice. However, allowing people to discover for themselves what to do early in practice before being shown what to do can have later benefits for skill retention. These so-called "retroactive demonstrations" are believed to aid cognitive processes associated with memory and self-evaluation of actions.

There is currently some debate about whether demonstrations can take the place of physical practice when interspersed in a learning paradigm with physical practice. This is of course important in a practical context where physical practice time might be limited and hence observational practice may be a valuable low-impact training opportunity. For example, if 200 trials of practice are given, does it matter whether 50 percent of those trials are watched rather than physically performed? In one study involving dyad (two-person) learning of how to make wide and fast movements on a ski simulator, alternating physical practice between the pair (i.e., 50 percent observation, 50 percent practice) was as beneficial as 100 percent physical practice throughout. Similar results were found in a study that required people to aim towards targets in a novel "virtual" type of environment. Mixed practice, where 75 percent of the practice was by observation, was as good as physical practice in terms of accuracy on a posttest. Interestingly, in measures of recalibration of the motor system to determine whether the relationship between motor commands and a person's intended effects had changed, the mixed practice group showed more recalibration than the physical practice group. Just observing, although beneficial with respect to first-time performance in the novel environment, did not lead to the same type of learning as physical or mixed practice (i.e., no recalibration). There are a number of studies which lead us to suspect that observational practice promotes a different, more strategic type of learning than physical practice but that interspersing physical practice with observational practice might alleviate these differences and potentially aid processes related to physically practicing. However, this is still quite speculative and further research is needed.

Finally, there is some evidence that watching demonstrations leads to gradually improved perceptions of ability, which might suggest an important affective component associated with observational practice even though it might not translate into immediate improvements in motor outcomes. Allowing people to view demonstrations when their abilities are low might foster a sense of competency which at the very least should aid motivation to continue to practice.

How much should I watch?

In terms of the amount of demonstrations to provide, as noted above, research has shown that the relative proportion of observation can be as much as 75 percent observation to 25 percent physical practice, with the same gains shown as 100 percent physical practice. Other researchers have reported that, when given the choice under time-constrained conditions, the preferred frequency of demonstrations to physical practice is about 10–20 percent of the overall amount of practice. People prefer "doing" more than just watching and it makes sense that this would be the case as physically performing provides the individual with self-generated feedback and a sense of their own action capabilities. However, it does appear that the more demonstrations watched during practice, the more likely it is that a desired movement form will also be adopted in addition to successful outcome attainment. Therefore, although giving athletes some control over how much they watch has some benefits, potentially having some base line levels associated with observation frequency might be useful if technique goals are important.

A variety of factors are likely to come into the determination of the relative percentage of observation to physical practice within a practice session. For example, some activities generate greater muscle fatigue, not allowing for extensive repetitions within a practice setting. Therefore, a greater amount of observation to physical practice may be required than in activities in which physical practice of the skills can be more frequent with little physical fatigue. Another factor to consider is whether the skill acquisition setting might involve taking turns. In this case, practitioners could optimize this practice scenario by encouraging those waiting to attend to their team-mates' performances and to listen to their corrective feedback. Given factors such as these, there are no specific rules concerning the optimal amount of observation to integrate into a practice but practitioners are encouraged to mindfully incorporate observation in what appears to be "dead" time in the practice.

CONCLUDING REMARKS

There are a variety of factors that practitioners can consider for optimally integrating observation into physical practice, such that the practice structure is designed to maximize the coaching outcomes. Based on the above review we have chosen to compile a list of our top 12 considerations for the effective use of observation for performance and learning. These considerations are detailed in Box 7.1.

Box 7.1 Top 12 list of considerations and guidelines for the effective use of observation

1   Observation should be combined with physical practice for maximum benefit.

2   Demonstrations should be interspersed with practice in a faded schedule (more at first, then gradually reduced) such that they are not relied upon and the learner figures out for themselves what they need to do to achieve success.

Box 7.1 Continued

3 The type of model should be dictated by the observation objective. If the goal is for the learner to feel more self-efficacious about their own capabilities to learn a new skill, a coping/learning model may work best. If the goal is for detection of critical movement information, a skilled (or mastery) model would be more effective.

4 Watching oneself perform a "future" behavior (through video editing) has more power to effect change, particularly during early learning, than positive review of current "best" performance.

5 Verbal cues can help guide observation. This is particularly useful for younger children and new learners.

6 Demonstrations work as performance feedback as well as prescriptions about what to do. Coaches should be aware that attempting a skill before being shown what to do can aid skill retention.

7 Demonstrations need to work to encourage change if they are serving a skill acquisition function. Differential emphasis on the action, the action end point, or the outcome goals should be considered to bring about change.

8 Observation serves a number of functions not only to improve skill learning and performance, but also for learning about strategies and modifying performance state variables (such as emotion, confidence, competitiveness).

9 Athletes should be encouraged to watch each other and to listen to the coaches' feedback during their own recovery or wait times to get the most out of a practice session. Taking turns in physically performing an action with a fellow athlete will afford opportunities for both physical and observational practice. This "mixed" method of interspersing observation and physical practice appears to be optimal for learning.

10 Allowing athletes to choose when they want to have a demonstration or see themselves on video can enhance the observation experience (although scheduling minimum amounts might be a good idea if technique changes are desired).

11 Demonstration effectiveness is enhanced through comparative information, such as self-videos.

12 Technique-focused demonstrations are best for practice and changing movement form. For optimal performance in competition, demonstrations that promote attention to the external action effects/outcomes are more likely to result in skill efficacy and efficiency (i.e., successful outcomes).

Nicola J. Hodges and Diane M. Ste-Marie

My first reaction on turning to the last page was "wow!" Doing less physical training and relying more on observation could prevent considerable wear and tear and prolong the life of an athlete by quite a few years. Why, then, are we not doing more of this kind of training? What challenges do specialists and experts encounter when attempting to apply this approach across the board?

I am fortunate to have worked with Olympic athletes as well as elementary school kids and everything in between. At the university, I have the luxury of instructing beginners and thus utilizing and testing various approaches to teaching basic volleyball skills.

I cannot dispute the findings of many studies supporting the validity of learning and training by observation. In fact, we have used these approaches with our varsity team throughout the years. However, I can list some of the additional challenges I have faced as I attempted to introduce this method, and offer some suggestions on how to make it better:

1 (a) What the brain captures and what it communicates to the muscles as actions to be emulated does not necessarily determine how the body will perform. The best evidence can be gathered by asking observers what they are doing; they may respond with different explanations for their performance. I will expand on this later.

2 (b) Elite athletes tend to be "doers." In fact, the culture of sport emphasizes and praises hard work as something essential for success in sport. There are two key points here: one relates to the mentality of elite athletes and coaches, and the second to the culture of sport.

Discussion

I will expand here on the point raised above – point (a) – about the ways in which watching translates into performance by sharing my experiences as a teacher of beginner, intermediate, and advanced athletes:

1 A discussion of the relationship between observation and performance should take into account the fact that the brain processes visual information on different levels. An athlete will not be conscious of everything he or she has taken in. We see proof of this by observing the performance of athletes who have watched a demonstration of movements and then attempt to copy them; often we are surprised by the fact that they do something markedly different. Their expressions of amazement after seeing themselves on video suggest that frequently there is a disconnect between what the eyes/brain computes and the physical performance. One of the methods I use to optimize the benefits of an observational exercise is to ask athletes to

execute the "wrong" action. I call this "Reverse Mechanics." Interestingly, once these athletes are made conscious of the wrong way to perform a movement, either they have difficulty doing it or they look at you strangely because they have been told numerous times by other coaches not to do it that way.

2 When athletes are asked to explain movements or demonstrate them for others, quite often their explanations do not correspond with the demonstrations.

3 It is always important to include a demonstration of the "wrong" way to provide observers with an image of actions to be avoided. Usually, I "clown around" exaggerating the typical mistakes so that students can see the difference between the correct movements and the incorrect ones. I have found this approach to be particularly effective with beginners.

4 Many theorists are committed to the "just doing it" approach. They believe in learning by playing with few additional cues. In other words, at the initial stages, coaching should be minimal.

5 Showing an athlete what an action "feels" like is another method I favor. This involves having athletes perform the action while limiting some sensory options (closing their eyes) so they can focus fully on how it feels to execute a particular movement. Some sports make frequent use of this approach (e.g., gymnastics and diving), but very seldom do we use it for instructing team sports.

In relation to my second key observation – point (b) – one of the other major challenges we face – and we do not see this addressed in this chapter – is how to arrive at a better understanding of the relationship between the mental state of athletes (particularly elite athletes) and the culture of sport:

1 Individuals become elite athletes because they possess traits that differentiate them from others. The ability to endure and enjoy hard physical work no doubt ranks high among those traits. Consequently, one can assume that elite athletes are keen on being active and that the opportunity to observe is not appealing unless it is accompanied by a systematic approach and compelling arguments.

2   The culture of sport has emphasized hard work to the exclusion of almost everything else. The idea of "working smart" has been introduced but, like all new ideas, it is gaining acceptance very slowly. If learning by observing is to become a key piece of the instruction and training of athletes, we must change the culture by convincing our coaches and athletes that there is now plenty of evidence that supports this approach and that it is both a better training method and better for the athletes.

Conclusion

This is a welcome contribution by Nicola J. Hodges and Diane M. Ste-Marie. They have gathered compelling evidence to steer the teaching and coaching of sports in a fruitful direction. If the challenges outlined in this commentary are addressed, the success of this approach is very plausible.

ACKNOWLEDGMENT

The first author would like to acknowledge funding from the Social Sciences and Humanities Research Council of Canada (SSHRC) in completing this project.

KEY READING

Bandura, A.J. (1997) *Self-Efficacy: The Exercise of Control*. New York: W.H. Freeman.

Calvo-Merino, B., Grèzes, J., Glaser, D.E., Passingham, R.E., and Haggard, P. (2006) 'Seeing or doing? Influence of visual and motor familiarity in action observation', *Current Biology*, 16: 1905–1910.

Carroll, W.R. and Bandura, A. (1982) 'The role of visual monitoring in observational learning of action patterns: Making the unobservable, observable', *Journal of Motor Behavior*, 14: 153–167.

Cumming, J., Clark, S.E., Ste-Marie, D.M., McCullagh, P., and Hall, C. (2005) 'The functions of observational learning questionnaire (FOLQ)', *Psychology of Sport & Exercise*, 6: 517–537.

Dowrick, P.W. (1999) 'A review of self-modeling and related interventions', *Applied and Preventative Psychology*, 8: 23–29.

Hodges, N.J. and Franks, I.M (2004) 'Instructions, demonstrations and the learning process: creating and constraining movement options', in Williams, A.M. and Hodges, N.J. (eds.) *Skill Acquisition in Sport: Research, Theory and Practice*. London: Routledge, pp. 145–174.

Hodges, N.J., Williams, A.M., Hayes, S.J., and Breslin, G. (2007), 'What is modeled during observational learning?', *Journal of Sports Sciences*, 25: 531–545.

McCullagh, P., Law, B., and Ste-Marie, D.M. (2012) 'Modeling and performance', in Murphy, S. (ed.) *The Oxford Handbook of Sport and Performance Psychology*. New York: Oxford University Press, pp. 250–272.

Maslovat, D., Hayes, S.J., Horn, R., and Hodges, N.J. (2010) 'Motor learning through observation', in Elliott, D. and Khan, M.A. (eds.) *Vision and Goal-Directed Movement: Neurobehavioural Perspectives*. Champaign, IL: Human Kinetics, pp. 315–340.

Ong, N. and Hodges, N.J. (2012) 'Mixing it up a little: How to schedule observational practice', in Hodges, N.J. and Williams, A.M. (eds.) *Skill Acquisition in Sport: Research, Theory and Practice*. London: Routledge, pp. 22–39.

Ste-Marie, D.M., Law, B., Rymal, A.M., O, J., McCullagh, P., and Hall, C. (2012) 'Observation interventions for motor skill learning and performance: An applied model for the use of observation', *International Review of Sport and Exercise Psychology*, 2: 1–32.

Wulf, G., Raupach, M., and Pfeiffer, F. (2005) 'Self-controlled observational practice enhances learning', *Research Quarterly for Exercise & Sport*, 76: 107–111.

CHAPTER 8

ORGANIZING PRACTICE

EFFECTIVE PRACTICE IS MORE THAN JUST REPS

JAE T. PATTERSON AND TIMOTHY D. LEE

Question: I know you had a practice session on Thursday, but how were the rest of them [practice sessions]? Was it just a problem with transferring of weight?

Tiger Woods: Absolutely. I can get it on the range, I can get it dialed in there, and we'll work on the same things and it feels really good, and I go to the golf course and I just don't quite trust it. It just means I just need to do more reps.

(http://web.tigerwoods.com/news/article/2012040828205704/news/)

For many people, "reps" (short for "repetitions") are the answer to any and all problems related to motor and sport skills; it is not just athletes such as Tiger Woods who believe this to be so. For example, physical therapists have been told that the memory representations that are responsible for the ability to perform movements (engrams) are formed only by repetition of the target movement. Forming engrams is believed to be achieved through thousands of repetitions and the perfection of movement patterns.

What exactly does a "repetition" mean and, more importantly, what purpose is served by repetitions? A long-held view is that a repetition is the replication of an ideal movement pattern and that its purpose is to "stamp" onto the central nervous system a memory of a correctly executed action. The idea here is that repetitions act like layers of clothing that protect a person from the effects of wind, rain, and cold – the more layers that are added, the more protection is provided. In the case of movement repetitions, we believe the commonly held view is that each correctly executed action in practice, such as a golf swing, will strengthen its memory and facilitate its reproducibility in a performance situation (e.g., in a competition). Therefore, the more "perfect" the repetitions, the stronger the memory of the correct action and hence the more effective the development of the motor skill. This is seemingly consistent with the idea expressed in the Tiger Woods quotation earlier with regard to his golf swing.

There are a number of implications that result from this implicitly held assumption about the role of repetitions. One implication is that movement repetitions and practice should be perfect (i.e., errorless; see Chapter 9). If this is so, then how can practice be organized to achieve perfect repetitions? Using the golfer on a practice range as an example, one way to achieve perfect practice involves repeating the correct swing over and over again so that it becomes "stamped" into the memory. However, golfers are often faced with the fact that they cannot make a perfect swing on successive repetitions. One common fix is the use of physical guidance devices that force the golfer to make the swing along a correct path or trajectory in space. Again the idea is to repeat the correct movement. Once an idea of the correct swing is attained, the guidance aid can be removed and the golfer should make many repetitions of the correct swing in order to better stamp it into memory. Some golfers seek instructors to help with their swings under the assumption that information provided from the instructor should be practiced as immediately as possible so that incorrect repetitions are no longer being made. These and other techniques designed to enhance the physical effect of repetitions emerge from a theoretical view that "practice makes perfect, and perfect practice makes more perfect." Research suggests, however, that nothing could be further from the truth.

In this chapter we take a different view regarding what makes an effective repetition, then provide evidence that practice of pre-movement planning and post-movement evaluation are as important as, if not more important than, the repetition of movement alone. Our goal here is to ask coaches and athletes to redefine their view of what makes an effective "rep" and the role that repetitions serve in the development of sport skill. To achieve that goal we ask the reader to consider the practice-related factors that serve to promote maximal involvement of the "3 Bs" in the skill acquisition process.

BRAIN, BIOMECHANICS, AND BEHAVIOR: THE "3 BS" OF MOVEMENT SKILL

We agree with Stephen Scott, who suggested the concept that movement skill consists of three fundamental components, which he called the "3 Bs": brain, biomechanics, and behavior. The process begins with the *brain* understanding the goal of the motor task, followed by the brain organizing a movement plan that is subsequently sent to the musculoskeletal system to achieve the goal of the task. The precision and coordination of the musculoskeletal system in achieving the goal of the task is referred to as the *biomechanics* of the planned movement. The success of the brain in planning the required movement and the characteristics of that movement (i.e., biomechanics) is inferred through the observable *behavior* of the athlete, that is, what happened in reference to the goal of the task (e.g., did the ball land close to the target?). The observable behavior is used not only by the coach to measure success of the practice context, but also by the athlete to assess the success of their motor planning (see Figure 8.1 for illustration).

Consider, for example, the "3 Bs" of movement skill in striking a golf ball. The role of the brain is to assess the situation (state of the environment such as wind, rain; state of the individual such as motivation, fatigue, anxiety levels) in order to decide a plan of action and to organize and channel a suitable movement plan for striking the ball. The biomechanics involve the response of the central nervous system to the movement plan including the output of the musculoskeletal

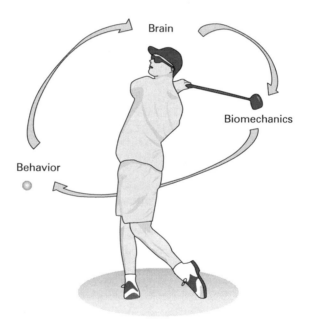

Figure 8.1 The "3 Bs" of motor control: the brain assesses the current state of environment (wind, rain, noise levels) and is impacted by the individual states (such as motivation, fatigue, and anxiety levels) of the performer; the biomechanics refers to the coordination of the motor action produced by the motor system; the behavior refers to what the movement felt like, sounded like, and looked like, and also includes feedback from others such as the coach.

134

system and resulting in the execution of the golf swing. The resulting behavior is the outcome of the golf swing – these are the sensory results of the action: what it looked, sounded, and felt like – plus feedback from other people or perhaps from an inanimate device such as a video recording (see Chapter 13). Feedback is then remembered and used by the brain in the preparation and planning for the next shot, starting the "3 Bs" cycle again.

To us, this description of movement skill provides a wonderfully simple yet accurate description of a repetition. More importantly, this conceptualization of a repetition lays down the framework for what we think is "perfect" practice. Quite simply, we believe that effective practice involves repeating the "3 Bs" of movement skill – maximal involvement of brain, biomechanics, and behavior – on each and every repetition.

Note that this emphasis on repetition as the involvement of all "3 Bs" is at odds with how most people practice and learn motor tasks such as golf. For most golfers, practice is typically undertaken (a) without a pre-shot routine (see Chapter 10), (b) under the same conditions, with the same club, and to the same target, and (c) without much reflection on the outcome of the shot. In our view, this style of golf practice, which Pia Nilsson and her colleagues call "scrape and hit," places too much emphasis squarely on the repetition of the swing, or just one of the "3 Bs" (biomechanics). In our view, such a style of practice is ineffective because it minimizes the involvement of the brain and evaluation of the behavior.

WHAT DOES THE RESEARCH TELL US? HOW TO ORGANIZE PRACTICE

Skill acquisition researchers suggest that it is not *how much* the performer practices (i.e., the absolute number of physical repetitions of the biomechanical pattern such as a golf swing), but *how* the performer completed each repetition (i.e., active involvement of the brain during planning and interpretation of subsequent motor behavior) as the practice factor that contributes most to the motor learning process. In fact, a famous work by the Russian motor behavior scientist Nikolai Bernstein suggested in 1967 that practice is "repetition without repetition" because it is not the physical repetition of movements (i.e., the movements required for a golf swing) over and over again that is most effective for learning. Rather, a repetition should require athletes to engage in the activities required by the brain to plan and interpret the outcome of their movement. Thus, a repetition should be viewed as an additive experience of all the factors responsible for movement production (e.g., the "3 Bs" of movement skill), such that the athlete has the opportunity to build upon past motor and cognitive experiences.

For each repetition, a strong link between the amount of effort the performer invests into planning a movement and the subsequent motor skill proficiency achieved is considered essential for skilled performance. Facilitating the relationship between efficient sport-specific cognitive processing and movement expertise is based on the following factors:

- the practice session must optimally challenge both the cognitive (brain) and motor (biomechanics) capabilities of the athlete;
- the practice session must facilitate the athlete's skill and efficiency at the cognitive processing requirements to plan a movement (brain);
- the athlete must be provided the opportunity to learn how to detect *when* errors have occurred in the movement, *why* they occurred, and *how* to fix them based on an understanding of relevant movement-related feedback from their own movements.

Therefore, a repetition (e.g., a golf shot) can be viewed as a problem-solving process in which practice reflects not only the movement component (e.g., the coordination requirements of the golf swing) of motor skill performance, but the cognitive processes as well (e.g., deciding on club selection, potential risks, assessing wind effects, and motivation levels). Emphasis on the cognitive processes required for movement planning and those processes required for interpreting the success of a repetition is consistent with the idea that motor skills are highly cognitive in nature. Many experts, in addition to their motor skill proficiency, also demonstrate superiority in the cognitive processes required for monitoring, planning (e.g., retrieval of information), and understanding (interpreting the results) of their motor performance (see Chapters 10 and 13).

Let us return again to the idea that "perfect practice makes more perfect." This misconception highlights an emphasis on the physicality (e.g., biomechanics) of the practice session, such that "errorless" physical repetitions are more desirable than repetitions with "error." Yet our current understanding of practice contexts facilitating skill learning challenges this myth by highlighting the importance of "training the brain" *with* the physical components of a repetition. For example, the information required by the brain to *plan* a motor skill such as a soccer kick and then to accurately *evaluate* the success of that skill is believed by many to be the steps required by the brain for skilled motor performance. However, for practice sessions designed to "train the brain" by requiring both planning and evaluation, there is a caveat: mistakes and errors. Practice contexts that ask the performer to think (plan and evaluate) more often result in performance that would be considered less *skilled* by the coach or the athlete (e.g., proper technique of a golf swing). Although more effective in the long run, this type of practice is accompanied by frequent movement errors early on that are gradually reduced over the duration of the practice session. However, as will be discussed later in this chapter, movement error is believed to be an advantage rather than a disadvantage to the athlete during the acquisition of persistent skilled motor performance, thereby challenging the notion that "perfect practice makes more perfect."

THE IMPORTANCE OF THE TIME BEFORE AND AFTER THE MOVEMENT

The organization of the practice session can be considered as two distinct events separated by the processes required by the brain *before* and *after* completion of a motor action. Before the motor action, researchers have identified such factors as how many motor skills are being trained in the same session, the order of practicing multiple motor skills, and the role of imagining the performance of these motor skills (e.g., motor imagery) as either positively or negatively influencing how the performer engages in the thinking processes required by the brain to *plan* a motor action. Once an athlete has completed an action such as a golf chip shot they must then engage in the thought processes required by the brain for understanding the success of the swing in reference to the task goal (reaching the green with little subsequent roll) and, if applicable, how to fix it on the next repetition. Practice factors such as the *frequency* as well as the *method* of presenting performance-related feedback have been found to positively facilitate the athlete's independence (i.e., ability to perform without the coach) and accuracy in detecting and correcting their own movement errors. Expertise and motor learning theorists agree that "perfect" practice contexts should be organized to facilitate performance of the skill at an appropriate level of cognitive and motor difficulty, motor performance should be augmented with informative feedback, and the athlete, within the organization of the practice context, must be encouraged to independently detect and correct their movement errors. Engaging the athlete in a practice context that optimally challenges their planning and error detection abilities has been shown to promote their autonomy and independence in performance essential for movement expertise.

Factors that facilitate learning before the movement

A practice schedule in which the skills are interspersed, rather than practiced in a predictable and blocked sequence (e.g., all drives, then all chips, then all putts) has proven to have a dramatic effect on learning and improving skills. A classic study by John Shea and Robyn Morgan in 1979 found that practicing three variations of a single motor task in an unpredictable repetition schedule (e.g., random practice) was superior for learning to a rote type of practice condition where the performer merely tried to repeat what was done on the previous attempt (e.g., blocked practice). Although the numbers of repetitions were the same in both blocked and random repetition schedules, for the blocked condition all repetitions of one motor task were completed before trials were undertaken on either the second or third variation of the motor task, as in the golf example above. In a blocked repetition schedule, athletes can plan a movement and then use this same motor plan for the remaining repetitions. In contrast, for the random repetition schedule, in which repetitions of all tasks are interleaved during practice, the performer is required to actively think about and construct a plan to achieve the current motor task goal as a unique experience.

The results of Shea and Morgan were rather surprising: performance in the blocked practice condition was superior to the random practice condition but during the practice phase of the experiment only. When learners returned later for retention and transfer tests (which provide measures of relative amount learned), the findings were reversed. Learning had been facilitated more by random than blocked practice.

The Shea and Morgan findings can be considered counter-intuitive to the traditional view of the value of a repetition suggested at the beginning of the chapter. After all, blocked practice allowed the learner to focus on just one task at a time and indeed produced far better performance during practice, compared with randomly ordered practice. So, by this view, how could a factor that depressed performance during initial practice be superior for skilled motor permanence? Clearly, the role of repetition as traditionally believed was challenged severely by the findings of this study; there was more to learning than just "reps."

Other research has generalized these effects outside the lab, to numerous sport settings. For example, Kellie Hall and her colleagues found that college varsity baseball players who received extra batting practice sessions to hit curveballs, fastballs, and changeups showed better batting success against these specific pitches when ordered at random than in a blocked order. Similar effects have been found in golf, badminton, and other sports. The benefits of *non-repetitiveness* in the practice sequence have been attributed to the active cognitive processes engaged in by the athlete during *motor planning* – in other words, the active involvement of the brain prior to the biomechanics. For example, the predictability of the repetition sequence determines the decision making required by the athlete to plan the upcoming movement. When the motor-planning requirements of the athlete are predictable, as found in a blocked repetition schedule, the decision-making demands are low since one motor plan can be used for many successive repetitions. However, if the motor-planning demands are unpredictable, as shown in a random repetition schedule, the cognitive demands required by the brain to plan the correct motor action on each repetition are much higher (see Table 8.1).

Another recently emerged factor to consider in designing practice is whether the session has been organized by the athlete or the coach. In fact, allowing the athlete

Table 8.1 Repetition predictability and degree of decision making during motor planning as a function of repetition schedule characteristics

Repetition schedule	Putting distance (feet)	Predictability in sequence	Decision making during motor planning
Blocked	8–8–8–8–8 15–15–15–15–15 22–22–22–22–22	High	Low
Serial	8–15–22–8–15–22 8–15–22–8–15–22 8–15–22–8–15–22	High	Moderate
Random	15–8–22–8–15–22 8–15–22–8–22–15 22–8–15–8–15–22	Low	High
Athlete-controlled	Athlete decides on repetition order (absolute number of repetitions equated)	High	High

rather than the coach the opportunity to individualize the repetition *order* of skills has shown positive effects for learning. For this type of practice session, the amount of physical repetitions for each motor task is the same (e.g., 20 repetitions each); however, the athlete is given the opportunity to control the order in which those repetitions will be completed. For example, the athlete is required to complete 20 putts to each of the following distances: 8 feet, 15 feet, and 22 feet. In this example, the athlete chooses the putting distance to be practiced before each repetition (e.g., two trials at 8 feet, then five trials at 15 feet, then nine trials at 22 feet). What the research shows is that expert and novice performers commonly choose a schedule that resembles a blocked repetition schedule early in practice where successive repetitions are completed of each motor task (i.e., five consecutive repetitions of the 8-foot, 15-foot, and 22-foot putt respectively). As practice continues, performers commonly show a preference for a repetition schedule that appears randomized (i.e., high movement-planning demands), where the putting distance switches on each successive repetition, thus requiring a different motor plan from the previous repetition, to the advantage of learning. These findings suggest that blocked repetitions early in practice allow the athlete to solve the *motor components* of the motor task goal (e.g., biomechanics), while at the same time placing low demands on the brain to plan the motor action (i.e., repeating the same putting distance goal for a series of repetitions). However, as practice continues, the athlete's preference to switch to a random repetition schedule highlights an understanding of the required biomechanics of the motor task, with an increased emphasis on training the *cognitive processes* required by the brain to effectively plan alternative motor actions on subsequent repetitions (i.e., alternating amongst putting distances on a series of repetitions). The benefits of an athlete-controlled repetition schedule are attributed to increase the motivation of the athlete to achieve the required motor task goals in their practice session. In summary, the findings from studies in which athletes control the repetition schedule suggest that athletes opt to understand the movement requirements of the skill first (i.e., biomechanics; preference for blocked practice), and then gradually increase the challenge on the required cognitive skills (i.e., motor planning) later in the practice session (e.g., random practice), to the advantage of learning.

A situation commonly experienced by athletes is a time delay between engaging in the cognitive processes required by the brain to plan a motor action and the opportunity to physically execute that action. This delay could be relatively short and within the competition, such as waiting for an opponent to complete their golf shot or waiting in the on-deck circle to face the pitcher. Longer delays could be hours, days, or weeks, such as those delays experienced by athletes between competitions or practice sessions or even during the off-season. The research suggests the time delay between movement repetitions can be utilized by the athlete to practice the cognitive processes required for motor planning, that is, "thinking" rather than "doing" in the form of motor imagery.

Motor imagery requires the athlete to engage in the cognitive process required by the brain to *plan* the required motor action (e.g., chip shot in golf) but, instead of following through with performance of that action, the athlete *imagines* completing the required motor action (i.e., biomechanics) and interpreting the expected sensory consequences of the imagined movement (i.e., what the movement would feel like, sound like, look like). Thus, in the absence of a physical repetition, motor imagery allows the athlete the opportunity to continue to practice the cognitive processes required by the brain to plan and interpret the expected sensory consequences of that motor action. In fact, research shows that motor imagery has a positive and additive impact on achieving skilled motor performance, compared with not providing the athlete the opportunity to engage in motor imagery (see Chapter 7).

The advantages of using motor imagery are shown in brain-imaging experiments. Experts required to imagine performing an action they are skilled at, such as a golf shot, have shown recruitment of the brain areas required for motor planning similar to those required to physically complete the motor action; the brain reacts similarly whether you are imagining a movement or actually doing the movement. In fact, skill acquisition researchers have recently shown that the athlete is effective at imagining not only the required biomechanics of the motor action but also the timing requirements. For example, Stéphane Champley and colleagues showed that alpine skiers asked to *physically* complete a downhill course and *imagine* completing the same course as fast as possible took similar amounts of time to complete both tasks. In summary, the results from motor imagery research with the expert

140

athlete offers the coach and the athlete an alternative and effective approach to training the brain in the processes required for planning a motor action and those processes required for the interpretation of the outcome of that motor action.

The pre-shot routine is yet another example of the athlete preparing their cognitive and motor system for an upcoming movement. During this routine, the athlete is believed to "test" their motor plan and get a "feeling" of the movement (i.e., bio-mechanics) by physically executing the motor plan in advance of the competition. Pre-shot routines are common in sports where the *initiation* of the motor action is directly controlled by the athlete such as a golf swing, a golf putt, or a free throw in basketball. In golf, for example, the pre-shot routine has been demonstrated by experts to be shorter in timing duration for a full swing than for a putt and is utilized more frequently than by novices. Research suggests that what the ath-lete practices in their pre-shot routine does not differentially impact performance between athletes, yet coaches should be encouraged that a pre-shot routine has proven to be a valuable performance tool for the athlete (if permitted by the sport context) (see Chapter 10 for more discussion on pre-shot routines).

Factors that facilitate learning after the movement: feedback

Every repetition results in two different yet complementary sources of feedback. Sensory feedback concerns what the athlete sees, hears, and feels during and after their movement (e.g., the different sensations that a diver becomes aware of when entering the pool). Augmented feedback is post-movement information provided by a coach to the athlete as a means of facilitating the interpretation of their sensory feedback (e.g., telling the diver that the upper body was slightly bent forward upon entry into the water). Augmented feedback provides information to the athlete regarding their success in achieving the movement goal. Augmented feedback pro-vided to the athlete regarding their actual movements (e.g., arm positions during a golf swing) compared with the required movements (e.g., required arm positions) is defined as "knowledge of performance" (KP), that is, the "how" of the movement. Providing the athlete augmented feedback regarding the outcome of their motor performance in relation to the task goal (e.g., ball landed 3 feet short of the hole) is defined as "knowledge of results" (KR).

As mentioned earlier, the myth of the role of a repetition is that it has a very spe-cific yet limited purpose for augmented feedback (i.e., KR, KP); in order to facilitate "perfect practice," augmented feedback is to be provided to the performer as often as possible (e.g., after every repetition) and as immediately as possible after the completion of a movement in order to *minimize* error. In fact, augmented feedback has been perceived as essential in the belief that, without it, skill acquisition would not occur. This is not entirely untrue – feedback is important for skill acquisition. However, what the research tells us is that "how" augmented feedback is presented to the athlete during practice has a dramatic impact on learning. In fact, frequent provision of augmented feedback has been shown to create athlete *dependence* on this form of information to guide error detection and correction. The consequence is that the athlete learns to depend on the coach for augmented feedback instead of interpreting their own sensory feedback from the just-completed motor performance to update a subsequent repetition; they do not know how well they have performed or, if it was less than optimal, why and what they might need to do to improve. Skill acquisition research has clearly shown that practice contexts organized to reduce the athlete's dependency on augmented feedback and engage the athlete in the processes required for interpreting movement-related sensory feedback train the cognitive processes required by the brain for independent error detection and subsequent correction. That is, when practice is structured to create a thinking athlete they can determine what they have done wrong and how to correct it independently.

Interestingly, Jack Nicklaus recently expressed these very sentiments about the augmented feedback that he received from his coach:

> Jack Grout taught me from the start. He said I need to be responsible for my own swing and understand when I have problems on the golf course how I can correct those problems on the golf course myself without having to run back to somebody. And during the years that I was playing most of my competitive golf, I saw Jack Grout maybe once or twice a year for maybe an hour. If I was in the Miami area or something, I'd run down and see Jack and we'd spend about an hour and we'd spend five minutes on the golf swing and an hour catching up. But he taught me young the fundamentals of the game. He taught me how to assess what I was doing. When I made a mistake, when I was doing things, how do you on the golf course fix that without putting yourself out of a golf tournament and then teaching yourself.
>
> (http://www.pgatour.com/tourreport/2012/05/
> nicklaus-on-bubba-tiger-and-arnold.html)

Considerable motor skill acquisition research supports the augmented feedback methods experienced by Nicklaus. Skill acquisition research examining various schedules of augmented feedback suggests that practice repetitions should be organized to require the athlete to engage in the cognitive processes required for independent error detection and correction – to think more. Therefore, each and every movement repetition must be structured to cognitively engage the athlete in the assessment of their motor behavior. Commonly used methods include decreasing the frequency or absolute amount of augmented feedback available to the athlete during the practice session. Compared with receiving augmented feedback on every trial, practice schedules that decrease the provision of feedback over trials increase skill proficiency (e.g., feedback on the first 10 trials, followed by feedback on seven of the next 10 trials, followed by feedback on three of the next 10 trials). Also, withholding feedback for a certain number of trials such as 5, 10, or 15 and then presenting the performer with a summary of the feedback (either verbally or graphically) on those completed trials – or presenting augmented feedback once after every five repetitions (reduced relative frequency) – has also been found to facilitate learning and independence in error detection and correction. The learning advantage of these different augmented feedback schedules is that, during the trials where the coach *does not* provide augmented feedback, the athlete is believed to engage in the cognitive processes required to interpret their response-produced sensory feedback, subsequently strengthening their ability to independently detect and correct their movement error (with an emphasis on the behavior of the motor action). On these trials, the athlete is problem solving. As a consequence, the *dependency* of the athlete on receiving augmented feedback from the coach is reduced and the athlete is provided the opportunity to fine-tune their interpretative skills of the resulting behavior. These effects are observable in superior motor skill performance when the augmented feedback is no longer available and the athlete is required to depend solely on their sensory sources of information from their movements to independently detect and correct movement error.

An augmented feedback schedule determined by how skilled the athlete is at the skill being practiced is one effective method of organizing an augmented feedback schedule within a practice session. For example, in a *bandwidth feedback* paradigm, a predetermined error tolerance is generated such that if the athlete achieves the task goal *inside* the error tolerance the performance is perceived as correct since no prescriptive feedback is provided to the performer. If the performance is outside the bandwidth (e.g., required golf shot distance is 30 feet) augmented information is then provided to the athlete regarding their exact movement error from the task goal. For example, in practicing a golf shot of 30 feet, a 5 percent bandwidth may be chosen whereby only qualitative feedback is provided if the ball lands within 1.5 meters ("that was a good shot"). Quantitative feedback is presented to the athlete if the ball lands more than 1.5 meters away. Theorists recommend that, in the early stages of learning, the athlete benefits from prescriptive quantitative information as a method of developing their early attempts at error detection and correction (e.g., "you were two seconds faster on your 10 kilometer run"). However, the strength of a bandwidth schedule is that once the athlete becomes more skilled at persistently achieving the task goal, the precision of the feedback changes from quantitative (e.g., prescriptive) to qualitative (e.g., verbally stating "good" to the participant).

Presenting qualitative feedback to the athlete suggests a "perfect" repetition has been performed and those motor-planning and movement interpretation processes should be repeated on subsequent trials. This method of organizing augmented feedback has been shown to effectively avoid an athlete's dependency on augmented feedback for error detection and correction and to subsequently facilitate independence in the processes required for performing and problem solving.

In addition to *performance-based* feedback schedules, skill acquisition research has also shown that empowering the athlete rather than the coach with the opportunity to control *when* they require feedback during practice context is also effective. The effectiveness of athlete-controlled feedback schedules has been described as a decision-making process that requires the athlete to be an active participant in the cognitive factors that support learning. This is where the athlete drives the training, and it is analogous to the previously discussed learner-controlled practice organization research. Results from research examining athlete-controlled feedback schedules have found that athletes prefer augmented feedback frequently in the early stages of the practice session but that it is gradually requested less frequently as they become more skilled at the motor-planning and biomechanical requirements of the motor action (i.e., similar to a coach-defined faded feedback schedule discussed earlier). More recently, the benefits of an athlete-controlled KR schedule have been shown in practice contexts where the athlete was required to control their KR when practicing multiple motor tasks in a single practice session. Skill acquisition researchers suggest the benefits of athlete-controlled feedback schedules are attributed to an individualized feedback schedule that is most beneficial to their specific needs and current level of information processing with regard to their independence at error detection and correction. That is, when athletes decide when they want to receive feedback, rather than anyone else, the requested feedback is suggested to match the needs of the athlete in regard to their interpretation of their movement success and confirm what needs and does not need to be corrected on subsequent repetitions.

The findings from athlete-determined KR schedules also highlight the importance of *when* the athlete prefers to receive KR. In fact, when queried after practice, performers indicated a preference for requesting KR after a perceived "good" rather than "poor" trial. Skill acquisition researchers have found that providing KR to the performer after only their most successful – rather than unsuccessful – trials facilitated skilled motor behavior. Providing augmented feedback based on successful motor performance is suggested to inform the performer of the movement (i.e., biomechanical) and brain (i.e., motor-planning specifics) requirements to successfully achieve the movement goal on upcoming repetitions. In addition, providing feedback on successful actions is suggested to heighten the *motivation* of the performer to continue at practicing the attainment of the motor task goal.

144

The positive impact of providing the athlete augmented feedback in reference to other athletes performing the same motor task is termed "social-comparative feedback." In this context, the athlete is provided with augmented feedback about their task performance and then told whether their motor performance was better or worse than a group of athletes performing the same task. As suggested by Rebecca Lewthwaite and colleagues, the mere perception that one is performing better than others in a comparison group has been shown to enhance skill acquisition. These benefits have been associated with heightening the motivation of the athlete to achieve the motor task goal.

The result from this research suggests that augmented feedback provided by the coach not only impacts the motor components of the skill (i.e., biomechanics) but also the athlete's perception of success and other task-related thoughts (i.e., motivation). Therefore, the coach and athlete must be aware that augmented feedback impacts not only what can be seen (i.e., the biomechanics) but also those activities that cannot be seen (i.e., processes in the brain such as motivational levels, perceptions of success). Yet both have an equally important contribution to sport expertise. Methods of providing task-related feedback to facilitate independent error detection and correction for the athlete are outlined in Table 8.2.

Table 8.2 Description of feedback schedules that facilitate independent error detection and correction processes in the performer

Feedback schedule	Description
Summary feedback	Augmented feedback about a set of repetitions (e.g., five) after the set has been completed. Summary feedback can be presented visually or verbally
Bandwidth feedback	Provision of quantitative feedback (e.g., 16 seconds too fast) only when performance falls outside an agreed upon criterion or bandwidth. Performer is provided qualitative feedback (e.g., "correct!") when performance falls within the bandwidth
Faded feedback	Decreasing the frequency of feedback provision over a series of practice trials. For example, augmented feedback is presented frequently at the beginning of practice and presented less frequently over practice trials
Performer-regulated	Frequency of feedback provision determined by performer's requests upon completion of a practice trial
Performer estimation	Performer estimates their error upon completion of an action. The coach then provides the actual error demonstrated by the performer
Content-based feedback	Performer is provided feedback based on a pre-established criterion (e.g., only good trials). Feedback after a series of "good" trials is suggested to enhance motivation of athlete to perform task

THEORY INTO PRACTICE: SUGGESTED APPLICATIONS FOR THE ORGANIZATION OF PRACTICE

The remainder of this chapter will provide the coach with an evidence-based approach to organizing a practice schedule to facilitate the physical and cognitive components of motor skill proficiency.

What is the role of biomechanical reps?

Until this point we have emphasized several key issues. One is that motor performance is a product of three processes: movement planning, movement execution, and movement evaluation – typified by Stephen Scott in 2004 as the "3 Bs" (see Figure 8.1). We acknowledge that motor skill learning requires physical repetition but further suggest that effective skill acquisition occurs only when the repetitions maximize the contribution of each of the three processes. In this chapter, we have considered a number of factors that impact on movement planning and evaluative processes and have ignored the impact of biomechanical repetition as a factor in the learning process. This was not unintentional. In fact, we go further and suggest that rote repetition of movement (i.e., repeating the biomechanics of a movement over a series of repetitions such as performing 30 drives on the driving range), in the absence of significant planning and assessment processing, has minimal or perhaps no role at all in skill acquisition. That is not to say that a biomechanical repetition serves no purpose – certainly there are biochemical and physiological factors that are impacted significantly by movement which will have important effects on performance. However, there is little research evidence to support *movement repetition* alone as the sole contributor to learning. We suggest that movement repetition supports motor skill learning only when accompanied by pre- (i.e., motor planning) and post- (i.e., error detection and correction) repetition processes. To put it very simply, moving without thinking will not provide the learning advantages that moving with thinking provides.

Practice factors facilitating motor planning: suggestions for the coach

A coach's challenge when organizing a practice session is to determine a balance between a practice context that ensures good performance by the athlete (e.g., blocked repetition schedule) and a practice context that emphasizes the cognitive processes required for independent motor planning. Some researchers suggest the practice session should be organized to encourage independent decision making with respect to retrieving the correct motor plan from memory, anticipating the action of an opponent, or planning an action under pressure (e.g., completing the movement in a limited amount of time). The decisions made by the athlete during the practice context should be similar to the decisions required in the athletic event. Further, the athlete should not simply be able to plan and accurately produce the correct action but also be cognizant of *why* they planned the action in that particular way (see Chapters 6, 12, and 13).

Recent theoretical ideas in the motor-learning literature suggest that a practice schedule should be organized to facilitate the cognitive processes required by the athlete for successful motor planning. During the initial stages of skill acquisition, the athletes are "getting the idea" of the cognitive and motor requirements to successfully perform the task.

For motor tasks that require a specific movement outcome, such as successfully scoring a basket from a basketball jump shot performed from three different distances on the court, a *blocked repetition schedule* may be considered an effective beginning strategy. In this context, the athlete practices planning the same action over a series of trials (e.g., shooting a jump shot 10 feet from the basket for 10 consecutive trials before progressing to a new distance). Athletes typically demonstrate quick performance success (e.g., the biomechanics appear adequate) during a blocked repetition schedule. To increase the cognitive demands required by the brain for motor planning, researchers suggest the transition to a *serial repetition schedule*. In this context, the athlete is required to plan a *different* motor action on each trial; however, the order of the repetitions is predictable (e.g., jump shots from 10 feet, then 15 feet, then 20 feet with this repetition order repeated). In a final progression, the athlete practices in a *random repetition schedule* where the upcoming required motor action is non-repeating and unpredictable. For example, the athlete practices a jump shot from 10 feet, then 15 feet, then 10 feet again, then 20 feet. In this context the order of the repetitions are non-repeating and unpredictable.

Once an athlete knows what to do (e.g., the biomechanics are understood), the problem-solving demands required of the performer to plan a motor action within the practice schedule should be adjusted to heighten the cognitive demands (i.e., processing required by the brain) necessary for motor planning. Importantly, the motor-planning demands required during practice should match the motor-planning demands required of the athlete within the athletic competition.

Providing the athlete with the opportunity to control the order of practice repetitions for a series of "to be practiced" motor tasks in a single practice session has proven to be an effective method in acquiring the required biomechanics and processes needed by the brain to plan a motor action. This practice context allows the athlete to determine, as a function of their individualized practice schedule, whether their focus will be on the biomechanics of the action (e.g., blocked repetition schedule) or the cognitive processes required by the brain to plan a motor action (e.g., random repetition practice schedule). In some instances, providing the athlete control for the duration of the practice context might not be desirable or possible. However, recent research has shown that providing the performer control for only a portion of the practice context (i.e., 50 percent of the total practice trials) is as advantageous to facilitating skilled performance as if control were provided for the duration of the practice context.

Scheduling augmented feedback: suggestions for the coach

Skill acquisition researchers recommend that feedback schedules should be organized to engage the performer in active error detection and correction upon the completion of *every* repetition. A commonly used method, which is opposite to the perfect practice view, is to reduce the *frequency* of augmented feedback during the practice schedule. Reducing the frequency (i.e., availability) of augmented feedback is suggested to be one method of avoiding the athlete's dependence on augmented feedback for error detection and correction. In one example, augmented feedback is presented after the athlete has completed a series of repetitions *without* augmented feedback (say, five). During the no-feedback repetitions, the athlete is instructed to estimate the success of their movement based on the interpretation of their own sources of sensory information (e.g., visual, auditory, proprioceptive, tactile) inherent within performance of the task (see Chapter 9). After the completion of the predetermined number of no-feedback trials the coach then presents augmented feedback about the just-completed repetitions. This method of scheduling augmented feedback has proven to be effective in facilitating the cognitive processes required for independent error detection and correction.

Gradually reducing or *fading* the availability of augmented feedback over a practice period is another effective method of facilitating the cognitive processes required by the athlete for independent detection and correction of errors. In this schedule:

- Augmented feedback is presented often during the early stages of practice to guide the athlete to the required motor behavior (e.g., biomechanics) and allows the athlete to experience what the movement should feel like, thus calibrating the error detection and correction capabilities of the athlete to the goal of the task.
- As practice continues, the frequency and availability of augmented feedback is gradually reduced, forcing the athlete to depend on their own error detection and correction mechanisms on trials where augmented feedback is not available. Interestingly, a fading feedback schedule is often demonstrated by performers in practice contexts where they are in *control* of when to receive augmented feedback (see Table 8.1).

148

■ The use of the performance-derived bandwidth feedback approach as detailed earlier in this chapter is a recommended faded feedback strategy.

In addition, practice contexts organized to provide augmented feedback based on "successful" rather than "unsuccessful" repetitions has shown to increase athletes' motivation and persistence at achieving the task goal of motor skill expertise and is preferred by athletes provided the opportunity to control their receipt of augmented information.

We suggest the coach be cognizant of the associated motivational impact of various practice variables (e.g., athlete-controlled practice contexts) on their athlete's long-term motivation in persisting at achieving motor skill expertise.

Verbal reports of perceived movement success

An effective method for the coach to infer the strength and accuracy of the athlete's error detection and correction capability is by utilizing verbal reports of the athlete's perceived movement correctness. In this context:

■ The athlete is first encouraged to provide a verbal estimate of their perceived movement correctness based solely on their interpretation of the various sources of sensory information such as the feel of the movement (e.g., the coordination of the upper body and lower body in a golf swing), visual observation of the movement effects (e.g., the trajectory of a golf ball), and the auditory consequences of the movement (e.g., golf club striking the ball).
■ The athlete's performance estimate must be presented to the coach *before* the athlete receives augmented feedback.
■ Once the athlete has provided an estimate of their perceived movement success, the coach must then provide augmented feedback to the athlete regarding their movement success.
■ Once feedback is received, the athlete can either confirm the success of their motor planning and subsequent biomechanics, or update their motor plan for the upcoming repetition based on the discrepancy between their perceived (verbal estimate) and actual movement success (feedback from the coach).

CONCLUDING REMARKS

To conclude, we offer a reinterpretation of the old adage "perfect practice makes perfect." We suggest that effective practice requires the athlete to actively engage in the cognitive processes required by the brain to effectively plan and accurately detect and correct movement errors. To us this represents "perfect practice." The significant contributions of organizing a practice context that are cognitively effortful during motor planning and error detection and correction are demonstrated when the athlete performs these activities, independent of the coach, in a game situation.

Recent findings from motor-learning research offer very specific guidelines for the coach organizing a practice context. Perhaps the most salient recommendation is that practice environments should be organized to encourage active participation of the athlete in the cognitive processes required for motor planning as well as error detection and correction. The decisions made by the athlete during practice in regard to motor planning as well as error detection and correction should closely approximate the decisions required of the athlete during competition. A consequence of organizing practice where cognitive effort is embedded within physical repetitions is that athletes are practicing the skills required to be autonomous in their motor planning and error detection and correction. The practice factors outlined in this chapter offer a specific evidence-based methodology for the coach

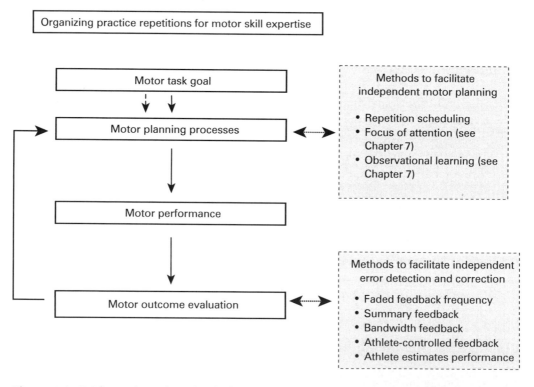

Figure 8.2 Evidence-based method of organizing practice repetitions to facilitate the attainment of motor skill expertise. The dashed lines represent optional methods of organizing practice for the coach.

organizing a practice schedule for the athlete just beginning to learn a motor skill or for the athlete who is considered an expert within their sport-related domain (see Figure 8.2).

To return to our original idea, the role of "reps" in the motor learning process seems to us to have achieved mystical status over the years, such that spending an enormous amount of time in the rehearsal of a movement pattern is the athlete's cure-all. One needs to wonder, however, if the concept of "reps" is merely another "snake oil" in the medicine cabinet of sports myths. We suggest that effective practice will be achieved only when the sport mind-set goes beyond reps to consider motor control and learning as part of a greater scheme of events that includes but, more importantly, precedes and follows movement.

COACH'S CORNER

Gary Bernard
PGA Professional and Chief Executive Officer, PGA of Canada

What repetition has traditionally meant to golf

Repetition in golf has, for more than 100 years meant "dig it out of the dirt and hit balls until your hands bleed." This mantra has been passed on to every competitive player who has ever tried to play golf at a high level, either as an amateur or as a touring professional. This idea has become so engrained in the culture of golf that it is now an integral part of the overall belief system that guides the game the world over. While this methodology was the staple of such greats as Ben Hogan and Moe Norman's training programs, in fairness to them it was the accepted modus operandi of the era and deeply embedded in the culture.

Any player not buying into this concept and perpetuating the idea was, and continues to be, looked upon as lacking in the area of commitment and work ethic. Some anomalies have surfaced from this group over the years, Bruce Lietzke, Ángel Cabrera, and Miguel Ángel Jiménez to name just a few. However, they have been labeled as gifted athletes who can get away with it or as players who might have reached their real potential had they pushed themselves and gone to the range to beat balls in a very stoic and monk-like fashion.

The use of technology

The current buzz and trend within the golf world is the analysis of the player's swing using launch monitors and video cameras in concert to review every minute motion the player makes during the swing action. One of the main challenges to this methodology is that it most often occurs in a range setting and not on the course where the player is forced to solve the problem they are faced with on each different shot. The manufactured range setting rarely allows for the competitive environment to be recreated, which is why so many players practice with perfect lies and more often than not in a blocked, scape-and-hit manner. This system of practice usually reflects great results on the practice range once the player gets into a groove and becomes comfortable with the shot at hand. Unfortunately, this never occurs on the golf course and the constant refrain of "why can't I bring the skill from the range to the golf course?" can be heard worldwide on any given day and any given course.

Feedback

It is probably fair to say that even today many players are fed a constant barrage of feedback after nearly every shot by a well-intentioned instructor or coach. It appears that some instructors and coaches are moving toward a more augmented approach to feedback and are attempting to utilize technology in this with video, launch monitor readouts, and numerous overlay systems to enhance the visual and empirical data feedback to the students.

Future issues

The future of instruction and coaching within the golf world may lie in a better understanding of how people acquire motor skills and the role that the brain plays in the entire process. I see golf instructors moving toward this knowledge base but there is still much work to be done to change the thinking habits of such a traditional sport and industry as golf.

The authors focus their comments on the beginning learner but what does the research suggest about the skilled or semi-skilled golfer who is trying to make changes to their swing and expecting high-performance results in competition? Some areas for consideration and additional research might be what kinds of practice conditions lead to better performance under stress and what kinds of practice conditions are most resistant to variability. The 2012 Open Championship held at Royal Lytham & St. Annes placed these concepts on a world stage. The golf world watched as the top-ranked touring professional Adam Scott's performance deteriorated down the stretch. His four bogeys on the last four holes occurred under what many would argue are the toughest conditions faced by touring professionals: the pressure of a major championship on a British links-style course. How did he prepare for this event? Was there a better way for him to have prepared?

How can coaches work with players to create training environments that better simulate the competitive environment? Clearly, the artificial training environments used by the vast majority of players around the world are not preparing them for the pressure of the competitive arena. It may be creating a comfort zone for the player and coach but that comfort zone quickly deteriorates under the physical and mental pressure of competing at the highest level.

Quantitative statistical information and research abounds on the major tours with data collected every week on fairways hit, greens hit in regulation, and putts per

152

round to name only a few categories that are tracked. This information is an excellent benchmarking system but what the game really needs is some deep mining of behaviors and some predictive intelligence on why players are breaking down under pressure leading to unacceptable variability in performance. Additional research within the game of golf is necessary in the area of qualitative data on what players think and feel when the intended shot produced the expected result, and when it did not, both in training and in competitive environments.

KEY READING

Guadagnoli, M.A. and Lee, T.D. (2004) 'Challenge point: A framework for conceptualizing the effects of various practice conditions in motor learning', *Journal of Motor Behavior*, 36: 212–224.

Hall, K.G., Domingues, D.A., and Cavazos, R. (1994) 'Contextual interference effects with skilled baseball players', *Perceptual and Motor Skills*, 78: 835–841.

Hodges, N., Edwards, C., Lutin, S., and Bowcock, A. (2011) 'Learning from experts: gaining insights into best practice during the acquisition of three novel motor skills', *Research Quarterly for Exercise and Sport*, 82: 178–187.

Kantak, S.S. and Winstein, C.J. (2012) 'Learner-performance distinction and memory processes for motor skills: A focused review and perspective', *Behavioral Brain Research*, 228: 219–231.

Kottke, F.J. (1980) 'From reflex to skill: The training of coordination', *Archives of Physical Medicine and Rehabilitations*, 61: 551–561.

Lee, T.D., Swinnen, S.P., and Serrien, D.J. (1994) 'Cognitive effort and motor learning', *Quest*, 46: 328–344.

Lewthwaite, R. and Wulf, G. (2010) 'Social-comparative feedback affects motor skill learning', *Quarterly Journal of Experimental Psychology*, 63: 738–749.

Louis, M., Collet, C., Champley, S., and Guillot, A. (2012) 'Differences in motor imagery time when predicting task duration in alpine skiers and equestrian riders', *Research Quarterly for Exercise and Sport*, 83: 86–93.

Schmidt, R.A. and Lee, T.D. (2011) *Motor Control and Learning: A Behavioral Emphasis* (fifth edition). Champaign, IL: Human Kinetics.

Scott, S.H. (2004) 'Optimal feedback control and the neural basis of volitional motor control', *Nature Reviews: Neuroscience*, 5: 534–546.

CHAPTER 9

PRACTICING IMPLICIT (MOTOR) LEARNING

RICH MASTERS

At the US Masters in 2012, Gerry Watson found himself in a play-off. Under immense pressure, he played a golf shot that no "weekend warrior" could play (at least, not intentionally). In the trees of pine debris, "Bubba," as his father nicknamed him, hit a 164-yard hook shot with a 52-degree wedge. The ball literally bent around a corner and onto the green. Bubba Watson's website states that he received a solitary golf lesson from his father when he was very young. After that the rest is history!

INTRODUCTION

Lion cubs at play in a pride acquire skills that are needed for survival. They stalk, pounce, and wrestle, oblivious to the fact that their competence at the skills will someday be the difference between life and death. Children at play in a yard, on a field, or by a court acquire skills for life too. They run, catch, and hit, oblivious to the possibility that their competence may someday be the difference between winning and losing. For some children, a day comes when winning and losing becomes all-important. Superstardom beckons. Playtime is over and the pressure is on to get skilled and win. Coaches, administrators, parents, and grandparents – even well-meaning friends of the family who confabulate that they too could have "made it" – offer advice and tips on how best to execute the shots or make the moves. Everything has changed!

Skill learning for the weekend warrior and the would-be superstar is very different. For the weekend warrior, acquisition of sport-related skills is about leisure, pleasure, and health. For the would-be superstar, acquisition of sport-related skills is about medals, media, and money. These very different motivational states shape the way in which skills are learned, modifying the knowledge that is built up to support movement. For the would-be superstar, skill learning becomes an active pursuit followed in earnest. Play is suspended, fun is forgotten, and for many years skill learning is dominated by the testing of hypotheses in order to establish the best way to move to achieve the desired level of performance. Correct hypotheses (e.g., "flexed knees mean more power") are stored as rules for future reference (explicit knowledge), whereas incorrect hypotheses are discarded or ignored (but not always forgotten).

The consequence of this aggressive search for effective skills is that, over time, the performer accumulates a deep pool of explicit rules and knowledge. With practice, the skills become expert and automatic but they are inescapably linked to an explicit, highly verbal mode of control. At inopportune moments (e.g., match point down in the fifth set) or when too much time is available in which to construct the necessary movements (e.g., a gently lofted catch to the outfield), verbal modes of control can sometimes cause the normally fluent skills of the expert to regress to the awkward, error-prone movements of the beginner. In essence, conditions such as over-eagerness to perform well or too much time to think can result in *reinvestment*: the tendency to consciously attend to knowledge that underpins the skill in order to control the quality of performance. Most athletes have, at some point in their careers, faced this problem.

SOME EVIDENCE, A QUESTIONNAIRE, AND A QUOTE

There is now evidence that shows that the larger the pool of explicit knowledge that a performer has accumulated about how to perform his or her skills, the greater the chances that reinvestment will occur, especially under pressure (see Chapter 10). Additionally, different performers have different psychological propensities to reinvest. Every club or team has at least one member who incessantly rehearses their technique and we all secretly admire (or envy) performers who are so "chilled out" that they seem never to think about what they are doing or how they are doing it. The propensity to try to control performance by consciously directing attention to knowledge that underpins the skills can be measured using a questionnaire called the Movement Specific Reinvestment Scale. The scale also assesses the propensity to be self-conscious about one's movements. Although these two facets of the human personality are related to each other, there is evidence available from the study of populations with movement disorders, such as Parkinson's disease or strokes, which shows that a strong predisposition to think about one's movements (i.e., a high score on the Movement Specific Reinvestment Scale) is associated with greater functional impairment of the movements. Additionally, anxiety to move effectively, which is a natural emotion in those who move awkwardly, can cause patients to consciously monitor the mechanics of their actions even more than they normally would in an attempt to reduce the awkwardness of the movements. Similarities exist in the sporting world, where athletes can occasionally become so conscious of flaws in their technique that they begin to display pseudo-clinical skill disorders, such as the "yips" in golf or "dartitis" in darts. These athletes are likely to have very high propensities for reinvestment.

The Movement Specific Reinvestment Scale consists of a series of questions, as presented in Table 9.1. Normally, the questions are presented in a random order and the performer is asked to rate the strength of their feelings on a six-point Likert scale that ranges from *strongly disagree* (one point) through *moderately disagree* (two points), *weakly disagree* (three points), *weakly agree* (four points), *moderately agree* (five points), and *strongly agree* (six points). The minimum score for each personality trait is thus five points and the maximum score is 30 points.

Modern coaches are subject to considerable pressure to nurture the skills of the learner to an expert level in the shortest possible period of time. These pressures may emanate from sports administrators and associations who are fiscally restrained to meet the costs associated with producing top performers – the sooner the performer is on the circuit the better the budget balances. Parents have their own budgets to consider and the performers themselves are often in a hurry too – time is short when you want to be a superstar and even today many sports propagate the adage that "if you have not made it by the time you are 16 or 17, you never will." In short, the coach comes under significant pressure to accelerate the learning process. In order to do this the coach will persuade the learner to adopt certain fundamental methods and techniques that may be in vogue at the time or that somehow have

Table 9.1 The Movement Specific Reinvestment Scale

Conscious motor processing
I reflect about my movement a lot.
I try to figure out why my actions failed.
I try to think about my movements when I carry them out.
I am aware of the way my body works when I am carrying out a movement.
I remember the times when my movements have failed me.
Movement self-consciousness
I am concerned about my style of moving.
I am self-conscious about the way I look when I am moving.
I am concerned about what people think about me when I am moving.
If I see my reflection in a shop window, I will examine my movements.
I sometimes have the feeling that I am watching myself move.

The scale is used to assess the propensity that an individual performer has for conscious motor processing (i.e., attention to the process of movement in order to control performance) and for movement self-consciousness (i.e., concerns about style of movement and about making a good impression when moving).

become embedded in coachlore as "best practice." The coach may even persuade the learner to adopt certain techniques simply because they worked for the coach.

Whatever the reason, the information is usually communicated in a manner that leaves the player consciously aware of *how* to execute the technique. Often the default for the coach is to use explicit verbal instructions simply because the coach knows of few other ways in which to bring about the recommended changes in technique. It becomes very difficult for the performer to carry out the skill without at some point exerting conscious control over the movements and it is this reinvestment that can lead to skill breakdown, particularly if the performer is highly motivated to perform well, which is not surprising given the huge cost and the intense and enduring commitment that is required to become an expert (not to mention the rewards that come to those who are victorious). As all performers know – and the Zen Buddhist teacher Daisetz Suzuki articulated – best execution of skills occurs when there is no interference from consciousness:

> Thinking is useful in many ways, but there are some occasions when thinking interferes with the work, and you have to leave it behind . . . It is for this reason that the sword moves where it ought to move and makes the contest end victoriously.
>
> (D. T. Suzuki, *Zen and Japanese Culture*, 1959)

MORE EVIDENCE, A RULE, AND A BIT ABOUT THE HISTORY OF IMPLICIT *MOTOR* LEARNING

Electroencephalographic (EEG) studies of brain activity have shown that the propensity for reinvestment can be discriminated by the synchronized nature of the communication (coherence) between two particular regions of the brain: the left temporal (T3) region and the frontal midline (Fz) region. The T3 region is thought to support verbal-analytical processes related to language processing and possibly hypothesis testing, whereas the Fz region is associated with the planning of movement. When performing motor tasks, high reinvesters display reliably more synchronized communication between the two regions than low reinvesters, suggesting that they have more verbal-analytical engagement in their movements. Coherence between the two regions has also been shown to increase under high-anxiety conditions, suggesting that performance pressure causes increased verbal-analytical engagement in motor planning and performance.

Neurological trauma appears in some cases to reduce verbal-analytical involvement in motor performance with striking outcomes. In one such case, a 53-year-old man presented with atrophy of the left frontal and temporal lobes, including the left hippocampus. These areas of the brain are involved in verbal aspects of motor control. The man displayed poor social skills; however, he showed no reduction in the ability to follow the complex rules that are so much a part of the traditions of golf. For example, Rule 12-1 of the Rules of Golf, stipulated by the Royal and Ancient Golf Club of St Andrews, states that:

> In searching for his ball anywhere on the *course*, the player may touch or bend long grass, rushes, bushes, whins, heather or the like, but only to the extent necessary to find and identify it, provided that this does not improve the lie of the ball, the area of his intended *stance* or swing or his *line of play* . . . [and] a player is not necessarily entitled to see his ball when making a *stroke* . . .

Although unable to explicitly report the rules and etiquette of golf, the patient was able to adhere to them. More importantly, the patient's golf handicap improved after the verbal control areas of his left hemisphere were damaged, suggesting that reduced verbal-analytical involvement improved his motor performance.

Although such a cure for reinvestment is undoubtedly effective, a less invasive approach exists. Considerable evidence now shows that reinvestment can be avoided if motor skills are acquired implicitly without recourse to hypothesis testing or instructions and thus the subsequent accumulation of consciously accessible explicit knowledge about the movements. After all, if athletes do not have access to explicit knowledge of how they move, how then can they use such knowledge to consciously control their skills?

The first efforts to bring about implicit *motor* learning of sport skills took place in 1992, some 20 years ago. A dual task approach (requiring the learner to complete two tasks at once) was deployed to prevent novice learners from testing hypotheses about the motor movements that they were making. The learners were asked to generate letters from the alphabet in a random order while they were learning to golf putt. The task is harder than it may seem because the learner must constantly monitor each letter to ensure that it has not been repeated previously or placed in a sequence of letters that makes up a real name or word. This early work showed that people who carried out a second task while learning to golf putt accumulated little or no conscious explicit knowledge of their putting skill compared with people who learned by self-discovery or by explicit coaching instructions. Importantly, the performance of the implicit learners remained stable under conditions of psychological pressure that normally is enough to cause the skills of an athlete to fail as a consequence of reinvestment. In the laboratory, a poor cousin to these psychological pressures is usually the presence of an audience, peer pressure, or financial enticements.

158

In the intervening decades since this work was carried out, a variety of implicit skill-learning approaches or paradigms have been proposed and validated. The work has included paradigms that encourage implicit motor learning by constraining the physical environment in such a way that performance mistakes seldom occur (we sometimes call this errorless learning) or by presenting analogies that guide learners towards effective movements without explicit instructions. Alternatively, visual feedback about the success of the movements during skill learning has been withheld in order to discourage hypothesis testing (and thus reduce accretion of explicit knowledge). For many skills, learning is compromised when visual feedback is withheld (not surprisingly) so an alternative approach has been to provide visual feedback that the learner is only marginally aware of. Learners tend to use such feedback without consciously realizing that they are using it.

From an applied point of view some of these techniques are difficult to maintain over the extended periods of practice necessary for expertise to develop. With the exception of analogy learning, which will be discussed shortly, these techniques also cause skill learning to be slower than normal, in the early stages at least. This can undermine a performer's perceptions of his or her competence or ability which tends to reduce motivation to continue practicing. As most coaches preach, but do not necessarily practice, anything that undermines the sense of self-competence (confidence) of an athlete should be avoided. Despite the significant challenges to the coach in overcoming these difficulties the advantages associated with learning skills implicitly are significant. Recent work has suggested that skills that are learned implicitly are performed better in front of an audience, create less interference when the performer has a complex decision to make, and even appear to be resistant to physiological fatigue. Beginners who learned implicitly to perform a rugby pass maintained their passing accuracy when significantly fatigued at an anaerobic or an aerobic level, whereas those who learned explicitly did not. Furthermore, one year later, passing performance remained robust under physiological fatigue, despite the complete absence of passing practice during the year.

Such advantages have been explained using an evolutionary framework which suggests that skills were learned unconsciously (or implicitly) far earlier in our evolution than they were learned consciously (or explicitly). Long before we could verbalize we needed to be able to run, throw, and hit with considerable competence. If not, we did not survive. Consequently, unconscious implicit processes evolved with a degree of resistance to psychological stress, distraction, and even physiological fatigue. The implicit motor-learning paradigms that have been developed for use in sport (and increasingly for other motor domains including rehabilitation, surgery, speech, etc.) are designed to increase the degree to which these fundamental implicit processes are utilized during performance of skills, often at the same time reducing the degree to which explicit conscious processes are utilized.

AN APOCRYPHAL STORY

If coaches are to exploit the advantages of implicit motor learning they will need to rise to the challenge of adapting the laboratory-developed implicit learning paradigms for the field. For some coaches this will require a pedagogical *volte-face*, perhaps even the sacrifice of a cow, as Luis Suárez, former manager of Ecuador's soccer team, told his players prior to the 2006 FIFA World Cup. Suárez recounted to his players the apocryphal story of a master and his servant who came upon a shack during their travels. The family that lived in the shack was extremely poor but nevertheless invited them into their home for food, drink, and rest. The master asked how such a poor family could provide such wonderful hospitality, to which they replied that they owned a single cow that provided for all of their needs from its milk and from the beef and hides of its calves. Many years later the servant returned to the area. The shack was gone and in its place stood a beautiful mansion surrounded by magnificent gardens. When the servant knocked on the door to ask what had become of the family he was amazed to find that they lived in the mansion. "How can this be?" he asked, to which they replied that many years earlier they had lived in poverty with only a single cow to provide for their needs. As luck would have it the cow had died, compelling them to take a new path in their lives – a path that led to fame and fortune. At the end of this story, Luis Suárez said to his players: "Gentlemen, we are going to play in the World Cup. It is time to kill your cows." Ecuador went further in the 2006 tournament than ever before in its history.

The coach who goes to the lengths needed to create an implicit motor learning environment will benefit by producing performers who can step up to the plate when it matters, but the coach who argues that he or she is paid to tell people explicitly what they are doing wrong may not. The "people" in this context are adults. Most of the work on implicit motor learning has been conducted using adults and it is not yet clear how well the findings generalize to children. Adults display self-awareness of their thought processes and their knowledge (metacognition), which develops only slowly through childhood. It is clear, however, that even very young children interact effectively with their environment using knowledge of which they are completely unaware. For example, children under the age of one year display surprisingly good understanding of inferential probabilities. When shown a large box full almost entirely of red balls, save for a few white balls, children tend to show the behavioral equivalent of surprise (longer looks) when a person reaches in and removes mainly white balls, but not when a person reaches in and removes mainly red balls.

Goal-directed movement abilities – such as walking, reaching, or grasping – develop before the language abilities of children develop so it seems probable that implicit learning is by default the primary means by which children acquire motor skills. What follows is a discussion of some ways in which implicit learning techniques

160

can be adapted for use outside the laboratory in the real world. The intention is not to provide a comprehensive list of implicit learning paradigms as alternatives to explicit practices, but rather to stimulate thoughts on how to create a unique environment for performers (adults or children) in which they learn their skills implicitly.

METAPHORICALLY SPEAKING

An analogy takes a familiar concept with underlying causal relationships that a learner already understands and relates it to an unfamiliar concept that is to be learned. Thus, a person who is familiar with the concept of a pump immediately understands the fundamentals of the heart. Most coaches have resorted to the use of analogy at some point when instructing an athlete. Often they do not even realize that they are using analogies when they tell their players to "swim like a fish" or "jump like a gator" (I made that one up). In fact, analogies are rife in sport. Listen to any sports broadcast and you will realize how common they are. You might hear a tennis commentator praising a player for "punching a volley" or a rugby referee warning a flanker to "go through the gate" rather than enter the maul from the side. The victorious captain might even claim that his team was "on fire" during the game.

Analogies can be used to present the key coaching points of a skill to be learned as a simple metaphor that can be reproduced by the learner without reference to, or the need for manipulation of, large amounts of explicit knowledge. This allows the coach to instruct the performer implicitly without resorting to the use of verbal instructions. Not only do analogy learners seem to quickly identify and mimic the fundamental form of the skill that they are trying to produce, but they do so without acquiring explicit knowledge of how they are producing the skill.

There is empirical evidence available to show that in tennis (and table tennis) a right-angled triangle analogy can be employed to teach beginners a topspin forehand shot implicitly. The learner is instructed simply to strike the ball by bringing the racquet (or bat) squarely up the hypotenuse portion of the right-angled triangle. It is vital, though, that the concept of a right-angled triangle and its hypotenuse is familiar to the learner. Strangely, tennis coaches often tell beginners to "brush up the back of the ball" in order to impart topspin. How meaningful is such a concept? With respect to the right-angled triangle analogy, most learners for whom Pythagoras's theorems are meaningful will automatically take a Western-style grasp of their racquet, accompanied by a stance that naturally allows the hips to rotate and the racquet to travel from low to high with the kind of force necessary to generate topspin and so on. The learner is unlikely to be consciously aware that he or she is using any of these important causal rules that underlie a topspin forehand.

Moreover, as studies have shown, the learner is likely to display performance advantages that are characteristic of an implicitly learned skill, such as stable performance under pressure or even when physically fatigued. Although analogy learning has not directly been examined with respect to implicit motor learning in children, a large literature demonstrates that analogy making is a powerful cognitive mechanism by which children gain understanding of their world so it is likely that the performance advantages of analogy learning in sport also hold for children.

The extent to which analogies are effective is perhaps best illustrated by the success of those who use them. Dr. Tom Amberry, from the USA, became the world record holder for basketball free throws in 1993. Remarkably, he was 71 years old at the time, which makes a mockery of the adage that "you must *make it* before you are 16 or 17 or you never will." Amberry, a weekend warrior who stopped playing basketball in his forties and only took up free throwing as a hobby when he retired, made 2,750 throws consecutively without missing over a 12-hour period. He is said to have stopped only because the gymnasium was booked for a college game. Importantly, the greatest basketball free throw shooter of all time advises that for each throw his arm is like an extendable limb which simply drops the ball through the basket. One wonders how effective such an analogy would be for learners if combined with instructions to "put your hand in the cookie jar," which research has shown also to be effective (see Figure 9.1).

Currently there is no sport in which a comprehensive directory of analogies exists for each movement or technique. Nor is there likely to be given the many-faceted complexity of ways in which each of us as individuals can manipulate our degrees of freedom, our muscles, joints, and so on. Coaches must, therefore, develop their own repertoire of analogies, taking care to confirm that the learner is fully familiar with the concepts underlying each analogy, yet not defeating the purpose of the analogy by accompanying it with an explicit lecture about the expected effect that it will have on the mechanics of the learner's technique.

Research has also shown that there are cultural differences in responsiveness to analogies. For example, the right-angled triangle analogy has been shown to be an ineffective method for teaching a topspin forehand implicitly to Hong Kong Chinese learners, who are often familiar with the physical principles of a right-angled triangle but are less likely to map the underlying causal principles to their movements. It is likely that the analogy conveys an inappropriate abstraction to Hong Kong Chinese learners that makes it difficult to translate the conceptual image into movement. In response to this problem, an alternative culturally relevant analogy has been developed and validated (i.e., "move the bat as though it is travelling up the side of a mountain"). The new analogy, although appearing to encapsulate the same fundamental geometric attributes of the right-angled triangle analogy, is perhaps more culturally decipherable. A very good example of this might be the

162

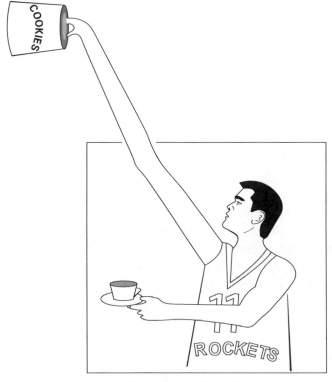

Slam 'dunk', Yao Ming!

Figure 9.1 An analogy for basketball shooting: putting your hand in the cookie jar.

wonderful "chase a chook" analogy narrated by Neil Craig when he was Senior Coach at Adelaide Football Club. Rather than present three or four coaching points to players about how to secure an erratically bouncing AFL ball (i.e., assume low body position, use soft hands, etc.), players were instructed to pretend that they were trying to catch a chicken. For those of us who have chased "chooks" in the past this analogy leaves an indelible image, but it is a safe bet that most people in Hong Kong are not familiar with chasing a chook.

The "chase a chook" analogy highlights one of the important advantages of analogy learning; it appears to allow many pieces of information about a skill (i.e., rules or instructions) to be presented to the learner in one manageable "chunk." This contrasts with traditional coaching methods which involve the explicit presentation of many individual bits of information about how to move. Considerable practice is required before the learner can integrate these pieces of information into a manageable chunk, as is clear when one considers the length of time that it takes for most tennis beginners to learn how to make a ball toss with one hand, scratch the back with the racquet in the other hand, bring the back foot through alongside the front foot, flex the knees, snap the wrist, and strike the ball. And that is only a first serve.

"Chunking" has been examined in depth with respect to its critical role in human memory facilitating the organization of very large amounts of information. Research that examines chunking as it relates to analogy learning in sport has not reached the same depth. Nevertheless, an advantage of chunking in analogy learning may be that considerably more information than normal can be presented to the learner in a short period of time. Presumably, analogy learning should therefore provide a faster route to expertise, although to date no empirical evidence exists to support such a claim. The implications for elite-performance development, however, would be significant and might have potential to take years off the 10-year rule of necessary preparation that has in the past been provided as a yardstick of the time it takes to become an expert (see Chapter 2). The duration of financial support required from sport governing bodies would be reduced, parents would come under less pressure to remortgage the house, dropout rates caused by loss of motivation would be lower, and failures under pressure reduced.

ERRORS OF THE PAST

John Wooden, one of America's great basketball coaches, was positive that "doers make mistakes," implying that winners are those who have made more errors in the past. But all those errors become learned – and then need to be unlearned. When people make errors during performance they have a natural inclination to try to correct them. For example, a cricketer for whom a long throw to the stumps is challenging is likely to practice long throws. The cricketer will actively test hypotheses about how best to make each throw successfully. In so doing, the cricketer will use conscious explicit processes to control performance, rather than unconscious implicit processes, so it may be preferable to set goals that are just easy enough to be achieved without recourse to hypothesis testing. For instance, the cricketer might first set a goal to consistently make a short(ish) throw to the side of a barn. Once that specific goal is achieved, the cricketer might progress to a slightly longer throw to the barn door and then to the barn window. Eventually, the cricketer will progress to the most challenging goal (to throw down the stumps from the outfield), but the overall process is likely to have involved less explicit hypotheses testing because fewer errors occurred along the way.

Many professional athletes probably continue to test hypotheses about their movements and accumulate knowledge about their sport throughout their career. In some sports this is more obvious than others. Well-known golfers at the top of their trade may publicly remodel their swing to gain an extra yard, or superstar swimmers may alter their technique to shave just a fraction of a second off their time. At

164

the upper limits of human ability, such goals are truly challenging and challenging goals indubitably produce better performance than easily achieved goals. The catch is that challenging goals by their very nature promote errors and errors encourage performers to actively test motor hypotheses to correct them.

It is not uncommon to see even great performers lose confidence because of the skill errors that they make and, for reasons that are not always logical but which by default are always mediated by their goals, make changes to those very skills that got them to the top. During one low point in his career, Severiano Ballesteros, who had won five major championships in golf, famously was persuaded to memorize 40 swing thoughts to think about when he played a shot. His confidence did not appear to profit.

This raises a compelling question: is it possible to relearn implicitly a skill that has been learned explicitly? Implicit skills can arise in two ways, either because the performer has never had conscious access to explicit knowledge of how the skill is performed or because the performer has gradually lost conscious access to the knowledge by forgetting.

For an athlete who wishes to relearn implicitly, the answer may be to carry out many trials using an implicit technique, such as errorless learning, until access to the explicit knowledge components of performance has been suppressed by the implicit ones. Errorless learning results in skills that are implicit because the absence of (motor) mistakes, meaning that the performer does not need to test hypotheses about the best way to move. For example, a basketball player who thinks too much when standing on the free throw line should be encouraged to carry out many throws in which performance is error-free (e.g., perhaps to an over-sized hoop or from very close distances that gradually increase). Case studies of the very best netball shooters have shown that this approach results in changes in movement patterns and even characteristic ball trajectories of which they appear to be unaware.

"The man who removes a mountain begins by carrying away small stones" (Chinese proverb – Confucius). An accompanying benefit of errorless learning is that it allows a very challenging ultimate goal to be achieved by gradual increases in difficulty. Far fewer errors therefore occur than if the very challenging ultimate goal were always practiced. Not only does implicit motor learning occur but, step by step, a performer builds a history of successful experiences. A history of successful experiences is the mainstay of self-efficacy, a performer's sense of whether he or she has what it takes to succeed. In short, completing many trials with few failures increases confidence in one's abilities.

Errorless learning is a form of implicit motor learning that has been examined with respect to children. Studies of typically developing children and children with disabilities that cause poor movement skills (such as cerebral palsy or intellectual disability) have shown that an error-reduced learning approach is more effective than an error-prone approach for acquiring fundamental movement skills such as throwing. Not only do they display some of the advantages of implicit motor learning, but an important sense of mastery is encouraged and the children are less inclined to be self-conscious about their abilities relative to other children if few errors occur when they perform.

A potential criticism that may be directed at errorless learning is that it tends to limit variability during the learning process, which is normally seen as a disadvantage by those who advocate development of skills that are flexible and adaptable (see Chapter 8). The jury is out on this one. Errorless learners may, in fact, have flexibility to be variable in the way that they complete the skill from trial to trial because the task is so easy – that is, they can succeed in many different ways without making an error. Whether a learner completes the skill with or without variation during errorless learning may be a consequence of individual differences or indeed level of expertise. An expert may quickly become bored with such an easily achieved outcome and thus introduce variation from trial to trial, whereas a beginner may decide upon a strategy and then repeat that strategy over and over. Alternatively, an expert might adhere rigidly, almost superstitiously, to a known strategy in the belief that no other will suffice, whereas the beginner stumbles from variation to variation.

For many sports, it is probably not even possible to design truly errorless forms of learning. A coach might therefore consider designing pseudo-errorless paradigms that create variability from trial to trial without sacrificing "errorlessness." For example, place-kicking in rugby union or rugby league might be practiced first from directly in front without a crossbar, then from an acute angle without goal posts, then from a greater distance with the crossbar adjusted to a very low height, and so on. Once again, it is for the coach with his or her specific expertise in a particular sport to find effective ways in which to articulate these principles on the field.

SEE NO EVIL, HEAR NO EVIL

An alternative way to learn or relearn skills implicitly might be to prevent access by the performer to visual outcome feedback during practice. In the same way that errorless learning makes hypothesis testing pointless because the movement is always successful, this form of learning renders hypothesis testing impossible because the performer *sees* no information with which to test hypotheses. There is a story of a Norwegian biathlon competitor who was so conscious of his poor performance in the shooting discipline that he could not sleep for thinking about it. His vastly experienced coach advised him to literally shoot for the sky whenever

166

and wherever he could, so he took to carrying his gun with him at all times and whenever the urge came over him he took potshots into the sky. Eventually, he became less conscious of his shooting and went on to claim gold at the Winter Olympics. Although this story may (or may not) be an urban sport legend, there are examples of legendary performers renowned for their stability under pressure, who somewhere in their skill-learning past have trained without feedback or practiced without error. Jonny Wilkinson, for example, kicked the winning goal for England in the final of the 2003 Rugby World Cup and is said to have practiced his kicking into a net for hours on end. Such practice would provide little or no feedback with which he could test hypotheses about his skills, nor would errors be apparent. Similarly, Tiger Woods practiced with his father at night as a youngster on a US Naval course where feedback was aided only by the peripheral lights of the base.

It is possible, however, that such dramatic remedies may not be necessary if skills are acquired implicitly during the early stages of learning. Brief initial periods of implicit motor learning have been shown to provide learners with advantages of stability under pressure or multi-tasking even if the performer later accumulates a large amount of explicit knowledge. It may be that the initial period of implicit learning propels a learner irrevocably down a motor control pathway that is dis-associated from explicit control of the skill. This finding is of particular applied value, given that it is impossible to restrict a performer to an entirely implicit learning environment. Control over the learning environment cannot, for example, be maintained during competition where an umpire (or an opponent) is unlikely to respond sympathetically to requests that the lights are turned off in order to remove feedback. Furthermore, it is very natural for a performer to endeavor explicitly to work out what is happening when skills go wrong. Indeed, many coaches argue that performers need to have a foundation of explicit knowledge of the rule structures underlying their skills to fall back on when things go wrong. It is appealing to consider that a bout or bouts of implicit motor learning very early in skill development might provide all of the positive advantages associated with non-conscious control of performance, and allows later accumulation of consciously accessible skill knowledge that can be used if necessary, but does not increase the likelihood of reinvestment.

THE CRAFTY COACH

A problem with removing visual outcome feedback is that people do not necessarily learn very effectively, although this may be less important for experts who already have developed relatively effective movement patterns. Nevertheless, even experts need to attune their movements to the demands of the environment, which in most cases is best achieved by processing visual information about the outcome of each movement attempt. One option is to present visual outcome feedback to the performer so that, although it is received, the performer is unaware of having perceived it. That is, the information has not reached conscious levels of awareness. As an example of just how sensitive the human perceptual system is, we have shown in a series of studies in our laboratory in Hong Kong that a goalkeeper can, simply by standing marginally to the left or to the right of goal-center, influence a penalty-taker to direct more penalties to the side that has more space. The goalkeeper can then dive in the biased direction to make a save. The importance of this finding is perhaps not obvious until one realizes that if the goalkeeper stands to the side by a mere 6 to 10 centimeters, the penalty-taker will not be consciously aware that there is more space to one side. In fact, when asked, most penalty-takers firmly believe that the goalkeeper is standing in the exact center of the goal. Nevertheless, they are much more prone to direct their shots to the side with more space.

In other studies, we have shown that it is possible to cause implicit motor learning by presenting feedback regarding the outcome of movements in such a way that performers *believe* that they have not seen what happened when they performed the skill. This is typically known as the subjective threshold of awareness and, although people will claim that they see no information about their performance, if forced to say what happened (e.g., where the ball went or the location of the target), they are usually very accurate. Sophisticated equipment is required to present information in such a way that it cannot be perceived consciously, especially since most people have slightly different thresholds of awareness. These challenges ensure that this subliminal approach to implicit motor learning is one that is not likely to be applied by the average coach, but there are crafty ways in which a coach can mimic the subliminal presentation of information to change movement patterns without the athlete necessarily becoming consciously aware that a change has occurred. For example, a volleyball coach may wish to get his players to extend the arm more when spiking. Rather than explicitly describing the changes in technique that he wants to see, the coach might consider increasing the height of the net during practice sessions in increments so small that the players are unaware of the increased extension of the arm that is required to make a successful spike. Eventually it will become obvious to the players that the net is higher than normal but by then the movement changes will have occurred implicitly and the coach will have achieved his aim without ever uttering an instruction.

In an alternative approach that achieves a somewhat similar outcome, the coach might consider a "*Karate Kid* method," taken from the film of the same name in which the wise old instructor, Mr. Miyagi, encourages his young protégé to spend many hours pointlessly waxing his car with the famous line "wax on, wax off." The same movement with which "wax on, wax off" is achieved is also that with which a punch is deflected. Researchers have shown that this incidental learning approach is also effective for learning anticipation skills implicitly. Players asked

168

to specifically concentrate on predicting the *speed* of tennis serves displayed more improved ability in predicting serve *direction* than players who were explicitly instructed with cues about what to look for in order to anticipate where the serve was going.

AN UNASHAMEDLY EXPLICIT CONCLUSION

Would-be superstars, weekend warriors, or seasoned sport celebrities aggregate explicit knowledge about how they perform their skills by testing hypotheses and taking instruction regarding the most appropriate way to move. Conscious access to such information is often disruptive to performance, especially when performers are highly motivated to succeed. There is evidence that practical advantages are associated with forms of implicit motor learning that avoid the accumulation of explicit knowledge about the mechanics that underlie the skill.

The coach has substantial influence over the physical and social learning environment of the performer, child, or adult. The willingness to use an implicit motor learning approach raises practical obstacles that a coach must navigate and, although he or she cannot always constrain the environment to provide a comprehensive implicit skill-learning experience, much can be done to bring forward the unconscious and push back the conscious during performance. Implicit motor learning theory asserts that, in particular, early skill-learning experiences should be maximally constrained to be *implicit*, the learning environment should discourage active testing of hypotheses about performance outcomes, and any form of instruction allowing *explicit* access to rule structures underlying the skills should be strictly rationed.

COACH'S CORNER

Tom Willmott
Head Coach, New Zealand's Winter Performance Park & Pipe Programme

Implicit learning: does it work in practice?

The cultures of the sports of snowboarding and freeskiing lend themselves to skill acquisition by way of *play:* informal progression in groups with individuals one-upping each other and learning together by trying new things and emulating maneuvers from the latest video releases. Riders in groups or crews push and help each other out with the odd piece of explicit instruction although feedback is mostly in the form of recognition of success and style.

Halfpipe snowboarding became an Olympic discipline in 1998; enter the coach, shunned by some exponents of the sport who are not keen on having an "instructor" tell them what to do and would rather let their own creativity, freedom, and artistic performance flow. Many coaches, especially at the developmental level, are most effective when they, rather than being the coach in the typical sense of the word, simply lead the pack and contribute and shape the direction of the group, allowing implicit learning to flourish rather than providing the classical ski instructor "bend the knees" approach.

I am currently working with two very different elite athletes. Aside from one being a skier and the other being a snowboarder, they learn and are motivated in completely different ways. One would be considered a high reinvester, has been coached from an early age in the sport, specializes in her discipline, and thrives on testing hypotheses. The other is self-taught, is new to being coached, has broad experience in the sport in a variety of conditions, has previously learnt in an implicit manner, does not respond well to explicit cues, and possesses limited hypotheses and explicit knowledge of the sport. They both have their individual strengths and weaknesses and, of course, present their individual coaching challenges! The former athlete has an ability to adjust her technique based on self-identified or coaching cues if things go wrong or a movement pattern is not effective in training or competition. The latter athlete benefits from the ability of being able to adapt to the environment "on the fly," can compete in a variety of conditions, and intuitively adjusts technique appropriately.

We (New Zealand Snowsports high-performance coaches) were fortunate enough to spend some time with Rich Masters at a spring training camp in New Zealand in October 2010, where we had an opportunity to put implicit learning theory into practice with our athletes.

Implicit learning strategies applied and tested during spring camp

Secondary tasks

Humming, counting backwards in threes from 100, and singing a song out loud were all introduced as strategies for athletes to use, particularly when frustration was rearing its head or if an athlete was simply over-thinking a particular skill. We found that a suitable level of complexity of secondary task must be aligned to the complexity/risk/stage of development of the primary task. With a new skill, humming was enough to distract the conscious process, whereas a minor modification to a learned skill required a more complex secondary task.

An athlete was building towards attempting a frontside 900 (two full rotations in the air, turning the front of their body to the bottom of the halfpipe) for the first time. In order for her to feel confident in her ability to land this complex maneuver she was keen to complete some frontside 720s (a prerequisite skill with a similar takeoff and just 180 degrees less rotation). On the first few attempts it was clear the athlete was not finishing the rotation with her head which, instead of looking over her shoulder to complete the trick, was looking down at her board. Rich suggested I move to a position on the opposite side of the halfpipe as a visual target and ask the athlete to tell me how many hands I had in the air (one or two) while she was completing the trick. On the first attempt following this intervention the athlete had not been able to look at me and therefore could not tell me how many hands were raised; she looked down at her board and the trick was unsuccessful. On the second attempt the athlete kept her head up and was looking for the landing earlier in the maneuver, but the trick was still unsuccessful. On the third attempt the athlete kept her head up and was looking for the landing earlier in the maneuver, she landed the trick successfully, and was able to tell me I had one hand up. After a further successful repetition the athlete had increased self-confidence and attempted a 900, and the following week landed it on her second attempt. A key piece of advice from Rich, when experimenting with secondary tasks, was to persevere with the secondary task, as it will often take a number of repetitions for an athlete to successfully incorporate the secondary task into what they are doing.

Errorless learning

Recently, and particularly in the push to the Vancouver Olympics, where the bar was raised with double-inverted maneuvers being commonly integrated into medal-winning competition runs, teams have been seeking safe environments and training tools to speed up safe skill acquisition, with foam pits and airbags (see Figure 9.2) introduced to the mountain environment formerly the domain of stuntmen and acrobats. The airbag setup allows experimentation and creativity in "real snow," with similar specifications to a competition halfpipe with the same takeoff, air time, and feel as the real thing, but "safer" skill execution than in a standard halfpipe. An errorless approach to a training session using the airbag can focus on getting one particular aspect of the skill such as the takeoff timing or grab-hold successfully completed without paying any attention to the quality of the landing.

Analogies

"Forming a pizza" with skis has been identified as a highly effective way of introducing kids in particular to the "snowplough" technique in beginner's ski lessons. Some of the complex movement patterns in snowboarding and freeskiing are fairly unique in nature and are therefore difficult to chunk entire movements into one effective analogy, although with perseverance solutions can be found.

An athlete was interested in developing an analogy for a new maneuver he was attempting to take from the airbag (see Figure 9.2) to the halfpipe for the first time: a double-inverted 1080 (spins on two planes including two flips and a half rotation) taking off backwards and landing forwards while grabbing the tail of his board. In a combination of explicit and implicit approaches, he established that success of the trick in the errorless context of the airbag (discussed below) was achieved by focusing on taking the trick "up" into the air at takeoff (to gain the required amplitude and air time to allow successful execution), to "grab" the board to help keep his body position tight, and to imagine he was being punched in the stomach by David Tua (New Zealand heavyweight boxer) to ensure he achieved the desired double flip. The athlete repeated to himself "up, grab, Tua" when imaging the trick prior to trials in the airbag and used

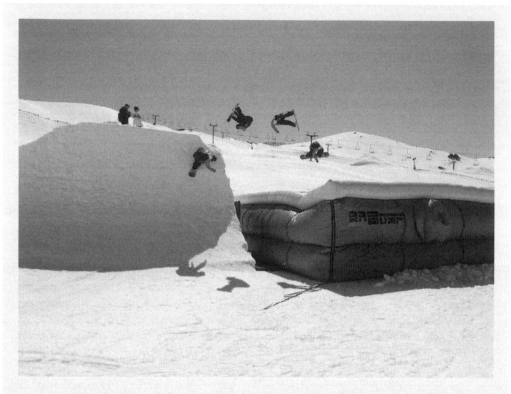

Figure 9.2 Attempting new maneuvers with reduced consequence (errorless practice) into an airbag.

the same approach to successfully transfer the trick to the halfpipe, landing it on his sixth attempt. The "up–grab–Tua" self-talk phrase appeared to be highly effective in developing the skill, not only by providing a vivid analogy of the desired body position the athlete needed to adopt in mid-air while spinning and flipping multiple times, but also by giving him supreme confidence that the movement would be successful and that he would probably land without injury when taking the trick to the halfpipe thanks to successful attempts in the airbag. Benefits of the "David Tua punch to the guts" analogy were that, during the first few attempts when the athlete was consistently under-rotating the flip aspect of the trick, I reminded him that he was being punched in the guts by David Tua and not by his sister; this effectively increased the extent to which he bent at the waist, increasing his flip speed, and allowing him to complete the trick landing over the top of his board.

Direct subliminal input

Priming an athlete on the chairlift with simple math (what's 2 × 5? what's 4 × 20?) has been one technique I have used to subconsciously persuade an athlete that it might be a good time to consider attempting a 1080 (when asked five minutes later on the side of the halfpipe what they want to do next).

Random practice

I have successfully employed random practice to reduce the impact of "paralysis by analysis," to prevent hypothesis testing from occurring, to enhance the quality of learning during a session with athletes constantly challenged to reconstruct movement patterns, and to reduce frustration from unsuccessful trials (but see Chapter 8). Strategies including "sno-dice" (where a rider rolls a dice to dictate which trick he/she attempts next) or simply tossing a coin to randomize the order of practice of two skills have been applied successfully. I have experimented on numerous occasions at taking a deliberate *random* rather than *blocked* practice approach and have more often than not achieved learning success.

For instance, in one session the goal was to perform a backside 900 in the halfpipe. We were taking full runs and there was enough room for two repetitions. The rider performed prerequisite tricks (backside 540s and backside 720s) in the pipe. Usually we would have blocked the practice by repeating these until the backside 720 was at such a stage of execution that, on the subsequent run, taking it to 900 would be considered feasible. Instead we opted to follow a run in the halfpipe by taking a run over jumps – attempting the backside 900 maneuver in a different setting and then going back to the halfpipe. Alternating between a run in the halfpipe and a run through the jumps seemed to assist learning mostly by preventing frustration. If an attempt in the halfpipe was unsuccessful there was no opportunity to get frustrated and reinvest on the subsequent attempt as the context had changed. Paralysis by analysis appeared to be prevented and a greater learning effect was achieved.

Session two and a fatigued athlete had been working on frontside 720s (one and a half full rotations) with varying success in two previous sessions. Rather than focus solely on the frontside 720 we made the practice session random by selecting the frontside 720 and one completely different trick (i.e., "alley-oop indy" – spins in the opposite direction to normal, rotating 180 degrees towards the top of the halfpipe). I flipped a coin – heads was the frontside 7, tails was the alley-oop. The first three flips were all tails, the fourth was a head, and the athlete was successful at the 720 on the first attempt, having landed prerequisite skills earlier in the session.

Summary

In the New Zealand Snowsports coaching community, awareness has been raised of the many times that we already use an implicit learning approach, of the benefits and further opportunities to develop this style as a functional coaching approach. Since Rich's visit we have continued to manipulate our training environments, and to test and consciously utilize implicit learning theory (alongside explicit approaches) for the skill acquisition of our elite athletes. In a sport which is subjectively judged based on criteria including how the performance looks from the outside and the quality of execution, automaticity and perceived effortlessness is sought by athletes and coaches. An implicit learning approach can therefore be beneficial for many reasons including avoiding robotic, mechanical, and awkward movement patterns. At times it is certainly not easy or suitable to implement an implicit approach, particularly in snowsports with their inherent high-risk nature. For example, in some circumstances an explicit cue may be required to meet a short-term requirement for confidence. However, we are all firm believers in the suitability and potential for the application of implicit learning theory as a facet of our coaching toolkit.

KEY READING

Capio, C.M., Poolton, J.M., Sit, C.H.P., Eguia, K.T., and Masters, R.S.W. (2012) 'Reduction of errors during practice facilitates fundamental movement skill learning in children with intellectual disabilities', in *Journal of Intellectual Disability Research*. DOI: 10.1111/j.1365-2788.2012.01535.x

Hatfield, B.D., Haufler, A.J., Hung, T., and Spalding, T.W. (2004) 'Electroencephalographic studies of skilled psychomotor performance', *Journal of Clinical Neurophysiology*, 21: 144–156.

Liao, C. and Masters, R.S.W. (2001) 'Analogy learning: A means to implicit motor learning', *Journal of Sports Sciences*, 19: 307–319.

Masters, R.S.W. (1992) 'Knowledge, knerves and know-how: The role of explicit versus implicit knowledge in the breakdown of a complex motor skill under pressure', *British Journal of Psychology*, 83: 343–358.

Masters, R.S.W. and Maxwell, J. (2008) 'The Theory of Reinvestment', *International Review of Sport and Exercise Psychology*, 1: 160–183.

Masters, R.S.W., Maxwell, J.P., and Eves, F.F. (2009) 'Marginally perceptible outcome feedback, motor learning and implicit processes', *Consciousness and Cognition*, 18: 639–645.

Masters, R.S.W. and Poolton, J. (2012) 'Advances in implicit motor learning', in Hodges, N.J. and Williams, A.M. (eds.) *Skill Acquisition in Sport: Research, Theory and Practice*. London: Routledge, pp. 59–76.

Masters, R.S.W., Poolton, J.M., and Maxwell, J.P. (2008) 'Stable implicit motor processes despite aerobic locomotor fatigue', *Consciousness and Cognition*, 17: 335–338.

Masters, R.S.W., van der Kamp, J., and Jackson, R.C. (2007) 'Imperceptibly off-centre goalkeepers influence penalty-kick direction in soccer', *Psychological Science*, 18: 222–223.

Maxwell, J.P., Masters, R.S.W., Kerr, E., and Weedon, E. (2001) 'The implicit benefit of learning without errors', *Quarterly Journal of Experimental Psychology*, 54A: 1049–1068.

Poolton, J., Masters, R.S.W., and Maxwell, J.P. (2005) 'The relationship between initial errorless learning conditions and subsequent performance', *Human Movement Sciences*, 24: 362–378.

Reber, A.S. (1993) *Implicit Learning and Tacit Knowledge: An Essay on the Cognitive Unconscious*. New York: Oxford University Press.

Rendell, M., Farrow, D., Masters, R.S.W., and Plummer, N. (2011) 'Implicit practice for technique adaptation in expert performers', *International Journal of Sports Science and Coaching*, 6: 553–566.

Zhu, F.F., Poolton, J.M., Wilson, M.R., Maxwell, J.P., and Masters, R.S.W. (2011) 'Neural co-activation as a yardstick of implicit motor learning and the propensity for conscious control of movement', *Biological Psychology*, 87: 66–73.

174

PART IV

EXPERT ATHLETE PROCESSES

CHAPTER 10

"CHOKING" IN SPORT

RESEARCH AND IMPLICATIONS

ROBIN C. JACKSON, SIAN L. BEILOCK, AND NOEL P. KINRADE

INTRODUCTION

> I was trying as hard as I could; I yearned for victory more intensely than
> in any match I had ever played; and yet it was as if I had regressed to
> the time when I was a beginner . . . My movements were sometimes
> lethargic, sometimes jerky, my technique lacked any semblance of
> fluency and coherence.
> (Matthew Syed, journalist and former international table tennis player)

Elite sport performers have attained their status by demonstrating an ability to
execute skills with a level of precision superior to their peers. What has intrigued
spectators, coaches, and psychologists, not to mention the performers themselves,
is how they respond to pressure situations. Some performers gain a reputation for
being "clutch players," others gain a reputation for "choking," that is, performing
significantly worse than expected in spite of being highly motivated to succeed.
Still others display instances of choking but subsequently display excellent performance under pressure. In 2011, the golfer Rory McIlroy led by four shots going into
the final round of the US Masters. The lead reduced to a single shot by the middle of
the final round, at which point his performance deteriorated dramatically. He went
on to take 80 shots, finishing 10 shots behind winner Charl Schwartzel. McIlroy
said, "I was leading this golf tournament with nine holes to go and I unravelled
. . . I just lost my speed on the greens, lost my line, lost everything for two or three
holes and couldn't really recover." However, in the very next of the four major golf
tournaments, the US Open, McIlroy maintained his composure over the final round
to win the tournament by a margin of eight shots and with a record score.

For researchers and practitioners with an interest in choking, it is important to distinguish between normal fluctuations in performance and instances that are significantly worse than expected. Scientific use of the term "choking" requires evidence, whether it be through introspective self-reports on the part of the athlete (such as the quotes from Rory McIlroy and Matthew Syed) or statistical analyses indicating that a given performance is unlikely to be explained by random variation.

In this chapter we present research that has attempted to uncover why choking occurs through examining ways in which pressure-filled situations change how individuals think about and attend to skilled performance. One implication of research in this area is that the way performers learn can influence how robust their skills are under stress. This is discussed in detail by Rich Masters in Chapter 9 of this book so it is not covered here. Our focus is on understanding how crucial moments affect the attentional processes supporting high-level skill execution and how this can be used to develop training regimens and performance strategies that alleviate skill failure. In the first section of the chapter, we summarize what researchers have revealed about the processes underlying choking in highly practiced skills. We then consider factors that might moderate or trigger this process. In the second section, we consider the implications of this research for designing strategies to prevent skill breakdown under stress.

WHAT DOES THE RESEARCH TELL US?

Evidence for choking

In sport there are numerous examples in which performers fail at crucial moments to successfully execute skills that have been performed perfectly time and time again in practice. Routine golf putts and rugby place kicks are missed, basketball free throws hit the rim, tennis players serve double faults, and soccer penalty kicks are ballooned over the crossbar. Although such instances grab the headlines, poor performance in high-pressure situations is far from unusual. Take the example of soccer penalty shoot-outs. In many cup competitions, a tied match is decided by five players on each team taking a penalty kick. If the score remains tied each team selects an additional player until one team emerges victorious. In researching the critical moments in these already high-pressure situations, Geir Jordet and Esther Hartman reviewed all 36 shoot-outs (359 kicks) that had occurred in the soccer World Cup, European Championships and UEFA Champions League tournaments. They found that success rates were considerably lower (61.8 percent) when players had to score to avoid losing the shoot-out than when they had a kick to win (92.0 percent).

Robin C. Jackson, Sian L. Beilock, and Noel P. Kinrade

Other researchers have identified pressure situations within baseball and found that hitting averages tends to be worse than the low-pressure equivalents. At the individual level there are several research examples in which participants were selected on account of their tendency to perform worse in high-pressure situations, for example, having lower basketball free throw shooting success in competition than in practice. Across many sports, it seems that, when the pressure and desire to succeed is highest, the performance of the very best athletes may be lowest.

Performers' experiences

Why does choking occur in well-learned and highly practiced skills such as the tournament winning putt or the all-important penalty shot? One important window into understanding choking is the performers' recollections about their experiences. Surprisingly, there is relatively little formal research in this area but a recent study of golfers underlines the different processes involved. Daniel Gucciardi and colleagues (2010) interviewed highly skilled players who had suffered three to six choking experiences over the previous two years. In describing the choking event they primarily referred to loss of attentional control, loss of emotional control, and departing from their normal pre-shot routine. The researchers also found that the golfers commonly referred to a negative interpretation of anxiety symptoms before the event (e.g., "I was anxious but it wasn't a good anxious because I think you have to be nervous to play your best but that's a positive anxious, but in this instance it was more of a negative anxious"). Alongside this, fear of failure was commonly cited, not least because they and others had invested so much in their sport. As one golfer said of the importance of performing well: "it validates my self-worth as a golfer."

In terms of the processes underlying choking, the loss of attentional control described by the golfers referred to being more distracted as well as exerting more conscious control over their actions. Thus, they referred to the distraction of thinking about an anticipated positive outcome as opposed to the processes required to attain that outcome: "all the simple things that get the job done and get you back to what you normally do well." It seems there is a fine line here between a positive and negative process focus. Focusing on continuing to do the things that have helped the performer get into the position to win was perceived as positive. Paradoxically, a process focus was also seen as a potential cause of choking if it triggered explicit monitoring of performance: "thinking too much about the processes and losing the automaticity that is there when I'm shooting at my best." Tellingly, micro-managing skilled movement is also evident in performers' descriptions of "yips" experiences. For example, one cricket bowler said, "I was literally saying to myself, jump, sideways on, coil, release."

Overall, the comments from these interviews point to the broad and complex nature of choking experiences with evidence supporting both conscious processing and distraction-based accounts. When these are coupled with the loss of emotional control and departure from their normal routines (usually speeding up) we see a cascade of events that are well beyond what is normally experienced by the performers. As one of the golfers said, "all of a sudden I fell out of my normal patterns and my normal game plan because I was thinking too much and couldn't control my emotions."

Explicit monitoring and skill-focused attention

In line with many performers' experiences of choking, several researchers have focused on how pressure situations induce self-consciousness in response to anxiety about performing well. This focus on the self is thought to prompt performers to turn their attention to the specific processes of their performance as they attempt to exert more skill control than would be applied in a non-pressure situation. For example, the basketball player who makes 85 percent of their free throws in practice may miss the game-winning foul shot because, in trying to ensure an optimal outcome, they monitor the angle of their wrist or the release point as they shoot the ball. After many thousands of hours of practice, these components of performance are not something that our basketball player would normally attend to. So, whereas many everyday tasks will benefit from slowing down and thinking things through logically, the paradox where motor skills are concerned is that trying to consciously control the step-by-step components of an action disrupts the smooth, effortless fluency of such skills. Again, performers walk a fine line between cue words that might help initiate fluent performance and thoughts that break down performance processes that normally run largely outside conscious awareness: "paralysis by analysis."

In support of the above ideas, work in our labs and those of others has demonstrated that, for well-learned and highly practiced skills, paying too much attention to task control and guidance (what we call skill-focused attention) does indeed disrupt skilled execution. Just as thinking about how and where we place our feet as we rush down the stairs may result in the disruption of well-learned walking movements and a fall, attending too much to skill processes that generally run off without conscious awareness can disrupt performance and cause skill failure in sport. For example, one study asked skilled soccer players to dribble the ball through a series of pylons while paying attention to the side of their foot that most recently contacted the ball. This instruction was designed to draw attention to performance in a way that does not normally occur. Dribbling performance was worse (i.e., slower and more error-prone) when the soccer players were asked to attend to performance than in a condition in which they dribbled without any instructions.

180

Similar results have been reported in research on baseball batting. When highly skilled baseball players were asked to perform a hitting task, while also attending to a specific component of their swing, their performance suffered. Here, baseball players heard a randomly presented tone and were instructed to indicate whether their bat was moving downward or upward at the instant the tone was presented. Biomechanical swing analyses revealed that performance failure was at least partially due to the fact that skill-focused attention interfered with the sequencing and timing of the different skill components involved in swinging. Interestingly, when participants were in a "slump" of poorer performance, their ability to report the position of the bat improved, supporting the link between explicit monitoring and poor performance.

This research suggests that paying too much attention to highly practiced skills disrupts performance. Nonetheless, there are probably well-learned components of sport performance that still require a significant amount of attention and effort for optimal performance and thus may not be harmed when performers attempt to control execution. For example, strategizing and problem solving can, at times, require considerable attention and memory resources to be performed at a high level. These skills may not fail when performers concentrate on what they are doing; rather they may instead fail if performers are distracted from the task at hand, possibly because they are worrying about the possibility of poor performance.

In addition, skill-focused attention may be necessary when making changes to a well-learned technique. High-level performers will most likely have to slow down and unpack automated processes in order to change their technique, which may result temporarily in poor performance. In highly technical, self-paced sports this can be a lengthy and difficult process with no guarantee of success. Tiger Woods is perhaps the highest-profile performer currently seeking to regain or surpass his level and consistency after a prolonged period making changes to his full swing and putting action.

Self-regulation and avoidance

Returning to the high-pressure situation of soccer penalty shoot-outs, Geir Jordet and colleagues have argued that players are responding to a breakdown in their ability to self-regulate, that is, to control their thoughts, emotions, and behavior in the face of the "ego threat" of the shoot-out. As we have seen, one response to pressure is to try to consciously control automated movements. A second response is evident in Jordet and colleagues' analysis: *avoidance behavior*. A particularly interesting finding of their research was that avoidance behavior was notably more pronounced in players or teams with high status. England players, for example, were much more likely than other teams to turn away from the goalkeeper after placing the ball and were also fastest in responding to the referee's whistle. This desire to "get it over with" is corroborated by a quote from the England player Steven Gerrard, discussing how he felt before a penalty attempt in the 2006 World Cup: "Jesus, I wish I was first up. Get it out of the way. The wait's killing me . . . Blow the whistle . . . get a move on ref! Why the wait? I was screaming inside."

Arguably, avoidance behavior can be seen in several other aspects of some teams' approaches to penalty shoot-outs: players turn their backs away from the action or avoid taking a penalty in the first place; team coaches and players describe the shoot-out as a "lottery," making the point that it is impossible to recreate the pressure of a real shoot-out, or argue that practice is of little use. Avoidance might also be seen in unwillingness to embrace findings from sports science research, resulting in limited understanding of factors involved with different penalty kick (and penalty-saving) strategies, and the role of disguise, deception, and anticipation skill. For example, England's relatively low success rate when the opposing goalkeeper dives in the correct direction (50 percent), combined with goalkeepers diving to the correct side more frequently against England than all but one other international team, suggests work could be done on helping players better disguise their intentions. More broadly, acknowledging that penalty shoot-outs are a real possibility in international soccer tournaments will foster an "approach" culture rather than one of avoidance. This, in turn, should enhance the likelihood of success.

Finally, it is interesting to note that, of all players who were studied in the shoot-outs, those who had won major individual awards scored less often (65.0 percent) than those who had received no award (73.6 percent). Moreover, players who went on to receive an award but had not done so at the time of the shoot-out scored 88.9 percent of their kicks. This body of work is important in establishing the behavioral impact of pressure and points to the importance of understanding the unique demands of different sports, and indeed different situations within a sport. For example, there is some evidence that minimizing thinking time improves golf putting performance; however, soccer players who took a split-second longer to compose themselves after the whistle sounded were more successful in penalty shoot-outs.

Triggers and risk factors

Now that we have attempted to describe why the failure of well-learned and highly practiced motor skills occurs in pressure situations, we turn to potential triggers of such failure.

Robin C. Jackson, Sian L. Beilock, and Noel P. Kinrade

Individual differences

The question of whether there are individual differences in how performers respond to pressure is an important line of research into choking. In considering whether certain individuals are more likely to try to consciously control their movements than others, Rich Masters and colleagues focused on self-consciousness and propensity to mentally rehearse emotional events. They devised the Reinvestment Scale (see Chapter 9), in which participants rate items such as "I'm aware of the way my mind works when I work through a problem" and "I'm concerned about what other people think of me." There is now good evidence that high scores on this scale predict propensity for reinvesting conscious control and choking under pressure in motor skills. Recently, Noel Kinrade and colleagues modified the scale to create a decision-specific version to investigate poor decision making under pressure. Results from basketball, netball, and korfball indicated that players with a stronger tendency to consciously monitor the decision-making process (decision reinvestment) and ruminate over previous poor decisions (decision rumination) were rated by their coaches as having a greater tendency to make poor decisions under pressure. Interestingly, recent research also shows that soccer referees who score highly on "decision rumination" make a disproportionate number of decisions in favor of the home team.

Task characteristics

The bulk of evidence supporting a conscious control model of choking has come from motor skills, whilst tasks that are more dependent on working memory (e.g., tactical planning in sport) have normally conformed with distraction-based accounts of choking. These suggest that pressure shifts attention towards task-irrelevant cues (e.g., worries about the importance of the outcome) consuming "attentional space" that is vital for successful performance. However, one facet central to both theoretical explanations is the role of task complexity. Choking has predominantly been observed in relatively complex motor tasks, such as golf putting, baseball batting, and soccer and hockey dribbling tasks, training for which is typically associated with substantial technical instruction. However, performance on simple motor tasks has proved more robust under stress. For example, performance on tracking, rod-tracing and card-sorting tasks was maintained and in some cases improved under pressure. It has been suggested that these might be considered "effort-based tasks" in which pressure can help maintain or increase motivation.

Imaging failure

Although one might assume that people in general (and most certainly highly disciplined athletes) are good at controlling their thoughts and performance-related images, it turns out that athletes *do* report thinking about the possibility of skill failure. Moreover, research has demonstrated that athletes' images of failure and even the mere mention of choking can result in less than optimal performances.

One of the first studies to examine this idea investigated the impact of negative imagery on dart-throwing success. It was found that combining dart-throwing practice with negative imagery (i.e., imaging the dart landing near the edge of the board rather in the center) led to a decrease in dart-throwing accuracy in comparison with combining dart throwing with positive imagery (i.e., imaging the dart landing near the center of the target). Additional evidence that pre-performance negative imagery can impair skill execution comes from recent studies exploring the effects of positive and negative imagery on golf putting. Golf putting accuracy declined when individuals employed negative imagery (e.g., thinking about missing the hole) prior to hitting the ball.

Thus, the ability to control one's thoughts and images prior to and during skill execution seems to be a crucial determinant of successful performance. Both negative self-talk and negative imagery immediately prior to performance may harm execution. Why? One possibility is that thinking about a negative outcome causes individuals to try and control their skill in an attempt to ensure that this negative performance outcome will not come to fruition. Ironically, as we have described above, such added control can backfire, disrupting well-learned and automated performance processes.

Heightened expectations

In contrast to the wealth of evidence for the home advantage, there is evidence that choking is sometimes more likely when performing in front of a supportive audience. For example, in 1984, Roy Baumeister and Andrew Steinhilber analyzed archival data from National Basketball Association (NBA) championships and Major League Baseball world series games. They found the home advantage reversed when the home team was one game away from winning the series. The home teams won just 38.5 percent of decisive seventh games in baseball and just 37.5 percent of basketball games in which they had a chance to clinch the championship.

Interestingly, after this research was published, home teams in basketball and baseball began winning these crucial games and the effect fell below statistical significance. Meanwhile, controlled studies painted a more complex picture. In one study, researchers found that the impact of a supportive audience depended on the

184

criterion for success. Participants were more prone to focusing on themselves and their skill execution in front of a supportive rather than neutral audience but this made performance worse only if there was a difficult criterion for success.

Overall then, there is some evidence that a supportive audience can adversely affect performance; however, it is likely to result from a combination of factors and the effect must be kept in perspective. A recent analysis of all the research on the home advantage showed that, overall, the advantage is slightly greater for championship (63 percent) than regular season (59 percent) matches. Since Roy Baumeister's research was published, the turnaround in NBA basketball has been quite remarkable: a run of wins in deciding matches means the home team now has the highest winning percentage in the final game of a tied series (game seven, 80.4 percent).

THEORY INTO PRACTICE: TECHNIQUES FOR PREVENTING CHOKING

If thinking too much can disrupt the fluent, automatic qualities of a highly practiced skill, a key issue is how to prevent this from happening. Clearly the solution is not easy because there remain many instances of poor performance under pressure. Nevertheless, there is a range of techniques that have proved effective in laboratory or field settings. While many of these studies are unlikely to recreate the levels of anxiety experienced in competition, they help provide the theoretical basis for interventions in the field.

Practicing under pressure

In military establishments, emergency services, aviation industry and medical practice, considerable time and money is spent on trying to simulate stressful situations. In these domains, as in sport, the aim is to have participants practice under the conditions they are likely to experience "in the field." One potential benefit of this approach is that it inoculates the performer against the negative impact of stress. Second, performers experience how they react under pressure and are able to practice coping strategies so they can better regulate their emotional, behavioral, and cognitive responses to stressful or high-pressure situations.

Recent research in sport indicates that practicing under pressure is effective. In one study, highly skilled basketball players practiced free-throw shooting over a five-week period when half of the players underwent acclimatization training, in which they were told their practice would be filmed and their technique evaluated by experts. They were also watched by the coach and other players, used individual and team sanctions for missed shots, and were told to imagine the free throws were decisive in a game situation. In total, each player in the acclimatization group practiced 96 free throws over the period while a control group took the same number of practice throws in the absence of pressure. After the intervention, the players' performance was re-evaluated under low- and high-pressure conditions. Interestingly, the levels of anxiety experienced by the players remained largely unchanged; however, the impact of pressure on performance differed markedly across the two groups. Prior to the intervention, both groups performed worse under high pressure (by about 5 percent). After the intervention, the control group again performed worse under high pressure (–5.2 percent) but the acclimatized group actually performed better under pressure (+6.7 percent).

Similar effects have been found in golf putting and in a study of handgun shooting using police officers. Those who practiced against an opponent who fired back (rather than using cardboard targets) subsequently performed equally well when tested in low- and high-pressure conditions. In these studies, it is interesting that acclimatization training does not seem to inoculate performers against experiencing anxiety in high-pressure situations. The fact that they continue to experience elevated anxiety under pressure yet no longer suffer poor performance suggests they are improving their ability to regulate their response to the situation. It seems practicing under pressure not only decreases the novelty of high-stakes situations but also enables performers to learn how to cope with their responses so that they retain a high level of performance. Whatever the underlying processes, the implication is clear. While we might not be able to recreate the levels of pressure (and anxiety) experienced in an Olympic Games, NBA Championship game, or soccer penalty shoot-out, having players practice under some degree of pressure serves as excellent preparation for performing to your potential when it counts.

Optimize your pre-performance routine

The more times one has to execute a skill the better the performance, right? We have all heard the adage "haste makes waste," but is this really true, especially with respect to the performance of well-learned and highly practiced skills? If thinking too much about how to perform a skill disrupts performance, then having a lot of preparation time to think about a technical skill performed with a small margin of error might actually result in a worse rather than better performance. For example, head coaches frequently take a time-out just before the opposing team kicker attempts an important field goal. This strategy of "icing" the kicker is effective: analysis of pressure kicks in the National Football League from 2002–2008 revealed that success was significantly lower (66.4 percent) for "iced" kicks than "non-iced" kicks (80.4 percent).

186

Coinciding with data on "icing the kicker," skilled golfers were found to putt better when instructed to execute their putts as quickly as possible than when instructed to take as much time as needed. This study used short putts of up to 1.58 meters so it is unclear whether the findings generalize to more lengthy, undulating putts that require more judgment of pace and direction. Nonetheless, minimizing thinking time might form part of an effective intervention for performers who suffer from "paralysis by analysis."

To give some context and perspective it is important to note that routine time and consistency per se are not strong predictors of performance. For example, in a study of rugby union World Cup goal kickers, neither concentration time nor physical preparation time was related to success. Indeed, large differences in concentration time between kickers were evident, with some spending just four or five seconds, while others spent over 20 seconds. There was also no evidence that better kickers had more *consistent* routine times. Instead, routine time varied systematically with the difficulty of the kick: the more difficult the kick, the longer the players took standing over the ball before running up to take the kick. Other researchers have found that the overall length of the routine is unimportant as long as the rhythm of the routine remains consistent. Taking the analysis to the individual level, a study of NBA free-throw shooting in 14 play-off games revealed that success was unrelated to routine time; however, when players did not follow their behavioral routine, performance dropped from 83.8 percent success to 71.4 percent. Interestingly, omitting elements of their usual routine did not degrade performance but adding one or more elements (e.g., taking a deep breath or an extra look at the basket) was associated with a much lower success rate (58.3 percent).

So what elements should be included in a pre-performance routine? It is evident that a routine should have at least three functions: helping the performer to (1) regulate their emotions and physiological responses to pressure, (2) deal with potentially distracting external (and internal) information, and (3) execute with a "quiet mind" under pressure. Accordingly, a pre-performance routine that included steps targeted at arousal regulation, behavioral consistency, and attention control (visual focus and cue words) was effective in eliminating choking in a study of ten-pin bowlers, who improved their performance under pressure by an average of 29 percent after the intervention. Their improvement in performance was accompanied by lower self-awareness and less negative self-talk in the pressure situation.

The sport psychologist Bob Singer proposed a five-step routine that consisted of readying (preparing for the act), imaging (visualizing the movement), focusing (on a meaningful cue), executing (with a quiet mind), and evaluating (the effectiveness of each of the previous steps). The readying and imaging steps are directed towards self-regulation and enhancing self-efficacy. The focusing and executing steps are clearly directed towards attentional processes: the focusing stage promotes a task-relevant, external focus, whereas the executing step is an attempt to prompt automatic, effortless performance free from conscious interference. For example, the rugby union goal kicker Jonny Wilkinson focuses intently on the precise point of the ball he wants to strike and has a very specific target focus in which he aims at a particular point in the crowd. Interestingly, many routines contain ritualized components that have no obvious function and it has been suggested that the mental effort directed towards, for example, counting the number of tennis ball bounces before serving might help dispel any distracting thoughts, cognitive anxiety, or thoughts about the mechanics of skill execution. Other performers incorporate strategies that help swamp the contested mental space that is working memory. The implication of the empirical and anecdotal evidence is that the mental component of a routine should involve conscious effort that helps promote an external focus. This is arguably more important as the physical routine becomes increasingly automated over time.

In terms of processes underlying the effectiveness of focusing strategies there is research evidence that distracting performers from the process of execution can aid performance under pressure. In one study, golfers listened to a series of words being played on a tape recorder. Every time they heard a target word, they had to repeat it out loud. The process of attending to a second task while putting drew the golfers' attention away from their own performance and benefited overall execution under pressure. Similarly, skilled field hockey players completed a skill test under pressure faster under dual-task conditions than under normal (single-task) conditions.

Overall then, there appear to be at least two elements to the successful use of pre-performance routines. First, there are components that help focus the performer's attention on a task-relevant activity (e.g., visual fixation on the target) (see Chapter 12) that in turn help block out distractions (e.g., crowd noise, thoughts about the consequences of success or failure). Second, there are components that direct the performers' focus away from the automated process of performance, allowing such skill processes to run off with minimal conscious involvement.

Primed for fluency

Priming refers to the influence of a stimulus on subsequent behavior or processing. There is recent evidence to suggest that performers can be primed to perform more fluently under pressure. In one study, skilled field hockey players attempted to dribble the ball through a set of cones as quickly and accurately as possible. The players completed the task under normal (control) conditions, a "skill-focus" condition, in which they attended to the position of their hands as they dribbled the ball, and a priming condition. The priming condition involved players re-arranging a series of scrambled sentences using four from five words. For example, the words "movement the smooth was could" can be re-arranged to form "the movement was smooth." Performance was found to be fastest and most accurate following the fluency prime, with primed performance under high pressure being at a similar level to normal performance under low pressure. In a follow-up study, the priming with negative target words (e.g., "breakdown," "poor," "slow") led to slower and less accurate performance than in the control condition.

The main implication of this study is that performance may be susceptible to subtle influences, whether it be words used by a coach, images used in a motivational video, or the numerous factors that make up the culture or climate of an organization. The sentence completion task was seemingly unrelated to the hockey task that followed yet significantly affected how players performed. Research in applying priming to sport is in its infancy so the extent to which it proves effective and practical requires further evaluation.

Strategy focus

Many skills require effective decision making as well as technical precision. This is particularly true of "open" skills such as open court play in racquet sports and open play in team sports such as soccer, basketball, and rugby. If skill failure is the result of trying to control well-learned motor skills then focusing on a "what to do" (strategy) rather than a "how to do it" (technique) might help prevent skill failure. Moreover, because strategizing generally requires one to take in and think about multiple pieces of information at a time, this type of focusing may have the added benefit of improving one's decision-making process.

In one study, skilled soccer players set themselves goals prior to completing a task involving dribbling the ball between a series of cones. The participants were told to choose a "process goal" that they felt would help maximize their success on the task. Participants set themselves goals relating to either their movements/technique (e.g., "keep loose with knees bent") or more strategic or positioning elements of the task (e.g., "keep the ball close to the cones"). Those who set themselves goals relating to movement or technique were subsequently slower whereas those who focused on strategy maintained the same level of performance. These findings were unaffected by pressure: participants focusing on strategy still maintained their performance under high pressure whereas those focusing on technique continued to perform more poorly. Again, this highlights the "paradox of control": performers may focus on things they believe will help or enhance their performance that in fact disrupt fluency and increase errors.

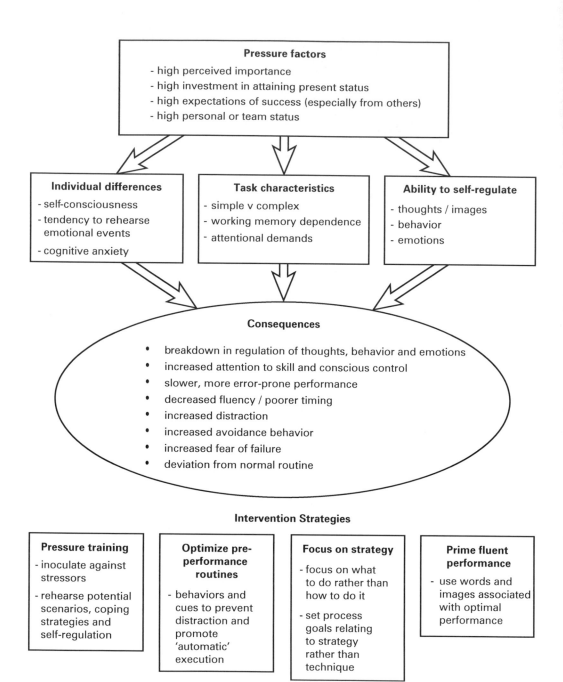

Figure 10.1 A schematic of the choking process and proposed intervention strategies. The consequences of situational pressure are viewed as being moderated by individual and task characteristics.

Robin C. Jackson, Sian L. Beilock, and Noel P. Kinrade

CONCLUDING REMARKS

There is a growing body of research examining skill failure under pressure in sport. We have given a brief summary of some of this research and have considered the implications of this work for developing effective intervention strategies (see Figure 10.1 for a schematic summary). Evidence from a wide range of studies points to the idea that the failure of well-learned and highly practiced motor skills occurs when performers try to consciously control elements of performance that normally occur automatically. This paradox of control, in which the desire to ensure performance does not fail actually triggers skill failure, provides a challenge to performers and practitioners alike. In addition, there is evidence that distraction plays a significant role, notably in tasks that place heavy demands on attentional resources. We have given a brief summary of some of this research and have considered the implications of this work for developing effective intervention strategies. Of course, while the science is good for providing a theoretical framework for interventions, no single intervention strategy is likely to be effective for all performers and all skills. The challenge for the coach, performer, and sport psychologist is how best to apply principles from the lab to design individualized interventions that are effective in the highly pressured competitive arena.

COACH'S CORNER

Scott Draper
National Coach, Tennis Australia

Experiences as a player

My experiences as a player have certainly influenced the way I now coach my athletes on the concept of handling pressure and importantly avoiding the dreaded "choke." While this chapter has focused on sport expertise, I feel we can all relive experiences where we have "choked," be it public speaking or trying to remember a person's name as they approach you.

The authors have done a great job in detailing the various mechanisms that may cause choking. From my perspective, I do not think failing under pressure is only to do with over-thinking; there are occasions where you become so anxious you go blank and cannot think at all about anything other than failing. Having competed at the professional level in both tennis and golf, I have had numerous opportunities to feel pressure and discover strategies to deal with it.

The four phases of focus

I used to consider that I played tennis in one of four attentional states. They are as follows:

- *In the zone* – this did not happen often but, like the textbooks tell us, when you are there it is effortless and you are playing great.

- *Typical "A" game* – this is your "7–8 out of 10" game. You are playing well but not in the zone.

- *Watching myself* – this is a fascinating and tricky phase. You are battling, feel like you are really focused on playing the game (trying to do all the right things), but you are not actually doing it but just watching yourself.

- *Capitulation* – a "1 out of 10" performance where you are totally overwhelmed.

In my tennis career I do not think I ever choked as per the textbook definition or as per tennis's definition: that of Jana Novotna unraveling in a Wimbledon final. However, I do remember one match where I was in the final at Queens (the traditional Wimbledon lead-up tournament) and I was winning and the score was 7–6, 4–3. At the change of ends (where I had time to think) my mind started racing about what could happen and I started to panic. Having had a long-term partnership with a coach/psychologist helped me considerably in this instance. I was able to change the score in my mind so that I was 3–4 down and coming out to simply hold my serve rather than going out to get to a 5–3 lead in the final. This mental shift in focus worked incredibly well and I went on to win. Obviously this story is a little different from the soccer penalty shoot-out success rates presented earlier in the chapter where kicking to win produced higher success rates. I think this is to do with the nature of the sports. Obviously in the shoot-out it is down to one kick whereas in my tennis example I am talking about a string of one-off executions or a game. I think this is also why we do not see the "choke" in tennis as we do in golf. In sports such as tennis, where there is an opponent, you may elect to play it safe (e.g., take speed off, hit the ball with more shape in flight). Similarly, if you are winning your opponent may throw caution to the wind and go for "winners," meaning it is no longer only down to you to control your destiny.

The McIlroy quote at the start of the chapter certainly brought back some similar memories for me during my golfing career. I was in the final round of the PGA Tour School and was scoring really well. I was in the Top 15 (Top 25 get their PGA card) and because I was doing so well I started thinking about making the Top Five, where I would get even more starts the following year. Not long after these thoughts I began "leaking oil": a bogey here, double bogey there. All of a sudden I was thinking not Top Five but missing out altogether. I lost the feeling of my swing and doubted I would even hit the ball. It was an awful feeling. I felt I had no ability to step back from the situation and pragmatically work through how to fix my swing. On the par-3 16th hole I hit my shot in the bunker. As I walked along the fairway to the bunker I drew on all my previous psychology skill-training experiences. When I got to the bunker I focused on where I wanted to land the ball and blocked everything else out of mind. I hit it so well that I holed it! From there I got back on track and got my card.

Robin C. Jackson, Sian L. Beilock, and Noel P. Kinrade

Coaching strategies

Practice under pressure

I totally agree with the authors that you need to try and replicate match conditions and pressure as much as possible. Importantly, this can be done in any competitive situation. If I was playing a less skilled opponent I would set a rule to win the two sets and cough up only 10 points to my opponent across the two sets. I remember playing where I was winning 6–0, 4–0 and had got tight and felt pressured because I had given up eight points and had not yet closed out the match. So, while any sort of training-based match practice is not necessarily the same visually or aurally as the real thing (e.g., no crowds lining the fairways or fans cheering between points) I think if you can put pressure on yourself to elicit the feelings you get in the real competition settings it helps immensely.

Routines

I have always been interested in the value of routines. The legendary golfer Jack Nicklaus did not necessarily have a routine. He might stand over his ball anywhere from 5 to 45 seconds until he felt completely ready to hit. At this point he would then have a trigger movement (e.g., two waggles of the club head) and then he would swing. I am a bit the same as Nicklaus: I do not believe you need a consistent routine. If you have one you can become too boxed into it. For instance, you see players such as Sharapova who clearly have a very defined routine. She walks to point A, flicks her strings three times, shakes her ponytail, and so on. It is very regimented. Similarly, the USTA (United States Tennis Association) promote a 16-second cure. Again the routine is broken into phases once a point is completed. For instance, turn your back on the net, place racquet into non-preferred hand, take a deep breath and reset . . . While all these aspects are fine, and many elite players have a routine, I feel you need flexibility. You need to be thinking about what you need to do to impact your opponent. For instance, you may want to speed up play between points to rush your opponent and maintain momentum.

I think more important than a routine is a trigger movement. The trigger may be different for each person but essentially it tells the body "I'm ready, it's time to go" and initiates the swing (see also the "quiet eye" concept, Chapter 11).

Play the percentages

I think a valuable strategy is to teach players about how to use high-percentage play to increase the probability of success. However, while this sounds simple, my experience is that it is not well understood. Although most players can articulate that high-percentage tennis is about playing into a safe zone and not missing, they do not understand that it may look different depending on the situation. For instance, high-percentage play will change depending on your opponent and game situation. While a serve–volley tactic is considered high risk in the modern game, it may be high percentage if you need to change up your game style to keep your opponent guessing.

Visualization drill

I ask my players to hone in on a target (e.g., the light tower at the tennis courts) and then I try to get them to hit the target with an overhand throw. I ask them to try and let their mind take a picture of the target and then just hit the picture. The resolution of your picture or, as I call it, "the megapixels" are better on some days than others. But the aim is to simply press "print" and let it go, let the body do what it does best. I think this is somewhat analogous to the theory on external focus of attention.

Summary

Pressure manifests in many different ways: anger, tanking, tears . . . not just in regard to skill choking. My experience has been that each player needs a different story to get them to buy into a strategy that will work for them. I think the authors have provided coaches with plenty of different strategies (stories) that can be trialed with different players depending on circumstances.

KEY READING

Ashford, K.J. and Jackson, R.C. (2010) 'Priming as a means of preventing skill failure under pressure', *Journal of Sport & Exercise Psychology*, 32: 518–536.

Beilock, S.L. (2010) *Choke: What the Secrets of the Brain Reveal about Getting It Right when You Have To*. New York: Free Press.

Gray, R. (2004) 'Attending to the execution of a complex sensorimotor skill: expertise differences, choking, and slumps', *Journal of Experimental Psychology: Applied*, 10: 42–54.

Gucciardi, D.F., Longbottom, J., Jackson, B., and Dimmock, J.A. (2010) 'Experienced golfers' perspectives on choking under pressure', *Journal of Sport & Exercise Psychology*, 32: 61–83.

Jackson, R.C., Ashford, K.J., and Norsworthy, G. (2006) 'Attentional focus, dispositional reinvestment and skilled motor performance under pressure', *Journal of Sport & Exercise Psychology*, 28: 49–68.

Jamieson, J.P. (2010) 'The home field advantage in athletics: a meta-analysis', *Journal of Applied Social Psychology*, 40: 1819–1848.

Jordet, G. and Hartman, E. (2008) 'Avoidance motivation and choking under pressure in soccer penalty shootouts', *Journal of Sport & Exercise Psychology*, 30: 450–457.

Kinrade, N., Jackson, R.C., Ashford, K.J., and Bishop, D.T. (2010) 'The development and validation of the Decision-Specific Reinvestment Scale', *Journal of Sports Sciences*, 28: 1127–1135.

Lonsdale, C. and Tam, J.T.M. (2007) 'On the temporal and behavioural consistency of pre-performance routines: an intra-individual analysis of elite basketball players' free throw shooting accuracy', *Journal of Sports Sciences*, 25: 1–8.

Oudejans, R.R.D. and Pijpers, J.R. (2009) 'Training with anxiety has a positive effect on expert perceptual-motor performance under pressure', *Quarterly Journal of Experimental Psychology*, 62: 1631–1647.

CHAPTER 11

EXPERT VISUAL PERCEPTION

WHY HAVING A QUIET EYE MATTERS IN SPORT

DEREK PANCHUK AND JOAN N. VICKERS

INTRODUCTION

The greatest athletes are not always blessed with the greatest physical attributes and, as a result, rely on other talents to set them apart. The great Canadian hockey player Wayne Gretzky once said, "I couldn't beat people with my strength; I don't have a hard shot; I'm not the quickest skater in the league. My eyes and my mind have to do most of the work." This quote illustrates how cognitive and, of particular relevance to this chapter, visual perceptual abilities play an important role in distinguishing good performers from great performers. From simple activities, such as throwing a ball, to complex tasks such as finding and passing a ball to an open team-mate, visual information is the primary driver of movement. In sports where accurate and precise control of actions are essential, the ability to direct the gaze mechanism (i.e., the eyes, the head, and the body) to appropriate areas of the visual environment at the appropriate time is what provides individuals with the information required for successful behavior.

Sport scientists have studied the role vision plays in developing perceptual–motor expertise for decades and have identified several factors that may (or may not) contribute to the expert advantage in sport performance. One variable that has been consistently found to discriminate elite performers from their near-elite and novice counterparts is the *quiet eye*. This chapter will provide an overview of the quiet eye phenomenon and its relationship to skilled performance. We will also explore the practical implications of understanding gaze behavior within an activity and how this understanding can be used by coaches and practitioners to improve performance.

WHAT DOES THE RESEARCH TELL US?

The eyes are commonly referred to as "the window to the mind," presumably because they provide insight into the internal thought processes that an individual engages in as they perform a skill. In sporting activities, performers attend to areas of the environment (e.g., objects, people, and spaces) that are relevant to their goals at that particular moment, such as a hockey goaltender watching the puck on an opponent's stick just before and as they take a shot. For expert performers, this gaze behavior is refined over time and is the consequence of learning not only *what* areas are relevant but *when* that area is relevant. The quiet eye is a reflection of both the momentary intentions of the performer and their experience with the task. From a technical standpoint, the quiet eye is defined as the final fixation or tracking gaze (with a minimum duration of 100 ms) held on an object or location in the performance environment (within 3 degrees of visual angle or less) prior to a critical, task-related movement. Put simply, the quiet eye represents the last *good look* an individual gets before executing a critical movement (the point of no return) within their skill domain. For example, during the basketball free throw the quiet eye period is the final fixation on the front, middle, or back of the hoop prior to the final extension of the elbow before release.

Before we discuss how the quiet eye relates to expert performance our description of the quiet eye needs to be defined in greater detail. First, the quiet eye is a stable fixation that must have an onset prior to the critical movement; this means it is necessary to record not only the gaze of the performer but their actions as well (see Figure 11.1 for an example of the coupled motor and gaze behavior). Second, the quiet eye must have a minimum duration of 100 ms and remain stable within

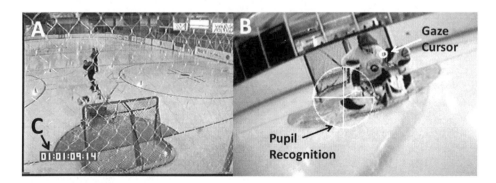

Figure 11.1 A coupled frame of video recorded with the Vision-in-Action (VIA) system, showing the motor image (A), the gaze image (B), and the frame counter (C). Also present in this frame are the gaze cursor (small circle) and the pupil indicator (large circle with crosshairs). Both images are synchronized perfectly in time.

Derek Panchuk and Joan N. Vickers

3 degrees of visual angle or less on an object or location within the visuomotor workspace. These parameters are important because they represent the minimum amount of time required to see with full acuity and process visual information prior to, and during, a simple action. Finally, the offset of quiet eye can occur before, during, or after a critical movement has been completed depending on the task. For example, during the free throw the quiet eye offset of elite players occurs prior to the extension of the arm/hand whereas in the golf putt the quiet eye offset occurs about 300–500 ms after ball contact. In the basketball free throw an early quiet eye offset is caused by the ball and hands entering the visual field whereas in the golf putt the extreme precision of ball/putter face contact requires a close relationship between neural centers responsible for planning eye movements and hand movements controlling the putting stroke.

Since the first quiet eye publication by Joan Vickers in 1996 an extensive body of research has focused on explaining the quiet eye phenomenon in different activities and how it relates to skilled performance. Through this work a number of general findings have emerged:

■ in elite performers the quiet eye occurs earlier and is of longer duration than that of near-elite and novice performers;
■ for a given task, the quiet eye of elite performers is of an optimal length which is determined by constraints within the task;
■ the quiet eye is earlier and of longer duration during successful performances than unsuccessful performances.

These findings have been replicated across a multitude of tasks including: golf putting, basketball free throw, volleyball, table tennis, rifle and shotgun shooting, goaltending, and locomotion. Taken together they illustrate how elite performers have developed optimal gaze and visual attention that allow them to extract the most relevant information under all the conditions encountered in a sport.

Along with basketball shooting, the golf putt is one of the most extensively researched tasks in the quiet eye literature and provides an excellent vehicle for demonstrating the fundamental findings related to the quiet eye, as well as the latest advances in the area. Even before the term "quiet eye" was first used by Vickers, she found that low-handicap (better) golfers used an efficient gaze strategy characterized by fewer fixations of longer duration on critical locations (i.e., ball, target, club) throughout the putt. In contrast, the high-handicap (poorer) golfers displayed approximately twice as many fixations of shorter duration, often on locations of no relevance to putting well. Prior to initiating the backswing (the critical movement in the golf putt) and during the stroke, the low handicap golfers maintained their gaze on the top or back of the ball. When accurate, they also maintained their gaze on the green after contact. This quiet eye dwell time was more pronounced in low-handicap golfers, who appeared to be better equipped to resist the visual distractions of the moving club head and ball after contact. Overall performance was more accurate when golfers maintained their gaze on the ball for approximately 1700 ms prior to contact and 200 ms after contact; findings that have been replicated since on both straight and breaking putts.

The quiet eye effect is not only limited to self-paced aiming and targeting tasks such as the golf putt; it has also been observed in externally paced tasks requiring interceptive actions and tactical decisions, such as ice hockey and soccer goaltending. When ice hockey or soccer goaltenders face shots, the speed of the puck/ball can exceed the physical capacity of the visual system to effectively track the projectile. In these situations, the goalie needs to position their gaze in a location that allows them to monitor the actions of their opponent and determine when to initiate their movement. Under these extreme conditions, where timing is essential, an early quiet eye duration of optimal duration is critical for successful performance.

Underlying neural and attention processes

Thus far we have seen that the quiet eye is critical in both targeting and interceptive timing tasks. An obvious question emerges from these findings: why is the quiet eye important? Although we are able to readily demonstrate a link between quiet eye, expertise, and performance across a range of activities, scientists are only now beginning to explain why an early and prolonged fixation and focus of attention is essential to high levels of performance. One of the most prevalent (and widely accepted) explanations is that the quiet eye represents a period of cognitive processing when movements are planned and the parameters set (e.g., force, velocity) prior to movements occurring. The quiet eye period essentially gives our brain the external spatial information it needs to know to decide *what* it is going to do and *how* it is going to do it based on our prior knowledge and the environmental information extracted by the eyes.

Measuring the quiet eye in tasks that become incrementally more difficult has shown that the duration of the quiet eye period is closely tied to the complexity of the task. The assumption is that, as task difficulty increases, the amount of pre-programming required increases as well and this is reflected in longer quiet eye durations. This behavioral evidence is supported by brain-imaging studies using electroencephalography (EEG) which measure electrical transmission on the surface of the brain. During the final few seconds prior to the putt there is a decrease in brain activity in the left hemisphere and increase in brain activity in the right hemisphere; the difference in activity between the two sides of the brain is larger in low-handicap golfers because of increased "quieting" on the left side of the brain.

198

In low-handicap golfers the quiet eye period is also highly related to an increase in brain activity called the "Bereitschaftspotential" (BP). An increase in BP activity is thought to be associated with attention allocation, movement organization, and timing. Because this activity is increased during the quiet eye period it suggests that quiet eye may be related to perceptual-motor preparation (e.g., planning the type of movement required given the situation the performer finds themself in).

The findings outlined above demonstrate strong links between quiet eye, cognitive processing, and movement planning. We have seen in the golf putt that not only does the quiet eye begin before the backstroke but it is also sustained through the stroke as the ball is contacted and for a period after. Online control reflects an individual's ability to make adjustments to a movement after it has begun (e.g., the ability to adjust the path of a putter after the start of the backswing). A long duration quiet eye before, during, and after the stroke may facilitate online control during the complete putt, supporting studies which show golfers are able to control parameters of the swing by monitoring how quickly the gap between the club head and ball closes. Although no research has specifically looked at how the quiet eye may facilitate online control during the golf putt, we have shown in ice hockey goaltending that disrupting the quiet eye by means of spatial occlusion creates difficulty in stopping the puck. In addition to suggesting the quiet eye may support movement programming and online control, we and other authors also suggest that an optimal quiet eye period facilitates the control of anxiety when under stress such that distracting thoughts are blocked out through a task-specific sustained focus.

Quiet eye and anxiety

Aside from the potential computational and online control benefits associated with the quiet eye period, a growing number of researchers have reported that quiet eye may also play a role in combating the effects of anxiety during performance. Changes in psychological arousal associated with anxiety-inducing situations are believed to alter the manner in which attention resources are allocated. When an individual becomes susceptible to the effects of anxiety it is thought that they switch from an attention system that is driven by goals, experience, and expectations (i.e., top-down processing) to one that is driven by salient, conspicuous stimuli in the environment (i.e., bottom-up processing; see also Chapter 10). For example, an anxious basketball player may become distracted by fans waving behind the hoop while taking a free throw. This switch impairs the underlying processes of attention inhibition (i.e., resisting attention capture by distracting stimuli) and shifting (i.e., the ability to direct attention to goal-relevant stimuli) which can be assessed by measuring gaze behavior. Measuring the gaze of anxious shooters, basketball players, and other athletes shows that accuracy is lower when the quiet eye duration is shorter. Thus, as an individual becomes more anxious, the manner in which they process visual stimuli becomes less efficient. Because one of the characteristics of the quiet eye of elite performers is that the final fixation is of an optimal length, the quiet eye period represents a behavioral measure of processing efficiency and researchers have assumed that a change in quiet eye duration associated with increases in anxiety represents a decrease in processing efficiency. Maintaining an optimal quiet eye duration during performance acts as a buffer that minimizes the likelihood that elite athletes will revert to inefficient or disruptive visual processing when confronted with anxiety-inducing situations. At the same time a long-duration quiet eye enhances an individual's ability to attend to appropriate spatial information (e.g., the back of the hoop) that is central to better performance.

Recent research has begun to tease apart the nature of the relationship between arousal, performance, and quiet eye. It shows that movement efficiency and hence performance outcomes are influenced by anxiety; for example, movement time and kinematic (technique) variability increases when individuals perform under high-anxiety (e.g., competitive) situations. These declines in movement efficiency are also associated with declines in quiet eye duration. For instance, Joe Causer and colleagues showed that, during competitive skeet shooting, both the quiet eye and the precision of gun barrel movement declined compared with a normal, stress-free condition. There is also evidence to suggest the quiet eye may also prevent elite athletes from "choking" under conditions of high physical exertion. Two athletes may perform equally well while rested; however, when performing after physically exhausting exercise, athletes who have a longer quiet eye are better able to maintain their performance. Growing research suggests that the quiet eye acts as a buffer against the potentially detrimental effects of psychological and physiological arousal (see also Chapters 9 and 10). Overwhelmingly, athletes who maintain longer (or more optimal) quiet eye duration perform better in situations where arousal (psychological or physiological) is increased.

It has been recently proposed that the quiet eye may promote a state of motor resonance in an athlete. Put simply, perceptual processes involved in the planning of actions (or imagining planned actions) have significant overlap with the motor processes involved in carrying out planned actions (i.e., perception and action are fundamentally linked). During a sport skill, if the gaze is located at the appropriate location at the appropriate time, then it is believed this creates the optimal transfer of information from the environment to the neural regions involved in perception and action and the motor system, resulting in performances that are significantly better. If less than optimal transmission of movement information occurs, the resulting motor performance suffers. For example, in golf putting, an optimal quiet eye on the back of the ball results in smooth putter movement through contact with an appropriate amount of force; whereas a non-optimal quiet eye results in ball contact that is variable and inappropriate for the current situation. When athletes display an optimal quiet eye period, the specific spatial coordinates required to organize the action are fed to the brain and this process occurs with seemingly little effort. The idea of motor resonance as a result of optimal quiet eye may also explain why arousal has less influence on individuals with an optimal quiet eye; when transmission occurs effortlessly, there is nothing else to worry about. The following section will explore how this knowledge has been used in applied settings and considerations for effectively training the quiet eye.

THEORY INTO PRACTICE: QUIET EYE TRAINING

A common perception is that elite athletes possess unique visual abilities that allow them to pick up visual information more effectively than their less skilled counterparts. Three decades of research have shown that this is not the case; there is little evidence to suggest that elite athletes have superior visual functioning (e.g., acuity, depth perception, contrast sensitivity). Instead the research shows that the expert advantage lies in differences in visual anticipation, attention, pattern recognition, problem solving, and decision making. As a result, perceptual-cognitive training programs have been used extensively to improve the anticipation and decision-making skills of athletes. A variety of techniques have been used to train perceptual-cognitive skills, including temporal occlusion (to improve a performer's ability to anticipate an opponent's actions using early kinematic information), pattern recognition (to help athletes identify common game situations in team sports), and spatial cueing (to draw the performer's attention to important stimuli in the environment during dynamic skills). Although field-based tests are becoming more common, perceptual-cognitive training protocols typically involve participants making some form of response to video-based stimuli. While this paradigm has its limitations, a number of studies have shown considerable benefits in improving the performance of athletes by using this approach (see Chapter 12).

Quiet eye training programs use a combination of modeling of expert quiet eye characteristics, feedback to the athlete regarding their quiet eye characteristics, questioning that probes what the athlete understands about their control of visual attention, and decision making. In traditional training environments there is a substantial emphasis on improving physical characteristics associated with performance whereas perceptual-cognitive aspects are often an afterthought. It is our contention that because gaze patterns represent learned behaviors they can be trained in a manner similar to physical skills. To this end, by following principled research-based guidelines, the quiet eye of an individual can be changed to more closely resemble the optimal quiet eye required for a particular activity. Quiet eye training has been used in a number of activities to improve the performance of athletes and minimize detrimental effects associated with anxiety. Table 11.1 summarizes the results from quiet eye training studies that included transfer trials or tests that occurred later in competition. Shown is the amount of improvement experienced by quiet eye trained athletes who had their quiet eye recorded and received feedback about how they controlled their gaze and focus of attention while performing compared with control groups (of equal entry skill level). Significant increases in performance by the quiet eye trained group are evident. In this section we will outline the process for developing quiet eye training programs and provide research evidence that demonstrates the efficacy of these programs.

A seven-step quiet eye training process has been developed to help athletes and coaches recognize the quiet eye characteristics of elite performers and apply this knowledge to aid the development of their sport expertise. The training process is based on Joan Vickers's decision-training model and shifts the onus of responsibility for learning back to the performer. Rather than being told what to do, the athlete has access to their quiet eye location, onset, offset, and duration – aspects of their performance that are not normally available – and a training environment where they can consciously improve their gaze and focus of attention. The seven steps are as follows:

1 *Research: the researcher identifies the quiet eye characteristics of elite performers during successful performances.* This is an essential first step because, as shown above, elite performers control their gaze and attention differently from non-elite performers, so is it important to establish what expert gaze behavior for a specific task looks like. Once this research has been conducted, the knowledge can be applied without the aid of an eye tracker, although it is recommended that all athletes be given objective information about their quiet eye location, onset, offset, and duration.

2 *Testing: the gaze and actions of the trainee are recorded in the field.* In step 2 it is important to collect quiet eye data from the trainee in a natural setting.

Table 11.1 Comparison of performance improvements in quiet eye (QE) trained and control participants in competition

Sport	Skill level	QE trained	Control	Authors
Volleyball	National team	+ 7%	0%	Adolphe et al., 1997
Basketball	University	+ 23%	+ 6%	Harle and Vickers, 2001
Basketball	Professional	+ 14%	0%	Oudejans et al., 2005
Golf putting	Low handicap	−1.9 putts/round	0 putts/round	Vine et al., 2011
Skeet shooting	Olympic	+ 5%	0%	Causer et al., 2011
Basketball	Novices	+ 34%	+ 23%	Vine et al., 2011

An advantage of quiet eye training programs is that they are field based or performed in conditions that simulate the competitive environment as closely as possible. This allows the quiet eye location, onset, offset, and duration of the participant to be determined when they are successful and unsuccessful.

3 *Modeling: the trainee is first taught the quiet eye characteristics of elite performers.* The quiet eye characteristics of the elite performer are shown on video and thoroughly explained to the performer. This allows the important aspects of the elite performance – such as the optimal location, early quite eye onset and long duration, and relationship to critical movements – to be highlighted at the outset.

4 *Feedback and problem solving: the trainee is then shown the video of their coupled gaze and motor data.* This step gives the athlete the opportunity to compare their quiet eye with that of the elite performer. Rather than simply telling them what the differences and similarities are, a questioning approach can be used to probe their understanding and guide them towards recognizing key differences. For example, when conducting quiet eye training for the free throw, asking questions such as "where were you looking prior to extending your elbow?" and "how does this compare with the expert model?" provides the player with insight into the critical location and timing of gaze behavior relative to the extension phase. The advantage of this approach is that it allows performers to observe exactly what they are doing during a task (many are surprised to see that their eyes are not doing what they think they are) and discover relationships between their gaze, movements, and performance outcomes.

5 *Decision making: the trainee decides what aspect of their quiet eye performance they would like to change.* Based on their assessment of their gaze behavior relative to the elite prototype the athlete makes a conscious decision about what aspect of their gaze behavior they would like to change (e.g., a more efficient gaze pattern, a specific quiet eye location, an earlier onset, or a longer duration). To prevent overloading the athlete, it is important to encourage them to focus on one aspect of their quiet eye to change. The selected behavior should also be gaze related with little to no emphasis on changing technique; as the visual information the performer uses begins to change, research has shown that their actions will begin to improve as they incorporate the new information.

6 *Blocked, variable and random practice: the selected skill should be practiced using specifically designed drills that promote the desired quiet eye focus.* In the beginning, blocked practice should be used whereby the same skill is practiced over and over. It is then very important to use a variety of drills that encourage the performer to adopt the gaze/quiet eye characteristics in the different challenges they will have to face in competition. By utilizing applied training principles that have strong support in the research literature – such as variable and random practice, bandwidth feedback, and questioning – the more successful the training will be (see Chapter 8).

7 *Follow-up testing and continued practice.* Changes in performance should be assessed in competition and additional quiet eye tests should be carried out to monitor changes in behavior. To ensure that long-term learning occurs, practice needs to be continued and adapted to the changing gaze and quiet eye characteristics of the performer as they evolve to increasingly more challenging environments.

Quiet eye training at work

The first study to use this training process focused on the skill of volleyball service reception and pass. In the study, athletes from the national men's volleyball team were invited to participate in a six-week training program that consisted of an initial consultation (steps 1–5) and five 30-minute training sessions (step 6), followed by a one-month posttest, where gaze behavior was recorded again, and a two-year follow-up in international competition (step 7). Initial testing showed that elite players were able to track the ball longer from the point of contact before making a stepping movement to receive the ball. With this in mind, the players involved in training were able to compare their gaze with the elite prototype and questioning was used to probe their awareness of differences in gaze behavior. To facilitate early detection of the ball and improve tracking, a number of drills were developed where players were asked to track small objects, identify numbers placed on balls as they were served, and identify numbers when less time was available (i.e., the server was occluded by a blackboard or the receiver had to turn 180 degrees after the serve). One month after completion of the training exercises, players had their gaze recorded on court and results showed that all of the athletes were able to track the ball earlier and for longer. Pass accuracy during competition also improved 7 percent over a three-year span following the study, whereas a comparison group of top international athletes who did not receive the training remained relatively stable over that period of time.

Although the example above demonstrates the effectiveness of quiet eye training in an interceptive task, the majority of quiet eye training studies have been conducted in targeting tasks where the actions of the performer are self-paced. For example, a similar training approach to that already described was used to improve the free throw shooting of a women's varsity basketball team over the course of two seasons. Players had their gaze behavior recorded at the beginning of season one and compared with the elite model. During the feedback session a number of points were stressed to the athletes and they were taught a three-step quiet eye routine to practice through the course of the season. The routine emphasized (a) taking their position on the line and orienting the gaze to the hoop as soon as possible, (b) fixating the hoop for about one second while holding the ball in front (this

204

was achieved by having the players say the words "sight, focus"), and (c) shooting quickly, using a fluid action. After training with the routine for one season, players had changed the timing of their free throw (longer preparation time and shorter shooting time), increased their quiet eye duration, and improved their free throw performance in an experimental posttest. The most significant finding from this study was the improvement in performance observed in competition over the course of two seasons; although there was no change in free throw performance in the first season, it had improved by an astonishing 23 percent in the second season.

Quiet eye training is not only effective in skilled performers; novice performers have been shown to benefit from exposure to it as well. For instance, it has been demonstrated that novice participants with little to no basketball experience can make 11 percent more free throws than a group who received training that focused on technical aspects of the skill. Although both groups improved performance, the results demonstrated a significant benefit for quiet eye training over and above technical training. The benefits of quiet eye training also extended to performing under pressure; when anxiety was induced by providing participants with a monetary incentive and comparing their scores with others, the group that received quiet eye training was able to maintain their level of performance whereas the technical training group's declined. This reinforces the role quiet eye training plays in insulating performers from the negative effects associated with anxiety and shows how training on appropriate gaze control strategies may act as a built-in buffer for withstanding high levels of pressure. For coaches, an awareness of the importance of the quiet eye and implementing techniques for training gaze gives them another tool in their coaching toolkit. Simple drills, such as having players identify the number on an approaching ball or the color of a marker under a golf ball during the putt, can promote effective quiet eye and be incorporated into practice with ease.

Although the number of quiet eye training studies is growing, there are still a number of questions that remain to be answered. Whereas numerous others (over 70 peer-reviewed papers) have consistently demonstrated improvements in performance associated with an optimal quiet eye, the mechanisms behind this improvement are not well understood. We have also seen that optimizing the quiet eye contributes to positive changes in technique. However, this area of research is in its infancy, as is research on the psychological factors (e.g., perceived control, confidence, motivation) that may be improved when an optimal quiet eye is used. We also know very little about the development of quiet eye. It is clear that quiet eye is an aspect of performance that can be trained over time but we do not know whether some individuals have inherently better quiet eye abilities at birth, whether it is a perceptual skill that is acquired over time, or whether it declines as we age. Changes in quiet eye behavior across the life span would be of great interest to individuals involved in developmental sporting programs as well as training master athletes.

CONCLUDING REMARKS

The aim of this chapter was to demonstrate the importance of the quiet eye to sports skill performance and the development of expertise, and to show that, like any other performance variable, it can be trained. The quiet eye is a variable that consistently distinguishes elite performers from their sub-elite and novice counterparts and discriminates successful from unsuccessful performances (see Chapter 12). What is apparent from the preceding sections is that optimal quiet eye control is essential for skilled performance; it can be trained but there is much we still do not know about why the quiet eye works.

COACH'S CORNER

Hayley Wickenheiser
Canadian ice hockey Olympian

"The eyes are the windows to the mind." My first real scientific understanding of what I had been feeling as an athlete for much of my career came in the third year of my kinesiology degree at the University of Calgary. This was *after* competing in four Winter Olympics in ice hockey and one Summer Olympics in fastball. I had the opportunity to take Dr. Vickers's KNES 251 course on the brain and the effects of the visual system on cognition and motor control. It began to answer many of the questions I had as an athlete and I was able to explore even more, through my own training, how important the visual system was to athletic performance. I immediately began to ask Dr. Vickers if there were ways I could improve my own performance as an elite hockey player. At my level, the smallest of improvements can lead to huge breakthroughs in performance. This curiosity led me to take part in quiet eye testing and training and to change the way I train for my sport of hockey.

Although hockey is a team game, it has a strong reliance on individual skill execution. What sets elite hockey players apart from the average, outside of pure physical ability, is the ability to anticipate and read the play ahead of anyone else, and to be able to change focus from broad (the entire play) to narrow (shooting on the goalie). Quiet eye training is not going to turn an average player into an NHL or Olympic superstar, but the merits of quiet eye training for both coach and athlete can be seen in areas of performance analysis, decreasing anxiety, and improving athlete self-awareness and confidence.

The research is really starting to demonstrate more and more how the eyes "turn on" the body. The visual system is a complex neural network under higher cognitive control. On average, it takes the brain 220 ms to consciously process visual stimuli and react to it, but the athlete is subconsciously aware of what is happening much sooner than this. The more disciplined pathways we can establish within our brains, the faster and more accurately we are able to react to our environment. Speed and efficiency are two main attributes to athletic success, regardless of sport. Better reaction times and coordination increase athletic performance. Similarly, understanding exactly where and when to focus our gaze and attention through deliberate practice and quiet eye training can improve performance. The best performers are able to attend to visual cues earlier and for longer than others. Dr. Vickers and colleagues demonstrate this in their literature and I agree with their findings.

What is it like to be quiet eye tested?

Prior to going on the ice, Dr. Vickers and I sat down to explore exactly why I wanted to be tested. My main purpose for doing the quiet eye work was to see if where I was looking when shooting at the goalie was the most effective place for scoring. She had me watch many of the top players in the world and determine for myself where I thought they were looking and the optimal style. From there we determined that, based on my game and style of play, there were three plays that repeatedly occurred over and over again in my game, the first being a direct attack on the goalie on both the forehand and backhand sides, the second coming across the top of the circles out of the corner, and the third being the penalty shot. The first two scenarios were done with other players pressuring me to make it as gamelike as possible against a highly skilled goaltender. For my sessions, Dr. Vickers and her staff set me up with a mobile eye tracker that filmed exactly what I was looking at while shooting. This device collected video data of my gaze at a rate of 33.33 ms per frame, way below the level of consciousness. An external camera was also set up to record my skating and shooting movements in the same time frame. Both the eye tracker video and external skating video were synchronized in the lab, coded, and analyzed, and my quiet eye while shooting defined. The mobile eye tracker was very easy to wear and non-invasive. Finally, the data was collected *in situ* or on the ice in order to replicate a game or practice situation as well as possible.

What was challenging was to complete the trials using either a "keeper dependent/ eyes up" or a "keeper independent/eyes down" strategy. Dr. Vickers explained that these strategies were based on research from Ice hockey and soccer (see Key reading below) that may explain the most optimal way for me to control my gaze and attention as I shoot. The purpose of the quiet eye testing was to determine which strategy was best for me – meaning, which was more productive in terms of scoring goals. In the "keeper dependent/eyes up" strategy, I was to keep my eyes on the net/goaltender all the time and shoot without looking down at the puck at all. In this gaze control strategy the idea is to play a type of cat and mouse game with the goalie and exploit any errors they make right up to the last moment. In the "keeper independent/eyes down" strategy I was to look at the net early as the play developed and determine in advance where I wanted to shoot and then keep my gaze down on the puck as I took the shot. In this strategy I needed to fixate the net early and make up my mind where I wanted to shoot and then concentrate on the shot while ignoring everything the goalie did.

Quiet eye testing results

Upon completion of the on-ice portion of the testing, Dr. Vickers and I met again to debrief and go over the results. Through a series of questions, she was able to determine my perception of how the testing went. My perception and the testing results were aligned; this does not always occur. I was also able to see on the gaze videos exactly what I was looking at as I prepared and took each shot.

The main results from my testing were as follows:

1   It took 3–4 seconds for me to execute the plays (forehand or backhand).

2   I used two "critically important" fixations during each play, with one on the net/goaltender and the other on puck/stick that together added up to about 500–600 ms.

3   I could perform both the "keeper dependent/eyes up" and "keeper independent/eyes down" strategy when I was asked to.

4   No matter what strategy I used, I always looked down at the puck as I shot, but the duration of this differed according to which strategy I used.

5   When I used the keeper dependent/eyes up strategy my first fixation on the net occurred late and averaged around 300 ms and this was followed by a final fixation down on the puck as I shot that was around 200–300 ms.

6   In contrast, in the keeper independent/eyes down strategy, I fixated the net early for about 400 ms and this was followed by a very brief glance down at the puck prior to the shot of about 150 ms. When I used this strategy my shot was actually faster and perhaps for this reason I scored more goals during the testing. I was also quicker picking up any rebounds that occurred.

Overall, I learned that it pays to use the keeper independent/eyes down strategy involving an early quiet eye fixation of about 400 ms on the net (prior to the backswing) followed by a very brief fixation of 150 ms down on the puck/stick during shot release. In the end, this results in a faster, more accurate shot and a better chance of picking up the rebound. This quiet eye strategy may also give the goaltender fewer clues about where I am going to shoot. In the next few months Dr. Vickers will be having me try out some training drills designed to increase my ability to see where I want to shoot earlier under all kinds of conditions.

How can coaches use quiet eye testing with their athletes?

It has been my experience training with some of the best athletes in the world that one common theme, regardless of sport, is that athletes are always trying to find ways to become better. They take a proactive approach to their development and, rather than waiting for someone to give them the answers, they seek them out. Many athletes intuitively "know" but do not "understand" how they learn or what they are actually "seeing" during competition. Quiet eye testing and training can help a coach and

Derek Panchuk and Joan N. Vickers

athlete look into this and formulate a plan of action for improvement. As a coach, it is important to help your athletes understand more about how they perceive the world they play in and find ways to improve their focus, be more independent, self-regulate, and make good things happen for themselves. Understanding your athlete and why they play/perform the way they do will enable a coach to understand how to communicate this more effectively to the athlete. Finally, the key to successful performance in high-pressure situations such as the Olympics for most athletes is controlling pressure and anxiety. Coaches can use quiet eye training with their athletes to focus on "seeing" what is really important in crucial situations, thus giving them greater confidence in being able to perform when the stakes are very high.

KEY READING

Adolphe, R.M., Vickers, J.N., and LaPlante, G. (1997) 'The effects of training visual attention on gaze behavior and accuracy: A pilot study', *International Journal of Sports Vision*, 4: 28–33.

Causer, J., Holmes, P.S., Smith, N.C., and Williams, A.M. (2011) 'Anxiety, movement kinematics, and visual attention in elite-level performers', *Emotion*, 11: 595–602.

Harle, S.K. and Vickers, J.N. (2001) 'Training quiet eye improves accuracy in the basketball free throw', *Sport Psychologist*, 15: 289–305.

Mann, D., Coombes, S., Mousseau, M., and Janelle, C. (2011) 'Quiet eye and the Bereitschaftspotential: visuomotor mechanisms of expert motor performance', *Cognitive Processing*, 12: 223–234.

Oudejans, R.R.D., Koedijker, J.M., Bleijendaal, I., and Bakker, F.C. (2005) 'The education of attention in aiming at a far target: Training visual control in basketball jump shooting', *International Journal of Sport Psychology*, 3: 197–221.

Panchuk, D. and Vickers, J.N. (2009) 'Using spatial occlusion to explore the control strategies used in rapid interceptive actions: predictive or prospective control?', *Journal of Sports Sciences*, 27: 1249–1260.

van der Kamp, J. (2006) 'A field simulation study of the effectiveness of penalty kick strategies in soccer: late alterations of kick direction increase errors and reduce accuracy', *Journal of Sports Sciences*, 24: 467–477.

Vickers, J.N. (1996) 'Visual control when aiming at a far target', *Journal of Experimental Psychology: Human Perception and Performance*, 22: 342–354.

Vickers, J.N. (2007) *Perception, Cognition and Decision Training: The Quiet Eye in Action*. Champaign, IL: Human Kinetics.

Vickers, J.N. (2009) 'Advances in coupling perception and action: the quiet eye as a bidirectional link between gaze, attention, and action', in Raab, M., Johnson, J.G., and Heekeren, H.R. (eds.) *Mind and Motion: The Bidirectional Link between Thought and Action* (Progress in Brain Research, Volume 174). New York: Elsevier, pp. 279–288.

Vine, S.J. and Wilson, M.R. (2011) 'The influence of quiet eye training and pressure on attention and visuo-motor control', *Acta Psychologica*, 136: 340–346.

Williams, A.M., Singer, R.N., and Frehlich, S.G. (2002) 'Quiet eye duration, expertise, and task complexity in near and far aiming tasks', *Journal of Motor Behavior*, 34: 197–207.

Wood, G. and Wilson, M.R. (2010) 'Gaze behavior and shooting strategies in football penalty kicks: Implications of a "keeper-dependent" approach', *International Journal of Sport Psychology*, 41: 293–312.

CHAPTER 12

THE RECIPE FOR EXPERT DECISION MAKING

DAMIAN FARROW AND MARKUS RAAB

The technical and tactical proficiency and physical prowess of an athlete is often used as a means of distinguishing the elite from their less-skilled counterparts in fast-paced interceptive and team sports. Not surprisingly then, a large proportion of training time is spent refining these qualities. However, there is also a less obvious quality that is of equal importance to performance that can distinguish between differing skill levels. Decision-making skill is the ability of a player to quickly and accurately select the correct option from a variety of alternatives that may appear before the ball is hit or kicked or as an opponent moves. Other terms such as "perception," "cognition," and "perceptual-cognitive skill" are also used to describe this process and are used interchangeably throughout the chapter.

Colloquially, decision making is often referred to as "reading the play." Some team sport coaches operationally describe a skilled decision maker as the player who is "a good driver in heavy traffic" – the player who seemingly knows what is about to occur two passes before it happens. While such players may not be the fastest around the court, their ability to accurately forecast a game's future means they always seem to have all the time in the world. While reading the play is a cinch for players such as the Australian footballer Chris Judd, ice hockey star Sydney Crosby, or soccer star Lionel Messi, for us mere mortals it is more like reading Latin.

This chapter is concerned with what research tells us about the key facets of decision-making skill and then, importantly, applying the theory in practice by reviewing how this skill can be improved through training. In order to outline the underlying key components of the decision-making process we discuss those components that separate the best from the rest. Second, we detail the common developmental pathways followed by expert decision makers as a means of identifying potential practice activities that may develop the key components of decision-making skill. Subsequently, two aspects of decision-making training are discussed: first, whether decision making can be enhanced through video-based simulation methods completed outside the usual training context; second, methods that can be used in a physical practice setting to increase the skill of players to make both *what* (what movement is to be carried out) and *how* (how a movement is to be carried out) decisions.

WHAT DOES THE RESEARCH TELL US? THE RECIPE FOR BECOMING AN EXPERT DECISION MAKER

What are the key ingredients to becoming an expert decision maker? From a scientific perspective there is a seemingly never-ending debate about the different perceptual-cognitive competencies an expert athlete should possess. The reason for the absence of a straightforward answer lies in the problem itself. An expert in sport needs to possess excellent perception, attention, memory, skill execution, and many more competencies. Before we discuss some of these concepts in more detail, however, it is necessary to outline the phases of the decision-making process. One model that is commonly used to describe the decision-making process is illustrated in Figure 12.1.

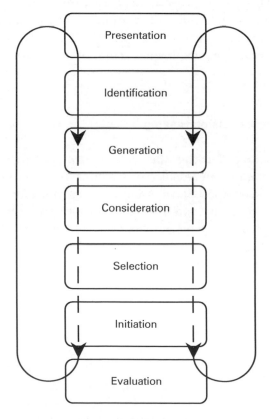

Figure 12.1 The route to decision-making skill in sport.

In order to describe this model we offer a brief example from basketball to illustrate each of the seven stages. Imagine a playmaker in basketball who is dribbling towards the basket and is approached by a defender. At this point, the decision problem has *presented* itself: what action should the playmaker take in response to the approaching defender? The striker *identifies* the constraints on his behavior (e.g., he cannot successfully throw from the midline) and prioritizes his goals (e.g., retain possession but score if possible). In light of these, he *generates* possible options that he may undertake, such as shooting at the goal, passing to a wing player, or dribbling away from the defender. He *considers* these courses of action, perhaps by ranking them according to their likelihood of achieving his primary goal (scoring). Then he *selects* an action; this is likely to be the one with the highest rank. He *initiates* the action by physically performing so as to bring about the action he selected (e.g., physically dribbling the ball to the right). In doing so, he buys time for the wing player to move towards the basket, where he passes the ball and assists in a shot to the basket that results in him positively *evaluating* his decision.

Expert decision makers have learned to progress through these stages very quickly and efficiently, resulting in intuitive performance in the most complex of situations under high pressure. How do they do this? To answer this question, we now describe some of the components that are acquired on the road to decision-making excellence.

Components of expert decision making

Expert decision makers differ from their less capable peers in a number of capacities as detailed throughout this book (see Chapter 3). Of particular interest to the current discussion is the expert player's ability to *read the play*, technically referred to as "pattern recognition and anticipation." Interestingly, pattern recognition skill was first investigated in the game of chess (see Chapter 2). Put simply, research demonstrated that chess grandmasters were able to sum up a board in one quick glance thanks to their ability to chunk the patterns presented. Sports science has subsequently demonstrated that elite team-sport players also possess the analytical mind of a chess master. Watching a team sport such as netball is a classic example of watching a continuously changing pattern. Interestingly, while the pattern may look meaningless to the untrained eye – that is, 14 players sprinting and dodging in all directions – to an expert player (or coach) it can all look completely logical and can inform them in advance where the ball is about to be passed. This is quite a handy skill to have if your job requires you to intercept as many opposition passes as possible. It is thought that elite players have developed the ability to rapidly recognize and then memorize patterns of play executed by their opponents.

212

Importantly, this capability to recognize an opposition team's attacking or defensive patterns is not because the elite players have a bigger memory capacity than the rest of us. Rather, their memory of sport-specific attack and defense strategies is simply more detailed than ours and can be recalled and used in a split second.

Research has also revealed that the ability to recognize patterns of play may transfer across team sports that possess a similar structure of play. Bruce Abernethy (Chapter 14) and his colleagues examined expert decision makers from the Australian basketball, netball, and hockey teams and compared their performances on a pattern recognition task with less-skilled athletes from the three sports. Consistent with previous work, the experts recalled patterns from their sport better than their less-skilled counterparts. However, of interest was that when the experts from one sport (e.g., netball) were tested on other patterns (e.g., basketball patterns), their recall was still better than the less-skilled athletes from that sport (i.e., the non-expert basketball players). Such findings imply that some elements of pattern recognition may be general in nature and can transfer between sports. This finding has been replicated in part for other conceptually related sports such as soccer and hockey and has important implications for the development of decision making, as discussed in the next section on the developmental pathways of expert decision makers.

It has been reasoned that superior pattern recognition skill provides a player with an awareness of what a team-mate or opponent is likely to do next. The outcome of effective pattern recognition is anticipation or the capability to prepare a response in advance based on the information provided early in an event sequence. The capacity to anticipate is particularly valuable in time-stressed sports for a number of reasons. First, in a situation such as the tennis return of serve it may be necessary to begin moving before an opponent has even struck the ball in order to successfully intercept it. Second, it provides a player with more time to prepare a response, which may increase the likelihood of executing a successful response. Finally, anticipation may also effectively reduce the expert's information-processing load. In sum, the net result of being an expert decision maker is to create the appearance of having all the time in the world with which to prepare and execute a response in time-stressed situations by efficiently traveling through some or all of the stages of the decision-making process previously described.

Developmental histories of expert decision makers

A commonly employed research strategy to understand decision-making skill has involved interviewing elite decision makers and asking them to detail retrospectively the types of activities they completed in their childhood and adolescent years. It is thought that such information may shed some light on the types of activities that should be practiced if one wishes to become an expert decision maker.

The same athletes that Abernethy and colleagues tested on pattern recognition skills also completed developmental history profiles. Although there are too many findings to detail them all there are a few of particular relevance to this chapter. Of note is that the athletes accumulated far less sport-specific practice (fewer than 4,000 hours on average) prior to reaching expert levels than the 10,000 hours that would be deemed necessary by the theory of deliberate practice (see Chapter 2 for more information on this theory). In explaining this finding, it is critical to note that the number of different sports these athletes participated in as juniors was inversely related to the number of practice hours required to become an expert player. For example, one netball player detailed only 600 hours of netball-specific practice before being selected for the Australian team. However, she had participated in 14 other sports as a junior.

Based on such findings it has been reasoned that participation in a variety of sports before specializing can be advantageous to one's development of expert decision-making skills. Importantly, as highlighted in some research on Australian football, it is not just any sport; rather, participation in sports that are conceptually similar to the one in which a child wants to excel is more likely to generate the transfer of pattern recognition skill previously described (as well as other capacities such as physical fitness). For example, expert decision makers in Australian football were found to participate in a significantly greater number of secondary invasion sports relative to non-expert decision makers. Invasion sports are those such as Australian football that involve players running freely on a field or court and being able in some way to directly challenge their opponents for possession of a ball. This includes sports such as soccer, hockey, and basketball.

Recent discussion has centered on the ever-increasing competition to become an elite performer, which in many sports has made it necessary to begin the process of specialization earlier. Some sport expertise researchers are now suggesting children must at least deliberately play in their preferred sport from a young age in both structured (formal competition and training) and unstructured (backyard play and other forms of the game) ways. While this evidence is still being accumulated, these recommendations will certainly change the current profile of participation detailed for expert decision makers.

THEORY INTO PRACTICE: DECISION-MAKING TRAINING APPROACHES

Now that we understand some of the capacities of skilled decision makers that separate them from other athletes, the key issue becomes how less-skilled performers

Damian Farrow and Markus Raab

can be trained to improve their decision making. The content of decision-making training depends on the theoretical perspective. For instance, one way to classify the content is describing the demands of the sport and the group involved (individual, group, or team training) defining competences (e.g., skills and abilities) to be trained as introduced above. Another way is to describe the different processes of choices and focus on training these components. Further, a more integrated training approach tries to describe simple heuristics that are the rules of thumb athletes use to make fast decisions. Such simple heuristics integrate rules of how to search for information, how to stop the search, as well as how to decide on and execute a choice. Finally, a distinction can be made between off-court and on-court training and this is used in the following section to provide an overview of what science informs us about how to train people in these two situations.

Off-court training

The time available to train players in team sports such as basketball and soccer is limited by their physical demands. Inevitably, these time constraints mean important skills such as decision making are not practiced enough. As a result, researchers have been interested in devising methods to both test and then, importantly, to improve the decision-making skill of athletes outside the normal training environment. In order for it to be considered a credible training approach, specific conditions must be adhered to:

- the decision-making skill to be developed must be a limiting factor to sports performance – that is, if it is not a quality that separates experts from the rest then there is little reason to focus on it in training (see generalized visual training section below);
- suitable training regimes are those that supplement (not replace) physical practice and selectively enhance the specific perceptual capacity;
- off-court training should be individualized to the training goals of specific strength and weaknesses of each athlete and provide active training with valid feedback;
- most importantly, any improvements in decision making arising from training must translate to improved sports performance.

The following section will review some of the training initiatives examined to date with the above criteria in mind.

General visual versus sport-specific training

A key issue when selecting off-court training programs is the notion of whether you are actually training the specific limiting factor to decision-making performance. A variety of training methods have been employed that have been broadly termed "visual perceptual training." The research literature investigating visual perceptual training programs in sport can be separated into generalized visual training programs and sport-specific perceptual/decision-making training programs. Generalized visual training programs have typically originated from within a clinical optometry setting, where behavioral optometrists in particular have prescribed visual training exercises designed to improve the vision of children with reading difficulties. The key tenet behind these training programs prescribed by behavioral optometrists is that improved visual capacity will translate into improved sporting performance. Alternatively, sport-specific perceptual/decision-making training programs have emerged from sport scientists seeking to train the visual perceptual capacities known to distinguish the performance of experts from novices in the specific sport of interest. These programs have typically involved video or computer-based approaches focusing on early postural cue identification or the reading of patterns of play. Both general and sport-specific approaches aim to increase the speed and accuracy of a performer's perceptual response to a situation, albeit by way of very different training stimuli and activities. This chapter will focus on sport-specific perceptual/decision-making training, as it is likely to provide a more fruitful avenue for the development of decision-making skill. Unlike generalized visual training methods (such as a player having to respond to a flashing red light on a screen as quickly as possible), sport-specific training attempts to closely replicate or simulate the decision-making conditions of the natural sport skill (typically through choreographed video sequences or actual game play footage).

Sport-specific decision-making training

Postural cue training

The solid empirical evidence demonstrating that expert performers use postural information sources such as an opponent's movement pattern to anticipate likely ball flight (e.g., direction of a tennis stroke or soccer kick) provided researchers with a logical starting point for the design of sport-specific decision-making training approaches. A popular method for training anticipation is through the use of video-based temporal occlusion training. This approach generally involves the video presentation of a performer executing a particular action from the player's perspective, with this vision then edited at a point just before the occurrence of a particular cue (Figure 12.2). Participants are asked to respond by predicting the

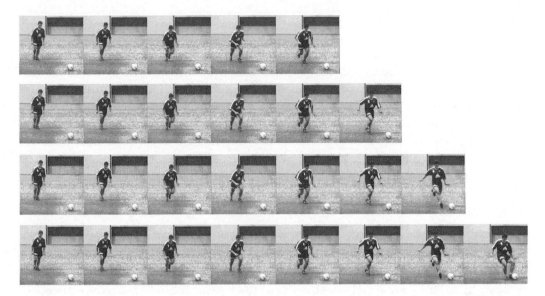

Figure 12.2 Temporal occlusion schematic depicting a progressive increase in pre-kick information for a soccer penalty kick.

outcome of the full play sequence. For example, players watch a tennis server from the receiver's perspective and as the server reaches the top of the ball toss, the vision is occluded or paused so that no more cues are provided. The participants then report their estimate of the direction and spin of the serve. The participant is then given feedback on his or her prediction either verbally or, more typically, by being permitted to view the post-occlusion action. This procedure has been used in an experimental setting and has in some instances successfully improved the perceptual speed and/or accuracy of sports performers.

In relation to interceptive skills, such as those seen in racquet sports, a number of studies has been conducted in which typically beginner to intermediate level participants have been perceptually trained. The training activities have involved a combination of temporally occluded video footage of particular strokes (i.e., tennis serve and passing shots) and specific instruction (guidance) concerning the relationship between the various perceptual information sources and subsequent ball flight direction (an instruction such as "a ball toss placed over the server's head indicates a topspin service is likely"). Improvements in perceptual skill have subsequently been examined through film or video-based tests that utilize movement initiation time or non-sport-specific perceptual accuracy measures (e.g., pen and paper response grids, vocal reaction time or a button press task, or touch screen response) as an indication of decision-making speed and accuracy. Results commonly revealed that the perceptual training groups made faster and/or more accurate responses relative to a control group and a placebo group.

Whereas postural cue training is more localized towards understanding the movement mechanics of the opponent, pattern recognition training is concerned with teaching players how to recognize and subsequently anticipate the outcome of familiar patterns of play as they evolve, as seen in a wide variety of team sports such as basketball. Although there has been less experimental work directed toward examining this issue relative to postural cue training, again the available evidence is generally positive. Improved decision-making performance has been reported in pattern-based situations such as defending or initiating offensive football (gridiron) plays, initiating offensive basketball plays, and selecting the best option in soccer situations.

A typical example of pattern recognition training can be highlighted using the sport of basketball (see Figure 12.3). Players' decision-making skill was examined by having them physically respond to near life-sized video-based simulations of typical offensive basketball situations presented from the player's perspective. Their task was to decide what to do next by choosing one of four available response options (i.e., pass to the top of the key, pass to the base of the key, shoot, or dribble). Training consisted of short sequences of play taken from professional matches that were frozen on screen at a critical decision point. Players were asked to imagine that they were the player in possession of the ball and make a decision whether to pass, shoot, or dribble as quickly and accurately as possible. They were then shown an unoccluded replay to provide knowledge of the result. The players' decision-making accuracy improved by around 15 percent. In comparison, a general visual training group and a control group did not significantly improve. In addition to highlighting the value of training players' recognition of common patterns of play, these data again confirm and extend previous research findings indicating that participants do not always require explicit instruction to promote the learning of perceptual regularities in the environment.

A recent evolution of pattern recognition training has involved the use of commercially available animated gaming packages (e.g., FIFA Soccer, Madden NFL by Electronic Arts). Based on the same principles as described for the pattern recognition training above, players interact with the games in an effort to enhance their decision-making skills. According to media reports, a number of professional football teams are purportedly using programs such as customized versions of Madden NFL to great effect. Similarly, individual athletes have commented on their value. For example, the professional soccer player Conor Chinn, as reported in *The New York Times* (April 2, 2010) spends an hour on the day of each real game in front of his Microsoft Xbox 360 playing FIFA Soccer by Electronic Arts:

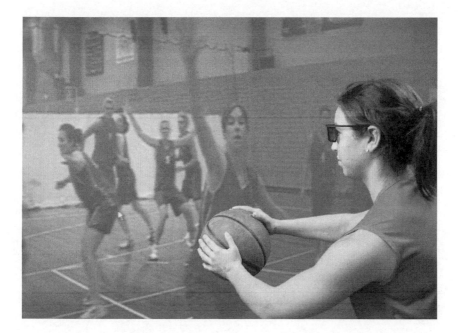

Figure 12.3 Example of a basketball player completing a 3D visual simulation training exercise.

> It gets your soccer brain started that day . . . each virtual player mimics the way a player moves, the way they shoot, the way they pass the ball in real life . . . You really get to see and experience the players' style of play.

Despite such glowing endorsements, published scientific evaluations of the impact of such programs are virtually non-existent at present and represent a logical future direction for researchers.

Future directions of off-court training

Recently a number of research activities have combined various measures such as eye tracking, self-reports, and physiological responses and related them to choices and decision time. Such multi-dimensional and multi-method approaches allow a fuller picture of the different processes involved before a final choice is implemented. A key issue that remains unresolved with video-based decision-making training is the degree to which the learning transfers to the on-field setting. Only a limited amount of research has focused on this issue; however, pleasingly, available evidence suggests transfer does occur although the exact conditions guaranteeing its success are not entirely clear.

One of the factors requiring further consideration is what specific features of the natural task need to be replicated in a simulation for any of the perceptual improvements commonly demonstrated in the laboratory to transfer to performance in the natural setting. When video- or computer-based decision-making training is considered, there are two areas that are of interest to scientists and coaches alike. First, whether such training is enhanced when linked in some way to the sport-specific physical responses and, relatedly, whether a virtual or immersive simulation is superior to the more traditional two-dimensional (2D) video- or computer-based simulation.

A small body of research has focused on the relative importance of linking decision-making training with on-court training. Some general recommendations can be made, albeit prefaced with the comment that further empirical work is required to substantiate these recommendations. First, it appears that perceptual learning can occur whether directly coupled to a physical response or not. Some perceptual-cognitive elements are transferred from the off-field decision-making context to the on-field task. However, wherever possible these perceptual learning activities should be reconnected with the physical task as regularly as possible. The relative importance of this connection with the physical response can be further defined by the specific nature of the task. It is likely to be more important to couple the perceptual and physical response in time-stressed interceptive actions – such as hitting a cricket ball or a baseball or receiving a tennis serve – as opposed to other contexts where the decision maker has (slightly) more time – such as option selection decisions in team-sport situations (e.g., a structured offensive play against a relatively static, zone defense in basketball). This recommendation is based on some researchers concluding that the requirement and/or opportunity to make bat/racket–ball interception is critical in demonstrating skill differences in anticipation. Such conclusions are further challenged with the training platforms now commercially available that have merged traditional video-based displays with sport-specific action responses (see ProBatter™ http://www.probatter.com). The lack of research to have investigated these newer technologies offers researchers a rich direction for future work and coaches a new avenue for perceptual training.

When the issue of virtual reality (VR) immersive simulation is considered, there is again a relative paucity of published work in the sport domain (but see the work of Cathy Craig and colleagues as an insight into the potential: http://www. qub.ac.uk/research-centres/PerceptionActionResearchLab/TechnologyWeUse/ ImmersiveInteractiveVR/). However, such tools have been used in other domains such as aviation, the military, and medicine that demonstrate they do have the capacity to improve the decision-making skills of the user. At a practical level, the key differences a virtual environment offers from more traditional video- or computer-based simulations are the two-way interactivity between the performer and the display, a first-person perspective able to be updated in real time, multi-sensory simulation, and complete control of the simulated variables. Which of these particular features are the most compelling additions to a simulation, particularly as it relates to sport skills, is currently not well understood. Further, such virtual reality simulations come at a significant resource cost that is beyond the scope of most sport program budgets and as yet are not necessarily embraced by many athletes as a legitimate part of their training.

Clearly, VR applications will continue to develop and offer researchers a means of addressing a number of the research issues identified and in due course provide more evidence-based recommendations on their suitability as decision-training devices.

Summary

Although there are many unanswered questions concerning the application of video- or computer-based simulations to develop decision-making skill, there is also enough evidence to support continued investigation and usage of such approaches. Unanswered questions include:

- What is the appropriate intervention length?
- What skill level of player benefits most from such training?
- What type of instructional approach is most effective (see Chapter 9), and how tight should coupling be to the physical response?
- Will a virtual reality approach provide further training benefits to those already gained through video-based approaches?

However, there is equally much evidence to offer encouragement to coaches in the field. In particular, video-based training simulations offer advantages that do not typically exist in the normal training environment. For instance, players who need to do extra decision-making training can do so without needing the remainder of their team-mates to be there to execute the team's patterns. Regular visual simulation sessions could be added to the usual practice week as a low-impact workout or simply to add a new and enjoyable method of training to enhance performance without increasing the physical demands on the player. Finally, the general opinion of athletes exposed to such training approaches is that they are a valuable addition to more traditional training methods.

On-field decision training

On-field decision training plays a key role in daily training. In this section we will demonstrate how decision training can be improved based on the current state of research. While the importance of decision-making skill in ball games is recognized by many coaches, what still needs to be resolved is how to optimally develop the quality of training to refine these skills.

We distinguish decisions about what movement is to be carried out ("*what* decisions") from decisions about how this movement should be carried out ("*how* decisions"). For instance, a table tennis player needs to decide between a forehand or backhand drive (*what*) and whether this stroke is played cross-court or baseline, short or long, with spin or without spin (*how*). *What* decisions are often trained in isolation in tactical training and, similarly, *how* decisions are trained in isolation in technical training sessions. In the following sections we will provide evidence for, and examples of, practical interventions for *what* and *how* decisions in isolation, as well as when integrated. The main conclusion we present is that *what* and *how* decisions should be combined quite early in the learning process or early in a season for more highly skilled athletes.

What decisions

Four factors that are important for the selection of movements will be discussed, namely, situation complexity, if–then rule use, creative choices, and option generation.

Situation complexity

Some tactical training approaches follow the logic of the traditional technical training model of a simple to complex progression of skill development. For example, basketball players are first presented with a two-against-two situation containing two choices for the ball player, such as pass or shoot. The situation is initially conducted with quite inactive defense and always from the same distance to the basket and then complexity is progressively added such as a more active defense, more variable situations, and the addition of more choices by increasing the number of players involved. Alternatively, some approaches propose to start quite complex so that players need to adapt quickly to the ever-changing situations such as those present in pick-up games two against two or three against three. This hard-first strategy seems of some advantage and is therefore recommended for more highly skilled players.

If–then rule use

Another important factor of *what* decisions is the use of "if–then" rules. For instance, in a two-against-two situation in basketball, coaches may present two if–then rules through verbal instruction or on a whiteboard. The first rule may be formulated as "*if* the defensive player opposed to you is too far from you, and your partner is closely defended, *then* shoot"; the second rule as "*if* your partner is in a good position, and the defensive player is too close to shoot, *then* pass to your partner." Of course labels such as "good position" or "defensive player is far enough away to shoot" depend on the skill level of the players in that situation. As an alternative, a coach could also implicitly develop more shooting opportunities by setting up a slower defensive player in one set of plays and more passing opportunities by setting up a good and fast defensive player for the ballplayer deciding between these options. Based on research conducted to date, it appears that in quite simple situations which involve two to four options, each defined by one "if–then" rule, better and faster choices can result from adaptive behavior that can be picked up directly by the player and may be interfered with or slowed down only if the if–then rules are coached explicitly beforehand. However, if the situation is more complex, such as a full five-against-five situation with a number of rules and cues that may require a player's attention to make a good decision, then coach instruction may be required to focus the player's attention on the key aspects of the situation.

Creative choices

A third and less-researched aspect of training *what* decisions is that of creative choices. Whereas training of if–then rules results in one good choice for a given situation or set of situations, it does not allow adapted choices to be made during the course of a game. Therefore, there are some methods that not only consider each choice in isolation but train choices in sequences and how people should react based on previous choices. One famous example is the "hot-hand" phenomenon that suggests that a player has a higher chance to succeed if she has previously been able to successfully shoot two or three hits than in a situation in which she previously missed the last two or three shots. However, the empirical evidence is not clear-cut that playmakers use such information for ball allocations. Using the belief that someone is hot can lead in some situations to better performance (e.g., if individual performance is variable) and in others to worse performance (e.g., if an opponent can gain an advantage from the more allocations to one player). Therefore, structuring training to require playmakers to remember previous hits/misses of their team-mates becomes a possible training activity. In sum, it is important to train the selection of different choices that can be conducted in the same situation so an opponent is left uncertain about potential changes in the play.

Another mode of training refers to the cognitive processes used when evaluating different choices within the same situation – called "option generation." For instance, one strategy used by coaches is to require players to play, within the same attack situation, the same option over and over again. Another strategy is to replay the same attack situation but using a different choice each time. For example, in basketball a specific routine for the playmaker may result in a pass to the left wing player, then a pass to the center player or to the right wing player. Research indicates that training with "option generation" results in better choices if players use a spatial strategy – that is, generate all options on the left side first and then options on the right side, rather than using a functional strategy that first searches for all passes over the court and then for shooting and dribble options. The advantage of a spatial strategy lies in the reduced number of options generated, which leads to a faster choice. Additionally, expert players are well guided if they rely on their intuitive first choice because this choice often generates the highest success given a specific situation.

How decisions

The *how* decision, for instance in tennis, is to choose the exact parameters of a backhand down the line return. The process of such a *how* decision follows the *what* (e.g., forehand or backhand drive) decision by only a matter of milliseconds and, as a result, it can be changed later than changing from a backhand to a forehand stroke, for example. There are at least three factors that are important for the production of movements: game-like situations, use of pre-cues, and the type of instruction (see Chapter 9).

Game-like situations

Practice sessions should replicate actual game events and phases of play with the coach ensuring players are educated concerning how the training activity used reflects the decisions and processing speed required in the competition environment. A well-known skill acquisition expert, Judith Rink, summed it up best when she said:

> Transfer of practice to the game environment depends on the extent to which practice or training resembles the game. If the athletes do not practice in game-like scenarios, they will not play the game well, yet, if

224

practice is too game-like, it may be too difficult to integrate and perform the emphasized skills. The resolution of this implication is that practice needs to occur at a level that incorporates as much of the game as the players can successfully manage.

The adoption of this philosophy is evident in well-publicized coaching approaches such as *Teaching Games for Understanding*, *Gamesense*, or *Play Practice*. A central tenet of all these approaches is that the decision-making elements of the task are given priority, at least initially, over the instruction of technique.

Use of pre-cues

Coaches use pre-cues to enable faster *how* decisions. For instance, they provide probabilistic information such as 80 percent of the opponent's topspin balls will be played to the backhand. As a result of such a pre-cue, the player can focus more on their backhand and then choose either cross-court or down the line based on the relative positioning of themselves and their opponent. Another technique is for the coach to direct their player to use perceptual information that changes very late in an event before conducting the *how* decision. For example, an opponent's movement to the left should result in an attack to the right. The time needed to react on such information in *how* decisions depends on the movement planned. For instance, in an attacking phase of play in soccer, information presented by the approaching attacker at the very end of his run will determine whether the goalkeeper should jump to the left or right corner.

CURRENT LIMITATIONS

We see systematic on-court decision-making training as still in its infancy and therefore we want to draw attention to some limitations that can be overcome by further research and best practice. In regard to coaching *what* decisions, further work is required to develop a method that allows coaches to know how to select between different tactical training methods to generate an optimal outcome given a specific team, situation, and task. The application of if–then rules as tactics seems a limited approach for teaching creative decision making and situation-based decisions. Furthermore, how to teach players about what kind of information to attend to when making their choice is not yet commonplace in real world training environments. For instance, in penalty situations such as in soccer the information that helps a goalkeeper distinguish between a left or right corner kick may be quite different when the kicker starts his approach from just before foot to ball contact.

In regard to *how* decisions, even in laboratory research where significant amounts of data are accumulated about instructions, feedback, and other parameters that influence performance, we still do not know exactly when to combine the *how* decisions with the *what* decisions in early learning or across seasonal training plans. For instance, coaches need to decide when in pre-season training an adjusted skill is ready to be tested in more complex tactical situations. Similarly, it remains unclear how to combine instructions and feedback of *how* and *what* decisions in complex training schemes. The individual limits of athletes' information-processing, emotional, and cognitive abilities are not yet integrated into guidelines for coaches.

CONCLUDING REMARKS

What does the research tell us about training decision making in the field of play? The best answer we are able to provide to coaches is that decision making is very (sport) situation specific and depends on both athlete abilities and the task at hand. Far from providing a comprehensive set of decision-making aids, we have presented some principles for the development of *what* and *how* decisions that are general enough to be applied across different sports and situations, yet specific enough to provide guidelines to choose between different training alternatives.

Expert decision makers are not born, but made through a combination of their developmental experiences as children and then through quality coaching that provides on- and off-court decision-making training opportunities. The on- and off-court training methods discussed here can be coupled with other learning approaches as detailed in the other chapters. A common question is how much each of these training types should be used. Naturally this question is difficult to answer in a general sense; however, our observations of current practice are that off-court training should be used far more frequently than is currently the case. Too often any off-court training completed is simply a coach-led preview and review of a competitive match which, although of some educational value, certainly does not proactively train the players' decision-making capacities. It is our belief that off-court decision-making training should be conducted in a similar manner to a weight-training program. That is, the training principles of volume, frequency, intensity, and overload are manipulated so that a progressive training effect is generated over time. The recipe for becoming an expert decision maker, in our opinion, is to systematically combine on-court training focusing on the execution of *what* and *how* decisions with off-court training. That is, all steps of the decision-making process, particularly the components of *generate*, *consider* and *select*, should be part of both types of training though not necessarily presented in an explicit manner.

I have worked with Damian Farrow for the past eight years on the training of decision-making skills for Australian rules football players. The fact that we have maintained a professional relationship for this period of time is indicative that I think there is some value in the methods discussed in this chapter. However, equally I think it is important to discuss the challenges experienced when employing such methods in a high-performance setting. Before a coach will utilize the services of a sport science provider such as Damian they will typically consider two questions: how much does it cost? and how much time will it take? (both in terms of programming and before a result will be seen). These two conditions need to be met for a new training direction, such as an emphasis on decision making, to be implemented. I will refer to these criteria in the following sections as I evaluate the successes of the methods we have used.

Off-field training approaches

I think the off-field training of decision-making skill is a significant area for future research and application. In the professional setting there are a number of reasons for this. First, training time continues to be reduced during the competition or in-season phase as the physical demands of the game increase and the need for recovery takes precedence. Off-field simulation approaches provide the opportunity to continue to develop decision-making skill with no associated physical cost. Furthermore, I think there is value in exposing injured players to this type of training to keep the decision-making processes engaged even though they cannot physically train.

We have used a number of methods that can be considered off-field decision-making training. The two approaches I am most familiar with have been the establishment of a video/web-based playbook and the use of interactive vision training. The video/web-based playbook is where we incorporate both video taken from the television broadcaster and added animation of team patterns and ask players to solve various tactical problems related to our game style. These could be related to the animated gaming approaches discussed in the chapter. Players solve the problems by way of multiple-choice responses, mouse clicks on the vision or pattern recall, or option selection as discussed in this chapter. I think such methods are a useful way of developing the player's game knowledge about our style of play and associated positional demands in all circumstances around the field. The other method we have used most is where a game situation is projected onto a large wall (so the image is nearly life sized) and our players are required to kick the ball to the player they think is the best decision-making option (see Figure 12.3 for an example of this approach from basketball).

I will focus on my observations of the interactive kicking task to highlight some of the challenges and benefits of this type of training. First, the players typically enjoy this training as they find it a nice change of stimulus but importantly feel they do get some additional decision-making training they would otherwise not have received. From my perspective there is both a cost and time investment in such training. A quality projector and projection wall is required to display the situations (cost), but more importantly there is a significant time cost. For instance, because video footage from the players' perspective was preferred to footage recorded by the television broadcasters (an aerial perspective), specific training drills/situations were created and filmed to provide the library of situations to be displayed. This took significant planning of our on-field physical training time to capture these situations in a realistic context and then there was a further time cost in relation to then selecting and preparing the situations for projection. This becomes an ongoing commitment as one of the strengths of such training is you can practice many decision-making repetitions in off-field training contexts in a short period of time (i.e., 20 situations may only take 5–10 minutes to complete), but on the flip side you need to continually update the situations displayed or players get too familiar with the content and some of the value is lost. Without an embedded staff member focused on this task, this training approach would quickly drop out of the program.

Last but not least is whether such a training approach actually works. Intuitively, I felt there was value but equally I required Damian to provide some assurances from the scientific literature, and subsequently from our on-field performances, that this would be the case. Based on the evidence accumulated I think there has been improvement in our players' decision making, particularly among the younger players in our squad. However, measurement of the improvements in the game situation, rather than just in the interactive simulation setting, is certainly a challenge. Decision-making skill is multi-faceted and interacts with factors such as our team rules and structure as well as with the player's technical skills/physical capabilities, such as kicking strength and physical conditioning status.

On-field training approaches

The on-field training of decision making is obviously more traditionally the domain of a coach. However, partnership with a skill acquisition provider can help to refine your approach and continually improve the quality of the training situations created. I think good on-field decision-making training is simply a matter of creativity in the development of different game scenarios coupled with assessment of the way players deal with or solve the situations presented. I am constantly evaluating factors such as player density. For instance, have we established the correct ratio of attacking versus defensive players? What is the correct amount of space to play this game? Have I overloaded the players appropriately? I find this particularly challenging when you have highly skilled decision makers where the usual training demands are not sufficient to challenge them. I think approaches such as dual-tasking the player (e.g., asking them to commentate the game out loud as they play) in an effort to challenge their skill further is valuable in this regard.

The cost benefit of on-field decision-making training is different from what I have detailed for off-field training. I think the cost on-field is not monetary but more related to your most precious resource: the player. Decision-making training games or drills are typically more physically demanding than more structured drills that require fewer decisions to be made. By virtue of the nature of the game, decision-making training involves a great deal of randomness and hence the risk of injury can increase. Consequently, the amount of this type of training has to be monitored to ensure players can get through the training load. Having said that, I think it is critical and will always err on the side of exposing players to more of this training than less. In terms of time costs, on-field decision-making training invariably takes longer than more closed down, structured drills. Coaching demands are increased as there is a need to observe and question players about their decisions and actions more than is the case if it is simply a kick to kick drill. Further, the relative number of on-ball decisions a player makes in such training is typically low. Hence there is a need for repetition of the games or drills so that players feel they have experienced enough decision-making practice. This issue is obviously why I think there is also value in off-field training approaches.

Summary

At present I think on-field training is where 90 percent of the improvements in a player's decision-making skills come from and the off-field training approaches are a nice top-up. This percentage may vary a little when you consider off-field training value for specific players such as those that are injured, young or new to the club, or the very poor decision makers. Perhaps as virtual reality approaches (e.g., those detailed in this chapter) become more commonplace and cost effective this may change.

KEY READING

Abernethy, B., Côté, J., and Baker, J. (2002) 'Expert decision-making in team sports', Research Report to the Australian Sports Commission.

Bar-Eli, M., Plessner, H., and Raab, M. (2011) *Judgement and Decision-Making and Success in Sport*. Oxford: Wiley-Blackwell.

Berry, J. and Abernethy, B. (2003) 'Expert game-based decision making in Australian football: How is it developed and how can it be trained?', Report to the Australian Football League Research Board.

Farrow, D. (2013) 'Practice-enhancing technology: A review of perceptual training applications in sport', *Sports Technology*.

Mann, D.L., Abernethy, B., and Farrow, D. (2010) 'Action specificity increases anticipatory performance and the expert advantage in natural interceptive tasks', *Acta Psychologica*, 135: 17–23.

Raab, M. (2012) 'Simple heuristics in sports', *International Review of Sport and Exercise Psychology*, 1–17. DOI:10.1080/1750984X.2012.654810

Ward, P., Williams, A.M., and Hancock, P.A. (2006) 'Simulation for performance and training', in Ericsson, K.A., Charness, N., Feltovich, P.J., and Hoffman, R.R. (eds.) *The Cambridge Handbook of Expertise and Expert Performance*. New York: Cambridge University Press, pp. 243–262.

Williams, A.M., Ward, P., and Smeeton, N.J. (2004) 'Perceptual and cognitive expertise in sport: Implications for skill acquisition and performance enhancement', in Williams, A.M. and Hodges, N.J. (eds.) *Skill Acquisition in Sport: Research, Theory and Practice*. London: Routledge, pp. 328–348.

Damian Farrow and Markus Raab

CHAPTER 13

DEVELOPING TACTICS

ADVANCES IN COGNITIVE PSYCHOLOGY AND TECHNOLOGY

STUART MORGAN AND SUE L. MCPHERSON

INTRODUCTION

Elite players who possess high levels of tactical skill are often described as the "playmakers" or "students of the game." Recent evidence suggests developing this type of brain power requires just as much effortful practice as other aspects of player development. For the most part, however, players' tactical skills are often reported anecdotally rather than examined in a systematic way. That is, most statistics about players' performance describe the outcome of behaviors, using such measures as ball speeds or averages of goals, errors, or assists, rather than the choice of behaviors themselves. We present some useful techniques that delve more deeply into the features of tactical knowledge in players at various age and expertise levels in a number of different sports.

Emerging technology-based tools, video analysis software, and sport data analysis systems also provide new insight into tactical performance, and recurring patterns of player behavior. In much the same way as biomechanical analysis techniques can inform coaches about important areas for attention in skill acquisition, new performance analysis techniques can inform coaches about what areas of tactical skill need to be addressed. We discuss some of these innovative techniques, and how they can provide coaches with a systematic knowledge of the tactical decision-making profiles of their own players, and also competitive insights into the recurring patterns of behavior in their opponents.

By studying the use of tactics and broader decision-making skill, sport scientists have begun to understand how athletes develop a knowledge base in their sport and what makes experts better than novices. Our experiences in high-performance sports also highlight the practical issues of providing tactical guidance and facilitating learning before, during, and after competition. The aim of this chapter is to:

- explore tactical skill and discuss how experts differ from novices;
- discuss new techniques for finding patterns in behavior;
- present activities designed to promote tactical skills of players.

We will begin by introducing terms and ideas about how tactical knowledge and cognitive skills develop. This section will be followed by a discussion of how technology aids tactical performance and finally we present activities designed to enhance tactical knowledge and cognitive skills.

HOW TACTICAL KNOWLEDGE AND COGNITIVE SKILLS DEVELOP WITH EXPERTISE

In tennis, the ability to interpret an opponent's serve tendencies may or may not lead to an accurate return of serve. Likewise, the decision to hit a forehand with topspin deep to an opponent's backhand may or may not lead to the ability to successfully execute this shot. It is important at this point to differentiate between being able to decide the right thing to do and being able to carry out that decision.

Decision and motor skills include two types of knowledge. One type is termed "declarative knowledge" and the other type is termed "procedural knowledge." Declarative knowledge is about knowing what to do or how to do something in step-wise terms. For instance, players know the rules of the game or that, in order to slice the tennis ball, the grip might have to change slightly to increase the angle of the racquet. Another example of declarative knowledge is recognizing when the opponents are playing a full press on a basketball court. Declarative knowledge is factual knowledge. Procedural knowledge, on the other hand, is the information required to carry out decisions: the knowledge of actions, skills, and operations. There is debate about how much a player needs to be able to verbalize how to do something in order to do it skillfully, but nonetheless experts have encoded the motor programming required to execute complex skills reliably and this knowledge is procedural. This complex interplay of knowing and doing is why it is important for coaches to examine players' overt behaviors and thoughts during real or simulated competitions.

A coach examining a player's declarative knowledge about decision skills might pause a game video and ask a player "would you pass, shoot, or dribble?" to determine if this player understands what to do or how to make a decision in

Stuart Morgan and Sue L. McPherson

this situation. However, often procedural knowledge can be encoded as highly automated perceptual-motor behavior and players may not be able to explain or rationalize exactly why they have made a decision. In this case the coach may continue to examine this player's decision skills in action by observing their decisions in similar situations during practice drills or actual bouts of competition. Motor skills may be examined by way of a similar process. For example, a coach could ask a player to critique another player's jump shot to assess their knowledge of how to do this skill. This coach could continue to examine their jump shot skills by observing their ability to execute jump shots during practice drills or actual bouts of competition.

Of course, the nature of the sport and the player's role (e.g., a goalie or forward) will influence the tactical demands on the athlete. A framework has been proposed (see Figure 13.1) to describe the various types of sport and performance contexts that need to be considered when we examine players' tactics and performance skills. For instance, in ball sports such as soccer or tennis, players need abilities in both areas of decision and motor skills. In soccer you need to be able to decide that the best option is a shot at goal and then be able to actually make that shot. In contrast, in sports such as gymnastics or figure skating, players need abilities that primarily involve motor execution skills. A gymnast, for example, has a set routine to perform and does not need to make any major decisions to choose what actions to perform. In Figure 13.1, the left to right arrow at the top represents the demands on the athlete, moving from the decision skills to the motor skills aspects of performance. For both decision skills and motor skills, the framework also describes the transition from knowing what to do (declarative knowledge) to knowing how to do it (procedural knowledge).

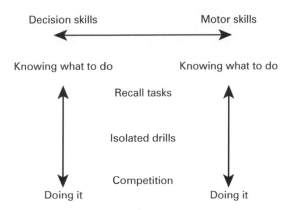

Figure 13.1 A framework depicting various levels of analysis and performance contexts in sports.

FROM KNOWLEDGE TO TACTICS

In order to understand a player's tactical knowledge and cognitive skills it is important to measure what they know about the sport, or their *sport-specific knowledge base*. Sport-specific knowledge bases can be thought of as a specialized system of units of information (or concepts) that are stored in the long-term memory (LTM) and accessed when needed. Sport-specific knowledge may also contain cognitive skills that help us read a play pattern, predict a pitcher's pitch, or gather and collect information about an opponent. For instance, skilled players create a profile of their opponent that is updated with information by watching how they behave in certain game situations. With practice and exposure to a variety of opponents, experts develop profiles about players' behaviors that are more efficient and effective than those of other players who do not have experience of doing this.

Another feature of the progression from beginner to expert can be seen in the types of sport-specific knowledge typically used during problem-solving or task performances. A beginner may be concerned with several general goals related to getting the ball over the net (e.g., hitting it over, keeping it in bounds), with minimal regard for anything else. In contrast, more advanced players become more concerned with selecting an optimal shot based on more specific goals, such as keeping their opponent behind the baseline, and they may use more detailed information, such as player and ball locations and the behavioral profiles of their opponent that they have established. Thus, to the advanced player, this situation is represented as a set of specific goals with solutions that make use of the current context and knowledge about an opponent.

Skilled athletes also manage to integrate many concurrent streams of information, including the current state of the game play, mental notes about the behavior profiles of their opponents, and pre-planned tactical blueprints for winning the point, game or match. Research by McPherson and colleagues has examined players' thought processes (using audio recordings) in a variety of performance contexts. This technique illustrates the knowledge they are using as they perform. Each player's thoughts are examined according to the concepts that they are linked to. Five major concept categories emerge from these studies relating to *goal concepts* (revealing the purpose of a planned action), *condition concepts* (recognizing the particular circumstances of the current play), *action concepts* (reflecting patterns of actions), *regulatory concepts* (self-monitoring the results of their actions), and *do concepts* (relating to how to perform an action).

Collectively, studies indicate all players regardless of competitive level utilize tactical objectives during competition that become more varied and specialized with expertise. Tennis players at more advanced levels utilize fewer execution goals, such as "hit it over the net," and more tactical goals that involve opponents, such as "keep him behind the baseline" or "force him to use his backhand." Solutions to goals become more tactical with expertise. That is, condition and action concepts become more sophisticated, varied, and related with expertise. At first, conditions primarily concern the current context (player formations, ball location) and become linked to actions; for example, "if this situation exists then I do this." Other concepts may be used together to form *condition profiles* that contain tactical information. For example, profiles are used to make decisions about shot selections or to update information in the profile that is currently being used, or in other profiles. These profiles are contained in players' thoughts at more advanced levels.

Athletes also combine the different concepts (i.e., goal, condition, action, regulatory, and do) to create more complex profiles in memory. Thus, *action plan profiles* and *current event profiles* develop with expertise. *Action plan profiles* are rule-governed prototypes used to decide the appropriate actions given the current match conditions. These profiles contain cognitive skills for monitoring current conditions such as player positions and ball placement, player formations, or coordination patterns of opponents to make accurate response selections. For example, coaches use diagrams and practice drills to develop players' knowledge and cognitive skills necessary to recognize and/or execute offensive and defensive play patterns. Research indicates that elite players recognize and recall player formations or patterns more effectively and efficiently than their less-skilled counterparts (see also Chapter 12). Often, sport-specific language or signals are used to communicate plays or situations. For example, in basketball players generate condition concepts such as "they are playing man-on-man," "that's a two-on-three zone defense," or "block her out" to communicate a complex sport situation or play. These kinds of expressions can richly encode large amounts of sport-specific knowledge and an important feature of tactical skill is the comprehension of these sport-specific languages.

Current event profiles are tactical scripts, used to keep relevant information active with potential past, current, and future events. A current event profile is built from past competition, or previous experiences prior to the immediate competition, and from cognitive skills used to collect information as competition progresses. Thus, elite players with well-developed profiles are predicted to have access to more effective and efficient tactical knowledge during competition than their less-skilled counterparts. Table 13.1 presents an example of how a condition profile about an opponent may develop with tennis expertise. In basketball, condition concepts reflecting current event profiles might be noted in such phrases as "I keep getting pushed out of bounds when I go for it, she is blocking me out under the basket" or "on the last two attempts we hung back too far and it is killing us on offensive rebounds." If players generate condition concepts that reflect only what happened, without any reasoning about why it happened, then the chances are they do not have any tactical scripts for diagnosing players or game events.

Table 13.1 Examples in tennis to illustrate how tactical knowledge and specialized processes develop with expertise

Level	Conditions about opponent	Specialized processes
1	Conditions about opponent not in problem representation; thoughts do not contain this concept	No need to monitor opponent; no specialized processes
2	Conditions about opponent reflect general or weak analyses; thoughts at times contain weak concepts about opponent	Monitor opponent occasionally reiterate events; no specialized processes
3	Conditions about opponent regard his/her position on court and/or prior shot; thoughts are in the moment thus reflect evidence of rudimentary action plan profile	Monitor player positions and shots; concepts about opponent linked to shot selection or reiteration of events
4	Conditions about opponent's position and shot tendencies updated on a regular basis; conditions about opponent emerge from action plan and current event profiles; profiles become more tactical and associated and linked to other profiles (e.g., about their own behaviors)	Analyses opponent's position and shot tendencies to update profile, develop tactics and shot selections; processes highly specialized and may be linked to other specialized processes in other profiles
5	Condition profile about opponent is highly tactical and based on prior knowledge of other opponents' style of play and preferences; action plan and current event profiles become more tactical and associated and linked to other profiles (e.g., about their style of play/preferences)	Same as No. 4: opponent profile is used to anticipate opponent's tactics

Note: Levels represent advancing levels of expertise (1, lowest level; 5, highest level).

EXPLOITING TECHNOLOGY TO IMPROVE TACTICAL PERFORMANCE: TIPS AND PITFALLS

Computers have become ubiquitous in sports and, more recently, smart phones, iPads, and other mobile devices have increased connectivity in ways that few could have conceived just a decade ago. The impact of mobile technology on sport has been profound. Not only can the viewing public access match video, player statistics, and other game details in "real time," so too can the coach. But the challenge for sports science is not to provide coaches (or players) with every bit of information imaginable but instead to distill vast sources of data into short and meaningful chunks that can improve tactical performance. In this section we consider some of the current trends and the implications for coaches who would like to enhance tactical skill without causing "paralysis by analysis."

As we have discussed in this chapter, skilled players in many sports demonstrate an ability to see the patterns in sport – information that informs decisions and tactical choices. Indeed, the ability to recognize patterns and structure in sport is a prevailing theme throughout many of the chapters in this book. As we have discussed above, developing sport-specific knowledge bases and cognitive skills such as maintaining profiles of opposition behavior is a cumulative process that may take many years. Modern techniques in computer machine learning (sometimes referred to as artificial intelligence) have tried to "learn" the behaviors of athletes in sport using information such as player positions, ball movements, shot locations, and other measurable components of a sport contest. For instance, software developed at the Australian Institute of Sport called "Pattern Plotter" gathers ball movements and other information about which players are in possession of the ball. A technique called "association rule mining" is then used to find recurrent combinations of certain ball movement patterns, game contexts, and specific players. Figure 13.2 shows an example of ball movements in field hockey that frequently occur when a certain set of players pass the ball among themselves. A minimum number of matching examples are used to filter the strength of possible patterns and to show more or fewer patterns. When a higher minimum threshold is used, only the most frequent patterns are shown. Coaches can refine the analysis to include any measurable combination of players and/or events (such as plays leading to goal shots or passing errors). This kind of information can also be presented to players in various visual forms to show how a particular opponent tends to play. Visual feedback can help players to create, affirm, or modify their current event and action plan profiles as we have discussed above.

Players and coaches tend to have a highly tuned eye for detecting tactical patterns in their sport and sometimes coaches prefer to trust their own judgment in preference to using statistics or data. There are, however, several advantages in using computers in notational analysis to supplement coaches' subjective judgments. Computers rarely feel the pressure of an important contest and they rarely allow their computations to be distorted by any emotional investment in the outcome of the match.

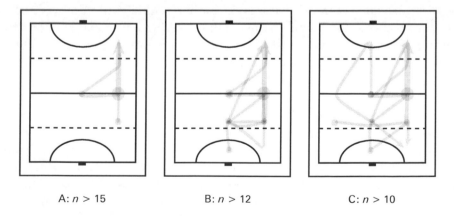

A: $n > 15$ B: $n > 12$ C: $n > 10$

Figure 13.2 Graphic association rules where the minimum number of instances (n) is greater than 15 (A), 12 (B), and 10 (C).

It is a common mistake amongst humans to attribute a performance level directly to the result: we won so we played well or we lost so we played poorly. Of course it is entirely possible to play quite badly and make tactical errors but to defeat an even poorer opponent, or otherwise to play extremely well and execute a tactically sound game but be defeated by a superior opponent. Computer-based analysis is generally immune to this kind of perceptual bias and allows performance and tactical trends to be measured in an objective, consistent, and reliable way.

Another perceptual trap for coaches is to miss infrequent but recurring patterns in tactical events because of the distracting influence caused by the most common events. For instance, a soccer team may use a particular ball movement strategy to penetrate their opponent's defenses and shoot for goal. Since soccer matches may include only a handful of goal shots throughout a game, the critical attacking pattern underpinning that play may occur only once or twice. Indeed, often scoring teams will save their most dangerous plays for the best moment to score when it is a surprise to their opponents. To the coach and player it can be easy to miss the systematic features of such a play if it happens very rarely. Computer-based techniques such as Pattern Plotter enable the coach to review data that are compiled over many matches so that even the most infrequent patterns become visible.

Although computer-based notational analysis has emerged in recent years, sport has a long history of manual notational analysis using a pencil and paper. In their foundation work of 1976, the researchers Reilly and Thomas began using written shorthand notations to analyze player movements in English first division soccer matches. This research focused on player work rates and showed that, contrary to the subjective opinion of many coaches, elite soccer players spent long periods of matches walking or jogging at slow speeds. This work highlighted the importance of objective measurement in guiding tactical performance and it led the way for an entire field of notational and performance analysis in modern sports science. This early work also demonstrated that it is certainly possible to perform very powerful analyses of tactical data simply by manually drawing ball movement patterns on sheets of paper. Let us consider the problem in soccer of finding the path of the ball leading to goal shots by an opponent team. Draw up a large map of a soccer pitch and manually trace the path of the ball into the attacking area for each scoring opportunity and then color code the movements based on the outcome (i.e., red for a successful goal shot, yellow for an unsuccessful goal shot, and green for a play that is defended before a goal shot). As these data accumulate throughout a match, color-coded patterns begin to appear that reveal the attacking tendencies of the team and this information becomes important tactical knowledge. This is a useful way to combine objective data with the perceptual expertise of the coach/ player. Skilled observers can view a ball movement graphic and then enhance their knowledge bases and cognitive skills to exploit the tactical insight provided by the objective visualization of the patterns.

238

Manual techniques such as this can be highly effective and inexpensive, but it can often be difficult to view data from more than a single match in this way. Computer-based methods, however, are especially well suited to managing very large data sets and are at the forefront of this problem because they allow for the compilation of many matches. Furthermore, it is not necessary to purchase expensive bespoke sport analysis software to achieve this aim. Much can be achieved simply by archiving important information from many matches and opponents in a "garden variety" computer spreadsheet. Some work in player-scouting analysis for baseball (recently highlighted by the book and 2011 movie *Moneyball*) has been a prominent example of the use of statistics and simple computer spreadsheets to evaluate player performances and guide tactical choices. Baseball is a professional sport that is played around the world; there are untold volumes of statistical data from baseball games that would be impossible for any person to filter through, or from which to find meaningful patterns or insight. The combination of a spreadsheet program and some relatively simple equations can be tuned for detecting patterns within very large data sets of the sort that are commonplace in baseball and more recently in many other sports.

Regardless of whether your approach to notational analysis is high-tech or low-tech, the most important feature of any tactical advice to coaches or to players is simplicity. It is well known that players who visually scan many objects in their visual field during game play tend to make comparatively poorer judgments, which indicates that they may not know what to look for and become overloaded with redundant information (see Chapters 11 and 12). It is certainly true that the same principle applies when presenting tactical information to players and that the availability of too much data can lead to the condition known as "paralysis by analysis." Therefore, instead of simply providing players with as much tactical information as possible, it is helpful to consider the cognitive frameworks discussed earlier in this chapter. We have described the way that skilled athletes possess knowledge from the declarative to the procedural and from the general to the specific. These knowledge bases and the cognitive skills that facilitate efficient access to knowledge are the integral components of tactical skill. Well-crafted tactical feedback to players should tap into these attributes by presenting information that is consistent with their existing knowledge frameworks. For instance, by showing the location of first and second serves on a graphical representation of a tennis court, that information can be contextualized to the perception of space on the court. This approach can be much more effective than reporting an arbitrary set of numbers and percentages to a player without any meaningful context. Studies have shown that when we learn new information we can recall it faster and more reliably when it is encoded within existing cognitive frameworks. Therefore, if players can integrate new tactical information into their sport-specific knowledge bases, then access to that information during competition is likely to be faster.

A final consideration in the presentation of tactical analysis to players is matching the appropriate content to the appropriate time. As an example, let us consider the timeline of tactical analysis undertaken for the Australian women's hockey team (the Hockeyroos) at the 2008 Olympic Games in Beijing. Performance analysis staff collected ball movement and player possession data using the computer program Pattern Plotter in real time during each match. At the half-time break, the coach would address the players to provide encouragement and guidance, and to reaffirm the team-based action and condition profiles. Just moments prior to the half-time address, the coach would have a short opportunity to review the tactical data that had been collected by his performance analysis staff throughout the game to that point. In fact, he had approximately three seconds. Time is a precious commodity in the "pressure cooker" environment of an Olympic games contest and, to be helpful, tactical information needed to be encoded within the well-established cognitive and perceptual frameworks of the coach and players. Therefore, only the most important information could be presented in this short time window and it needed to be shown in a graphical format that compressed complex patterns into a familiar and perceptually meaningful framework. We call this the "three-second rule." At other times of course it is possible to spend much longer in review of statistical, graphical, and video information. Nevertheless, one should always remain cognizant of the need to match tactical information with an appropriate timeframe for use and to maximize the cognitive links between the data and the knowledge profiles of the coaches and/or players.

WHAT TYPES OF PRACTICE AND OTHER ACTIVITIES PROMOTE THE DEVELOPMENT OF PLAYERS' TACTICAL SKILLS?

These concepts of knowledge bases, cognitive skills, and tactical profiles based on historical profiles provide a framework for guiding coaches in designing productive practice sessions that enhance tactical decision making. The following ideas should help coaches to work within their existing practice structure to modify activities rather than add length to practice. Several activities may be performed outside practice as well.

- When designing practice environments or developing other activities, consider what aspect of the knowledge base you are focusing on.
  - Are you attempting to develop action plan profiles, current event profiles, or a combination of both? Document what you do in practice and why. Record activities designed to promote tactical knowledge and skills. Is it possible that some drills and activities could be performed outside practice?

240

- The framework introduced previously (see Figure 13.1) may be used to organize practices. This is useful when considering tactics since they are influenced by the performance context, sport, and player position. This framework is also useful for assessing players' tactical skills and performance skills.

- Keep in mind that a "one size fits all" model may not be a suitable approach for developing players' tactical skills and, where practical, tactics can be individualized for each player. Of course there will be instances when tactics may not vary drastically between players. Let tactics emerge from players as much as possible. Players are more likely to invest in the process of developing tactical knowledge and cognitive skills if they have ownership.

■ Analyze players' performance skills periodically during practices and competitions.

- Use videotapes of practices and competitions to analyze decision skills. These provide important statistics for you as well as your players.

■ Reward and reinforce good decision making, not just good skill execution.

- Make good decision skills a priority.

- Alter scoring systems to reward decisions. For example, in tennis, a point may be replayed if the shot selected was weak or not the type of shot the player was assigned to work on. Also, performance skill tests should assess tactical skills as well as motor skills.

■ Design practice activities that allow (or force) players to make decisions in the context of game play.

- Develop drills that allow players to make choices regarding their shot selections. Make sure the context simulates game situations that promote the use of tactical knowledge and skills.

  As an example, in tennis, have players practice second serves in game situations with an opponent returning serves. This develops their monitoring skills concerning current context (players' positions and ball location) and decisions about shot selections (based on game situations, opponent's strengths and weaknesses, etc.). In baseball and softball, players should practice with runners on base, different pitch counts, and number of outs. This develops their visual search strategies to monitor runners and encoding and retrieval strategies to keep track of pertinent information to use in planning future responses, anticipating actions, and modifying plans based on changing game conditions.

■ Help players develop current event and action plan profiles during practice activities or while watching videos or scouting opponents.

- Have players develop profiles of their opponents. What are their opponent's strengths and weaknesses? How could I capitalize "my game" to counter the opponent's strengths? How could I protect "my own weaknesses" against this opponent?

- Have players determine play patterns in the context of game events or have them determine error detection and correction strategies, etc. What play did they run in this situation? When did you recognize the pattern? How? Did you use any cues? Why did you do better on that attempt?
- During practice interact with players:

  Apply the "stop, look (both ways), and listen" approach. That is, stop telling them what to do, assess tactical as well as motor skills, and listen to their thoughts. Using this process, you may gain useful information about what players are processing and what they are not processing. Stop play at various points to ask players what they are thinking. Just asking questions can focus attention toward thinking about tactics. Ask open-ended questions. Neutral and open-ended questions are more likely to reveal the problem-solving activities athletes engage in.

  Listen to what information athletes are attending to. What environmental cues do they attend to? Do they plan in advance? Are they paying attention and remembering what tactics their opponent may be using during play?

  Use specific probes to reinforce tactical knowledge and cognitive skills. For example, to assess a player's error detection and correction of a motor skill you might ask the following questions: How did you do that? Why did you do better on that attempt?

- Help players develop their own solutions; provide feedback during the previously mentioned activities only when necessary to ensure profiles are developing appropriately.

- Provide opportunities for players to learn how to analyze their own (and others') tactical behaviors during performance and how to practice for improvement.
  - Establish a mentoring program to pair players who use more advanced tactics with players who use less advanced tactics to work on diagnosing an opponent and/or team. Mentoring may be useful among beginners as well.

- Embrace and utilize technology. Coaches, players, and scientists continue to gain access to equipment that is transportable, low in cost, and user friendly (e.g., digital video and audio recorders/players, telemetry devices, virtual reality, editing software). For example, a professional baseball team in the US recently began using hand-held video devices in the dugout to review game clips.
  - Present players with only the most important information and keep it simple. Too much information can hinder rather than help.
  - When designing tactical feedback charts try the *three-second rule*.

242

- Have players record their responses or videotape competition. Use walkie-talkies or cell phones with this feature to obtain players' thoughts or communication among players and coaches. Players could develop and store daily logs (using digital recorders) to map their progress. Also, they edit their own video clips for motivation and reinforcement of tactical and motor skills. Overlays on video clips that contain probes or reminders to reinforce tactical knowledge and skills may be developed as well (e.g., identifying a type of skill). Several sports science centers or institutes and universities have access to more expensive equipment (e.g., virtual reality training programs) for training. Encourage players to take advantage of such opportunities (see Chapter 12).
- It is important to note that players will require guidance and training when utilizing technology to reinforce tactical skills. Merely watching videos or talking does not necessarily lead to better knowledge. Also, small notebooks and pencils work well for some players and are used by several professionals in a variety of sports.

CONCLUDING REMARKS

Developing tactical skills in sports is a challenging domain for coaches and sports scientists alike. Trying to develop players' knowledge too fast or just telling them what to think is not the solution. Knowledge bases are not built overnight. Using new technologies in tactical analysis is also a challenge for many coaches and players. Opportunities to experience activities related to tactics must be promoted and built into practice sessions to adequately develop tactical knowledge and cognitive skills. Research examining instructional interventions suggests what is learned depends on what is emphasized. Thus, much of the aspects of knowledge base development in sport domains will be in control of the coaches and their respective programs. Currently, several player development programs are embracing new ways to create opportunities to develop tactical skills in a variety of sports. Of course other factors (e.g., biological, physiological, psychological, sociological) addressed elsewhere in this book will influence the acquisition of sport expertise. Also, coaches' domain-specific knowledge bases and structure of practices, as well as other age-related issues, are predicted to impact the development of players' sport expertise. Thus, several factors should be considered when designing practice and other activities.

My knowledge development

My playing history meant that I developed an understanding of tactics from a relatively young age. By the age of 14, I think I was an astute observer of the game. Being the team's captain also meant I was the coach and would organize team practice. This meant I had to be thinking about our capabilities relative to our opponents and working out ways to beat them. As my playing skill developed and I competed in our national league, and then as an Australian representative in test matches, I would regularly come up against the same direct opponent. If a particular player beat me in a given game, I would pride myself on going away and learning from the experience and making sure it never happened again. I think this is a common trait of elite players: that they develop extensive knowledge about their opposition and do not just play against them but try to understand them. I try to develop this quality in my players by asking them to tell me about their opponent's strengths and weaknesses. I am often surprised by how many players do not even remember whether they have played against someone before, let alone have a detailed understanding of how they play.

How do you coach tactical knowledge?

I think the critical issue in developing knowledge is repetition. Players pick up information at different rates, which means you need to ensure everyone has enough exposure to be confident they know what to do in a specific situation when it arises. My role as a coach is to identify where there is a weakness in the opposition and then develop a strategy that will take advantage of that weakness. We then develop a drill or mini-game that will allow us to practice this over and over again until the team become familiar with it and can handle the situation under competitive pressure. In netball, being able to handle a team that shifts from playing a "man-on-man" to a zone defense is critical. Recognizing when it happens and then changing your style of play to overcome it requires large amounts of practice and repetition.

Another coaching strategy we used with the national team was to divide the players into their playing areas (e.g., defense, mid-court, attack) and get them to develop a solution to a tactical problem that may have arisen against a specific opponent. Although we as coaches may already have a strong idea about how to overcome the issue, we have found it valuable to let the players have some ownership of this process. If the players feel that they have significantly contributed to developing the solution, they are more likely to implement it with success in a game.

Another issue that arises when coaching an elite team is that you ultimately recruit/ select players from all over the country. Different regions have different coaching approaches and consequently produce players with specific styles of play. Combining

244

these different styles within the one team becomes a challenge. For instance, the linkage between the shooters and the center-court players that pass them the ball is one of the most important relationships on a netball court. If a shooter has been conditioned to lead in a particular direction and the center-court player is not used to passing to that type of lead, problems can emerge. Hence, a lot of preparation time is focused on getting players to understand each other's playing styles and finding a way to take advantage of that in a tactical sense.

Using technology to develop knowledge

One advantage of working in a high-performance setting is the opportunity to utilize some of the latest technological advances on offer. One tool I have found extremely beneficial in developing the tactical knowledge of our players has been a software program called Pattern Plotter. This software allows us to chart the movement of the players and ball throughout the course of a game. Then importantly from a coaching perspective we are able to generate reports that summarize the key elements of the game. For instance, we can compare ball movement that results in goals with ball movement that is unsuccessful. This information can be presented visually to players and can summarize a great deal of detail in a very simple but powerful manner (see Figure 13.2).

A second technology we have utilized in a variety of formats is video feedback and analysis (see Figure 13.3). On the training court we are able to have a plasma screen set up next to our court that feeds to a camera recording training. At any moment I wish to reinforce a particular coaching point I can get the players to come to the side of the court and watch an instant replay of our movement. Being able to use video during

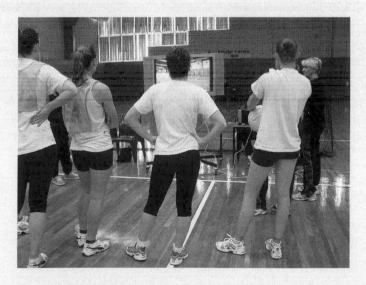

Figure 13.3 Norma Plummer coaching with the help of on-court video feedback.

training is an excellent way of maintaining players' attention and providing a different medium in addition to verbal instruction for providing feedback or giving direction. While you may have been yelling at a player from courtside to reposition in a particular way, it is often not until a player sees the incorrect movement that they believe you and make the change.

Another way we use video is through the use of large screen projections. We ask the players to watch specifically selected patterns of play that we pause at critical moments and ask them to write down what they would do next. We find this is another way of developing their court knowledge but in an off-court environment. Doing this type of training as a group is also valuable as players can share their responses with the squad and debate/discuss why they picked the option they did. I think it is important once you have completed a video session to then get on the court and reinforce the key messages that have been highlighted.

KEY READING

Baker, J., Horton, S., Robertson-Wilson, J., and Wall, M. (2003) 'Nurturing sport expertise: Factors influencing the development of elite athletes', *Journal of Sports Science and Medicine*, 2: 1–9.

Ericsson, K.A. (2003) 'Development of elite performance and deliberate practice: An update from the perspective of the expert performance approach', in Starkes, J.L. and Ericsson, K.A. (eds.) *Expert Performance in Sports: Advances in Research on Sport Expertise*. Champaign, IL: Human Kinetics, pp. 49–83.

French, K.E. and McPherson, S.L. (2004) 'Development of expertise in sport', in Weiss, M.R. (ed.) *Developmental Sport and Exercise Psychology: A Lifespan Perspective*. Morgantown, WV: Fitness Information, pp. 403–423.

Gallagher, J.D., French, K.E., Thomas, K.T., and Thomas, J.R. (2002) 'Expertise in youth sport: Relations between knowledge and skill', in Smoll, F. and Magill, R.A. (eds.) *Children in Sport* (fifth edition). Champaign, IL: Human Kinetics, pp. 475–500.

Hughes, M.D. and Franks, I.M. (eds.) (2004) *Notational Analysis of Sport: Systems for Improving Coaching and Performance in Sport*. London: Routledge.

McPherson, S.L. (1994) 'The development of sport expertise: Mapping the tactical domain', *Quest*, 46: 223–240.

McPherson, S.L. and Kernodle, M.W. (2003) 'Tactics the neglected attribute of champions: Problem representations and performance skills in tennis', in Starkes, J.L. and Ericsson, K.A. (eds.) *Recent Advances in Research on Sport Expertise*. Champaign, IL: Human Kinetics, pp. 137–167.

Oliver, D. (2004) *Basketball on Paper*. Dulles, VA: Potomac Books Inc.

Stuart Morgan and Sue L. McPherson

PART V

EXPERT COMMENTARY

CHAPTER 14

RESEARCH: INFORMED PRACTICE

ARE WE NEARLY THERE YET?

BRUCE ABERNETHY

THE JOURNEY THUS FAR

The first edition of this book provided a rich set of examples of how theory and research from the field of sport expertise offers promise as a means of providing new approaches and improvements to the practical issues surrounding practice and performance that are encountered every day by elite sport performers, officials, coaches, trainers, and sport administrators. However, the journey to fully understanding expertise in sport, and using this to develop research-informed practice, is likely to be a long one and not one for the impatient. Answering the concrete questions posed by practitioners to the standards of proof expected by science is necessarily a long-term, time-intensive venture, and one that as a journey is inevitably plagued by multiple crossroads, blind alleys, and potential false turns. Reminiscent of the standard question of the child on a long road trip, I wish to ask in this brief commentary on applied sport expertise research "are we nearly there yet?" Since the first edition of the book five years ago, have we moved demonstrably closer to, and within reach of, the goal of being able to provide evidence-based answers to the practical skill acquisition questions of relevance to coaches, athletes, and other sports practitioners? I will address this question within the framework of the three key organizational themes for sport expertise that I identified in my introduction to the previous edition of the text, namely:

1 determining what specific skill attributes essential for expert performance distinguish the expert from the non-expert;
2 determining what experts have learned that non-experts have not that permit the experts to control their actions in a more effective and efficient manner; and

3 determining what essential conditions need to be present during the developing years to support the emergence of expert performance.

This commentary is best read in conjunction with the original (Chapter 1, first edition), which outlines both the theoretical and practical importance of these three themes in some detail.

WHAT SPECIFIC ATTRIBUTES ARE ESSENTIAL FOR EXPERT PERFORMANCE?

Much of the existing research work on sport expertise has been concerned with determining those specific components of performance that reliably differentiate expert performers from non-experts. One of the key practical benefits of research identifying the limiting factors to performance is the potential that the knowledge of what factors do and do not limit performance can help provide a principled basis for determining what factors to focus upon in training and practice. With time available for practice being necessarily limited it makes more sense for coaches and athletes to use practice time improving factors that are demonstrably linked to superior performance (i.e., factors that reliably distinguish experts from everyone else) than in trying to improve aspects of skill that are not linked to expertise.

Over the five years since the publication of the first edition of this text there has been the accrual of further evidence of the expert advantage on established characteristics such as anticipation, pattern recall and recognition, multi-tasking performance, and the use of task-appropriate tactics. There has also been some increased clarity of the linkage between these characteristics (e.g., increased awareness of the role that anticipatory/predictive encoding plays in expert pattern recall), but relatively little by way of discovery of new facets of expertise. Similarly, with respect to properties such as visual acuity that have been previously established as poor differentiators of experts and non-experts, the past five years have seen some additional evidence related to the tolerance of sport performance to sub-maximal acuity (e.g., see the work of David Mann and colleagues) but no evident reduction in the frequency of practical attempts to enhance sport performance through a focus on improving simple visual properties such as acuity.

What is still lacking from the sport expertise literature is detailed identification and determination of paradoxical effects where the performance of experts is systematically poorer than that of non-experts. Some cases of this are evident in the cognitive skills literature and this approach has a long tradition in the ergonomics/human factors literature. Understanding the shortfalls of expertise (such as the reduction in the capability to consciously self-report on movement strategy or non-processing of particular information through selective attention) offers potential as an alternative pathway to understanding how the skill learning of experts deviates fundamentally from that of non-experts. As Itiel Dror notes, expertise is not necessarily a function of being uniformly faster or more efficient on all task components but rather more about doing the task in a different way from non-experts. The different approach of the expert can result in improved performance on most but not necessarily all aspects of performance. The trade-offs made in producing expert performance, and the functional degradations that may be consequently evident in some aspects of performance, potentially offer an important window into understanding the skill of experts but one that has not yet been utilized to any real extent in the study of sports experts.

Although knowledge of the defining characteristics of experts continues to consolidate, there still remains a significant paucity of evidence on the development of these attributes, how much they can be changed by practice, and the extent to which adult levels of exceptionality on these key attributes can in any meaningful way be predicted from performance at a younger age. Whereas this evidence is clearly challenging to obtain it is precisely the evidence that is needed to address, in an informed way, practitioner questions regarding talent identification and development. Without such evidence, talent identification programs worldwide remain surprisingly poor in their predictive efficacy and capability (see the work of Roel Vaeyens and his colleagues). In the absence of systematic, longitudinal data on key skill parameters, programs aiming to identify and nurture sporting talent remain dominated by physiological and anthropometric measures and assessments of skill that are based on subjective rather than reproducible criteria. What is clearly needed – though not yet evident – are systematic studies that track the development of key components of expertise longitudinally and not simply over days or months but over years and decades. Although such studies will be time-consuming and resource-intensive, and will take a long time to reveal answers, they are paramount to providing a step change in the quality of evidence and advice that sport expertise researchers can provide to practitioners. In other fields of human development such studies have proven pivotal to evidence-based practice. For instance, much of what is now known about the development and prevention of major chronic diseases derives from longitudinal cohort studies – the Framingham Heart Study (1948–) provides a quintessential example.

In terms of the journey of having practices in sport informed by research on the distinguishing attributes of experts, there is still clearly a long way yet to go.

WHAT HAVE EXPERTS LEARNED THAT NON-EXPERTS HAVE NOT?

Research identifying differences in the information (or "cues") that experts and non-experts use within their sport-specific tasks is important because it has the potential to help determine what must be learned in order to become an expert and this in turn may be valuable in a practical sense in helping the coach to decide how best to structure learning sessions, instruction, and feedback. Although development of a comprehensive, practically applicable theory of learning for sport remains as distant as ever, over the past five years there has been a pleasing growth in both (i) studies that examine the efficacy of novel practice approaches to the learning of the skills known to characterize experts (e.g., Savelsbergh and colleagues) and (ii) studies that use advanced imaging techniques, such as functional magnetic resonance imaging (fMRI), to seek out brain correlates of expert learning (e.g., Wright and colleagues). The increase in learning-type studies is an especially important step closer to the provision of the kind of knowledge about practice approaches that is constantly sought by coaches and athletes, although the majority of studies are still too short in duration, or not equipped with robust enough measures of sustained learning, to provide the kind of guidance to permit practical training decisions to be made with confidence.

Comparison between the kind of evidence available to practitioners in the health field from biomedical research and clinical trials and the kind of evidence that sport expertise researchers are currently able to provide coaches and athletes presents some particularly salutary lessons and highlights the distance we still need to go as researchers to satisfy the everyday needs of sport practitioners. The learning studies to date undertaken in the sport expertise field do not approach the rigor of the randomized control trials (with double-blinded methodologies) that are the gold standard for determining the efficacy of different drug treatments, for instance. Until such approaches become the norm for learning/intervention studies in skill learning, expertise researchers are going to be necessarily constrained in what they can tell an official, coach, or athlete in response to the key question of what type of practice is best for improving a particular facet of skill performance. Many of the more recent approaches to perceptual-motor learning that have been examined in the literature are based on an attempt to promote more implicit types of processing but advance is also constrained in this area by the absence of a systematic, objective means of determining if the engagement of the learner is indeed implicit as intended. Brain-based imaging approaches may provide an avenue to address this concern but such approaches are far away from the practicalities of the sports field or court and to date imaging studies have tended primarily to simply confirm rather than necessarily extend what has already been established from more traditional behavioral measures.

In terms of the journey of having practices in sport informed by research on the selective learning of expert skills, we are still a long way from the journey's end.

WHAT ESSENTIAL CONDITIONS ARE NEEDED FOR THE DEVELOPMENT OF EXPERTISE?

Studying the developmental histories and practice experiences of experts can aid in identifying those conditions that are necessary during the developing years for nurturing the emergence of expert performance. At a practical level, knowing those conditions can then provide an important evidence base for the design and formation of training and practice support systems.

As noted throughout this text, it is increasingly evident that, although enormous amounts of practice are necessary in order to attain expertise, not all practice is equally beneficial (see also Chapters 2, 8, and 15). While learning can accrue in a variety of different ways, and expertise can be acquired through a number of different pathways, generating a detailed understanding of the practice precursors to expertise requires more than simply counting hours and instead a more detailed understanding of the micro-structure of practice. This latter point was also made emphatically by Jan Starkes in the concluding chapter of the first edition of this book. Over the past five years more empirical evidence has been accrued highlighting the contribution of contextual factors – such as relative age and place of birth/development – in the development of expertise. In addition, more evidence has demonstrated the strong link between engagement in deliberate practice in the developing years and the eventual adult expression of expertise.

Overall, although the work on developmental sport expertise has helped identify a range of developmental and contextual factors that are in at least some way associated with the successful emergence of exceptional adult performance in sport, we still remain some distance from being able to fully describe to coaches and athletes both the developmental predictors for success and (importantly) the developmental risk factors for failure. To date very little is known about those athletes who practice extremely hard but fail to become experts – systematic data collection from such participants would seem to be an important step to balance the data collected to date on experts and to reach a more complete picture about the constraints to success. Established sport talent systems worldwide are a potentially rich source of data for retrospective assessment of these developmental differentiators of experts and non-experts. Without such evidence it is difficult, if not impossible, to provide sport practitioners, especially sport administrators, with a balanced assessment of the risks as well as benefits associated with different types of talent development systems.

A clear weakness in the existing evidence based on the development of expertise in sport is the almost exclusive dependence on retrospective data to determine the antecedents to the emergence of expertise. While efficient as a data collection methodology (especially given the relative scarcity of experts), retrospective data are always open to question with respect to their reliability. This is the case given the well-known fallibility of human memory, especially for daily events that may have occurred decades prior to the time of data capture. As the research on sport injuries, for instance, has clearly shown, prospective methodologies are more desirable whenever they can be applied and, if utilized in the study of sport development, would probably provide more insight on factors such as talent hotspots, relative age, age of specialization, deliberate practice, and deliberate play than has been possible using retrospective methodologies. As was the case with the examination of progress on the other key thematic areas of research on sport expertise, evidence of the highest quality on the developmental factors underlying sport expertise is still lacking and this necessarily limits the extent to which the available research can effectively inform practice. There is still some distance to go to bridge the gap between available evidence and the practical questions of principal interest to athletes, coaches, and other sport practitioners.

SOME FINAL THOUGHTS

In the long journey to genuine research-informed practice have we come some distance? Yes. Are we heading in the right direction? Yes, but the need for at least some changes in direction are looming fast. Are we nearly there yet? No. The journey to genuine evidence-based practice is likely to be a long one with incremental rather than quantum gains for both researchers and practitioners along the way. As per the standard advice to impatient children, it may be best to enjoy the trip rather than anxiously awaiting the final arrival.

KEY READING

Abernethy, B. (2008) 'Developing expertise in sport: How research can inform practice', in Farrow, D., Baker, J., and MacMahon, C. (eds.) *Developing Elite Sports Performers: Lessons from Theory and Practice*. London: Routledge, pp. 1–14.

Dror, I.E. (2011) 'The paradox of human expertise: Why humans get it wrong', in Kapur, N. (ed.) *The Paradoxical Brain*. New York: Cambridge University Press, pp. 177–188.

Gorman, A.D., Abernethy, B., and Farrow, D. (2012) 'Classical pattern recall tests and the prospective nature of expert performance', *Quarterly Journal of Experimental Psychology*, 65(6): 1151–1160.

Hecht, H. and Proffitt, D.R. (1995) 'The price of expertise: Effects of experience on the water-level task', *Psychological Science*, 6: 90–95.

Mann, D.L., Abernethy, B., and Farrow, D. (2010) 'The resilience of natural interceptive actions to refractive blur', *Human Movement Science*, 29: 386–400.

Memmert, D., Baker, J., and Bertsch, C. (2010) 'Play and practice in the development of sport-specific creativity in team ball sports', *High Ability Studies*, 21: 3–18.

Reason, J. (1990) *Human Error*. New York: Cambridge University Press.

Savelsbergh, G.J.P., Van Gastel, P.J., and Van Kampen, P.M. (2010) 'Anticipation of penalty kicking direction can be improved by directing attention through perceptual learning', *International Journal of Sport Psychology*, 41: 24–41.

Starkes, J.L. (2008) 'The past and future of applied sport expertise research', in Farrow, D., Baker, J., and MacMahon, C. (eds.) *Developing Elite Sports Performers: Lessons from Theory and Practice*. London: Routledge, pp. 193–206.

Vaeyens, R., Gullich, A., Warr, C.R., and Phillippaerts, R. (2009) 'Talent identification and promotion programmes of Olympic athletes', *Journal of Sports Sciences*, 27: 1367–1380.

Wright, M.J., Bishop, D., Jackson, R.C., and Abernethy, B. (2010) 'Functional MRI reveals expert-novice differences during sport-related anticipation', *NeuroReport*, 21: 94–98.

CHAPTER 15

THERE IS NO EASY ROUTE TO EXPERTISE

GEERT J.P. SAVELSBERGH

THE "FLYING DUTCHMAN"

In recent decades, the study of expertise has gained in importance and has become established as a field in its own right within and beyond sport sciences. As a result, more and more studies have been carried out, and we now know more about expertise. However, maybe even more importantly, these studies have also had a positive impact on practical approaches in sport and the development of talented and elite performers. The current book chapters are a spin-off of this emerging or better expanding field of study. It is also not surprising that Australia, especially the Australian Institute for Sport, acts as a catalyzer in this respect. The systematic collaboration between practitioners and scientists started there about 30 years ago and since then several other countries have followed this model. Coaches and elite sport people know how to make better use of sport expertise knowledge, and researchers know how to (and have the means to) address practical questions.

In this section, I will try *not* to follow the "Flying Dutchman" approach. What is this? According to Wikipedia, "The *Flying Dutchman* is a legendary ghost ship that can never make port, doomed to sail the oceans forever." So, it is not that I ignore the content of the several chapters (port) and sail around in circles. However, I acknowledge that I briefly touch on each chapter instead of discussing the reported finding extensively in order to ensure that I allow scope to offer some thoughts and suggestions for future research. Bruce Abernethy (Chapter 14) asks the relevant question "can research inform practice?" and, I would like to add, can practice inform research? I will try to answer this second question. For that purpose, first I consider and discuss some of the findings of the chapters, followed by a "reorganization" of the presented chapters into the practical setting through the use of the "Teaching Games for Understanding" model, and I will end with future challenges for researchers as well for coaches.

THOUGHTS FROM HISTORY: BACK TO THE FUTURE

In Part I, three chapters (Chapters 2, 3, and 4) reported on research centered on the topic of expertise with respect to deliberate practice and talent development. It is not surprising that one needs a large volume of practice in order to become an expert. For many years, the notion of 10,000 hours of practice has been promoted as the minimum amount necessary for becoming an expert. The danger of this type of rule is that it is (too) easy for coaches to apply this rule without consideration of why. That is, research demonstrates that it is not simply the amount of practice but also the *type* of practice that is critical. One such example is the concept of "deliberate play," introduced by Côté and others. Deliberate play consists of such activities, especially in the developmental years, as spontaneous and unsupervised playing in the garden or the streets. An important implication of deliberate play is that repetition in practice is not the main issue; rather, children will spend repeated time in practice under very different environmental circumstances, even away from the original intended sport skill. The question that now arises is whether this type of deliberate play enhances the route to expertise. My answer would be yes. Recent research from Daniel Memmert and colleagues shows that creative basketball, football, handball, and hockey players conducted similar amounts of deliberate practice to others, but that the difference in achieving expertise is the number of hours accumulated in "play." These findings suggest that a combination of deliberate practice with (unstructured) play activities is likely to be particularly beneficial for the development of players' creativity. Maybe deliberate play should be not only part of early development but somehow incorporated in "late" development too.

In addition, expert players are also characterized by having had a very broad-based experience of a range of different sports before specialization. For instance, in a recent study by Fransen and colleagues, athletes were found to achieve the same level of performance when a combination of different sports and fewer training hours were undertaken in comparison with the combination of one sport and more training hours. These findings suggest that the former combination leads to an improved quality of the training hours. Perhaps such findings exemplify the role of deliberate play in learning.

The step from concepts such as practice and expertise to the concept of talent development is a small one in theory, but a huge one when aiming to conduct research in this area. As discussed in Chapter 2, several parameters seem to be identified, such as self-regulation, tactical game insight, and some anthropometric parameters. Also, an increasing number of studies have aimed to address the more longitudinal question of how expertise is acquired, for example, by means of retrospective studies. However, we as scientists still encounter many methodological problems, which we will have to overcome in the future. Expertise is sport specific (otherwise it would not be expertise), which implies that researchers may need to carry out longitudinal research for each individual sport (e.g., tennis) or at best classes of sport (e.g., racquet sports) separately. Puberty (about 10–15 years old for girls and about 11–16 for boys) can cause considerable changes in an athlete at the cognitive and physical levels. There is also a huge dropout in sports at this age.

A most difficult question to address is: what is optimal talent development? The benchmark is not static, that is, the exceptional expertise level of today is not the one required tomorrow. So how can one solve this? I have no definitive solution, but maybe the most practical approach is to study expertise over a shorter period of time but still longitudinally. For instance, within one particular sport, one could study a group between 7 and 11 years of age, a group within puberty (11–16 years of age), and groups at the sub-elite and elite level (over 16 years). Thus, the utilization of a mixed experimental design that is both cross-sectional and longitudinal could allow examination of both short- and long-term athlete development. Such an approach may allow the identification of some of the common background characteristics of experts and the nature of their developmental (different) experiences and practice histories. Even though such research is clearly very tough it is essential that such programs of work are carried out.

Part II started some with some very interesting chapters on the topic of the official (Chapter 5) and coach (Chapter 6) development. As with the development of talent in different phases, in this topic early, middle, and late years of specialization are proposed in combination with the hours spent at each respective phase. The authors consequently consider whether it is most appropriate to specialize early or late as a function of different sports. At present, there is no scientific basis for the idea that a top-level athlete can easily become a top-level coach. Likewise, there are numerous instances of world-class coaches who did not compete close to the top level as an athlete. Similar reasoning and examples are applicable for referees and officials. Together, this suggests there is not one clear route to becoming a top coach or official. The model proposed and discussed in the chapter by Côté and colleagues is a nice starting point for mapping the development of coaching. It is suggested that a coach undertakes a developmental phase, which emphasizes a wide range of experiences in coaching different types of sport before specializing in one field. Examination of coaching hours, which is not the same as the hours spent supervising practice sessions, will provide a clearer picture on what, when, and how the coach develops. For instance, this may encompass multi-tasking skills to very specific skills. As a beginner, a coach may be expected to do everything (multi-task) – including be the manager, fitness trainer, and coach – before later specializing in one of these roles. Or perhaps a developing coach may gain experiences in different but related sports activities before later specialization. Or the other way around, specialize first in one aspect, for example, in on-field training, and then move on to team coaching. In future work, it is important to establish whether coaches and officials should develop a broad set of skills in different

258

sports before specialization in one sport, or whether there are other, alternative routes to expertise. Clearly, much work is needed in this area, but identification of the expertise required in these respective domains would provide an excellent research contribution. However, I must emphasize, there is still much to be learned before we get there.

In Part III, several "tools" for coaches and athletes were discussed. Some chapters focused on instruction and observation (Chapter 7), the organization of practice (Chapter 8), and implicit learning (Chapter 9). A rich history of literature exists for the topics considered in Chapters 7 and 8. Although many of these experiments in this domain have been conducted in the laboratory setting, they do offer some insight into the learning processes and offer suggestions of what should work and what may not. Furthermore, contemporary neuroscience – for example, the mirror neuron hypothesis – offers interesting implications for research such as observational learning (and learning by imitation). A recent and important event in the domain of learning was the translation of Nikolai Bernstein's work, which emphasized, and indeed demonstrated, that not every movement is exactly the same. This and related findings raise the question of repetitions and practice. What is effective? And, maybe even more important, is there an ideal movement model for a specific task? In Chapter 7, the finding that a self-modeling video can provide performance enhancement was further complicated when individual differences and the stage of development in coordination were considered. That is, what may be "optimal" for athlete X may not necessarily be the case for athlete Y. An aspect that makes the discussion even more complex is whether a movement model that is considered most appropriate at an early stage of learning is also applicable to a later stage of learning. Furthermore, how can we clearly separate or define the stages of learning? These questions are still very difficult to answer.

With his 1992 paper, Rich Masters (Chapter 9) succeeded in applying the concept of implicit learning to the study of motor skill. Now, 20 years later, a flow of papers has demonstrated the effect and applicability of this concept. The idea that the influence of stress or pressure on movement execution and performance is less when a task is learned implicitly should be very appealing to coaches and athletes (see also Chapter 10). In this regard, implicit learning (or minimalized explicit instruction) and the body of related research including Gaby Wulf's external focus of attention (Chapter 7) should be considered further in practice by coaches. By way of example, Chapter 10 also discussed several methods which may be used to simulate pressure alongside implicit learning interventions. Integration of these ideas in combination with research implications from the external focus of attention literature will provide a step forward for coaches with respect to the quality of the practice.

The final three chapters contributed to the topic of "decision making" and expertise. Chapter 12 connected the quiet eye chapter (Chapter 11) with the chapter about enhancement of tactical performance (Chapter 13). As has been demonstrated across many experimental studies, the use of gaze behavior measures as a window into the process of decision making is an important matter. The quiet eye is a putative "optimal" gaze behavior strategy which is starting to attract much research interest. Despite the research on this measure, which indicates that expert athletes may benefit from fixating a target for a lengthy duration during aiming tasks, we still know little about the function and underlying mechanisms of the quiet eye. In this regard, much work is needed to unravel the relationship between movement execution, performance, expertise, and quiet eye. For instance, the study of Matt Dicks and colleagues demonstrates that, if task constraints change, the gaze behavior alters too. This would imply that we need to know what gaze behavior is needed for not only a specific sport but also under which circumstances. And the question arises whether the same "optimal" gaze behavior is necessary for all athletes at the elite level. That is, in line with the argumentation that an optimal model for movement performance does not exist, there may be no optimal gaze behavior. It is highly plausible that the specific movement execution of an athlete goes hand in hand with a specific gaze behavior for a particular task.

Making a tactical decision, if one talks to coaches, is one of the most important aspects for peak performance, especially in team sports. As Chapters 12 and 13 have shown, there is some suggestion that decision making and pattern recognition appear to differentiate between levels of expertise. The huge challenge for future research in this respect is to capture the tactical expertise of athletes in more dynamic situations. How performers utilize information in the guidance of movement during evolving match situations is extremely difficult to study. If we succeed in doing so, this would be a massive step forward for learning research in the domain of decision making as well as talent identification and development (Chapter 3).

CAN PRACTICE INFORM RESEARCH?

The answer to this question is yes. Commonly, scientists' discussions with coaches and athletes do not easily translate into straightforward research questions that can easily be addressed experimentally. This challenge is not only applicable for sport scientists, but also many societal issues. However, with technological innovations we are succeeding more and more in formalizing good research questions and methods based on coaches' questions, as the chapters of the current book demonstrate. In this regard, sport scientists succeed more and more with providing answers to coaches and athletes; for example, why should certain training methods be preferred over others? With this quality of research, it is no longer an enormous step for coaches to apply and incorporate such research findings into their training

260

sessions. An alternative way of enhancing sport performance through research is by utilizing frameworks that stem from practical domains in order to ascertain how scientists (in small part) can contribute to sport. By way of example, I have utilized the "Teaching Games for Understanding" framework that is illustrated in Figure 15.1. The figure illustrates how the different research aspects play their role, how they are connected, and, consequently, how one can teach them. If we take the chapters of this book and fill them into the appropriate places in the framework, one can obtain a nice overview. The teacher or coach who makes use of such a framework in her/his teaching can see where and in what ways sport sciences (e.g., the content of the current chapters) can contribute to their work. As we can see from the figure, nearly all aspects of knowledge are available, but they do require integration with one another.

For scientists, the framework demonstrates where knowledge lies and where gaps in knowledge are present. Furthermore, from an applied view, if a sport scientist can consider research questions from a coach and athlete perspective, it is likely that the applied scientific contribution will be greater as the gap between theory

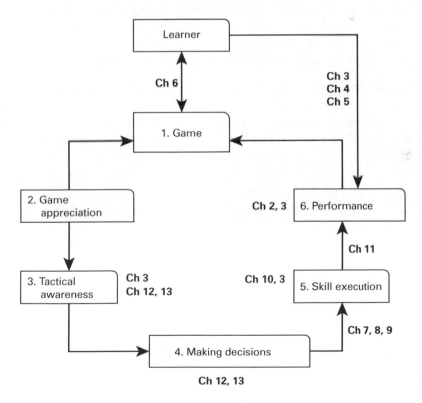

Figure 15.1 "Teaching Games for Understanding" with the chapters of the current book positioned in the framework. (Adapted from Bunker and Thorpe, 1982.)

and application is closer. If not, it is clear where more applied research is required. By using these types of practical approaches, with input from coaches, the research agenda is guided from a practical point of view. In order to have the most fruitful payoff, I expect that multi-disciplinary research will benefit greatly from this kind of approach.

FINAL THOUGHTS: THERE IS NO EASY ROUTE TO EXPERTISE

In order to avoid being the "Flying Dutchman" that never makes port, I will suggest some concrete issues for the study of expertise. Specifically, what are the future challenges for sport scientists for the practical application of scientific findings with respect to the development of expertise? First, it is my belief that, when discussing the implications of research with coaches, scientists may benefit from putting aside their respective theoretical backgrounds. Although such discussions are fundamental to any scientific work, theoretical topics are not always accessible for coaches and athletes. One challenging but potentially fruitful avenue may be for scientists to seek to integrate different theoretical perspectives in order to inform practical implications. That is, rather than emphasizing opposing theoretical views in discussions with coaches and athletes, it may be more worthwhile to focus on the complementary aspects of different theoretical perspectives.

An example of a recent integrated approach is that provided by John van der Kamp and colleagues, who brought together the ecological approach of James Gibson and the neuroanatomical perspective of David Milner and Melvyn Goodale. Milner and Goodale distinguished two neuroanatomically separate but interacting visual pathways underlying perception and action: the ventral (vision for perception) pathway is thought to be primarily involved in perception (i.e., perception of object, events, and affordances of the environment), whereas the dorsal (vision for action) pathway is engaged mainly during action (i.e., guiding movements). From an ecological view, the two systems can be conceived as complementary but exploiting different types of information across different time scales. When this perspective is considered alongside research in perceptual skill and decision making, van der Kamp and colleagues argued that many experimental paradigms impede upon the complementary function of the two visual systems or mutually influencing functions of perception and action. This view shows how the integration of theory and research findings from seemingly opposing scientific perspectives (e.g., indirect versus direct perception) can lead to the establishment of a promising new research agenda. Advances in different sport science domains may benefit from aiming to integrate different theoretical perspectives to inspire applied practice and future research.

262

Second, as considered above, we need frameworks based on practical applications (e.g., Figure 15.1) that guide research agendas. What would be interesting research topics for the very near future in order to unravel the route to expertise further? Inspired by the chapters in this book, I will now offer a few suggestions that are a reflection of my current thoughts on these topics of research:

- Quality of practice hours: while the amount of hours is of importance, everybody can reason that too much training may lead to over-training injuries and burnout. Research is scarce with respect to the effect of practice volume and practice quality for different sports in the development of expertise. Some existing research suggests that many elite athletes have taken part in several sports before 14–15 years of age, with a relative focus on deliberate play rather than deliberate practice. An important consideration is how to understand the interaction between hours of play and practice along the pathway to expertise across different developmental phases.
- Mapping adaptive behavior in relation to expertise: in relation to the previous point, it has been demonstrated that adaptive behavior is a characteristic of expertise. However, how is adaptive behavior acquired during the development of expertise? If we unravel this issue, it could help to reveal the necessary contribution of practice and play in the development of adaptive behaviors.
- Practice under pressure: an interesting next step in training interventions aimed at enhancing performance under pressure would be to consider the most appropriate pressure that different athletes are exposed to during the development of expertise. That is, should the simulated pressure that 10- to 12-year-olds are trained under be different from 16- to 18-year-old athletes? It is also important to ascertain whether the necessary simulated pressure differs between sports or even for different people within sports. For example, it would be interesting to examine the benefits of training under simulated pressure on the performance of officials and referees.
- Decision making in talent identification: we know that decision making can differentiate between different levels of expertise. However, the decision-making processes between sports are also likely to be sport specific. If we want to move forward in decision-making research, we have to capture the dynamics of this process. On the one hand, the dynamics of the game (thus not using static slides) have to be emphasized to study how performers adapt their decisions online to cope with the complex and variable structure of games. For young players the complexity of decision making is likely to differ at each stage of the development pathway. Therefore, how can measures of decision making that are sampled with a child at age 12 predict the quality of decisions taken by the same player at 18 or 25 years of age? Clearly this is a huge challenge, and, in this regard, there will be a big step forward if we can get some "fingerprints" on this issue.

- The further development of a model (phases) for coaches and officials with research aimed at examining the route to expertise for these groups. If we want to improve sport performance, we need to know how we can improve the expertise of experts. For instance, questions such as "what do coaches learn when working with athletes of different abilities?" appear to be most relevant as the field progresses.

To summarize, the study of expertise has established a field in its own right within and beyond sport sciences. As a consequence, positive impacts on practical applications have been achieved. The chapters in this book demonstrated this nicely, but the content in this book has also shown that there is no easy route to expertise, which applies to officials, coaches, athletes, and scientists. Expertise is still difficult to catch, like the "Flying Dutchman."

KEY READING

Dicks, M., Button, C., and Davids, K. (2010) 'Examination of gaze behaviors under in situ and video simulation task constraints reveals differences in information pickup for perception and action', *Attention, Perception, & Psychophysics*, 72(3): 706–720.

Fransen, J., Pion, J., Vandendriessche, J., Vandorpe, B., Vaeyens, R., Lenoir, M., and Philippaerts, R.M. (2012) 'Differences in physical fitness and gross motor coordination in boys aged 6–12 years specializing in one versus sampling more than one sport', *Journal of Sports Sciences*, 30(4): 379–386.

Latash, M. and Turvey, M.T. (eds.) (1996) *Dexterity and Development (with On Dexterity and Its Development by Nicholai Bernstein)*. Mahwah, NJ: Lawrence Erlbaum Associates.

Memmert, D., Baker, J., and Bertsch, C. (2010) 'Play and practice in the development of sport-specific creativity in team ball sports', *High Ability Studies*, 21: 3–18.

Milner, A.D. and Goodale, M.A. (1995) *The Visual Brain in Action*. Oxford: Oxford University Press.

van der Kamp, J., Oudejans, R.D.D., and Savelsbergh, G.J.P. (2003) 'The development and learning of the visual control of movement: An ecological perspective', *Infant Behavior & Development*, 26: 495–515.

van der Kamp, J., Rivas, F., van Doorn, H., and Savelsbergh, G.J.P. (2008) 'Ventral and dorsal system contribution to visual anticipation in fastball sports', *International Journal of Sport Psychology*, 39: 100–130.

Geert J.P. Savelsbergh

INDEX

Abernethy, Bruce xiii, 6–7, 213, 214, 249–55, 256
action concepts 234
action plan profiles 235, 240, 241–2
adaptive behavior, mapping of 263
after movement, factors facilitating learning 141–5
AIS (Australian Institute of Sport) 40, 56, 58–9, 109–12, 237, 256
Amberry, Tom 162
ambiguous actions 88, 90
analogies: cultural differences in responsiveness to 162–3; effective use of 161–4
analysis levels and performance contexts, framework for 233, 241
anxiety, quiet eye (QE) and 199–201
assertiveness skills 85
athlete outcomes, "4Cs" of 97–8, 101, 108
athletes, development of expertise in 2–3, 4–5, 13–29; competitive play, provision of 27–8; deliberate play in sampling years, focus on 21–2; deliberate practice 13, 14, 15–16, 17, 18–20, 25, 27, 28; deliberate practice in investment years and beyond, focus on 22–3; Developmental Model of Sport Participation 18, 22–3; expert perspective on 26–8; *General Adaptation Syndrome* (Selye, H.) 16–17; genes responsible for performance-related outcomes 19; HERITAGE Family Study 19; intrinsic motivation 21; perceptual-cognitive differences, between experts and non-experts 14; play and practice, determination of amounts of 26–7; play and practice for specializing years, integration of 22; play versus practice

in athlete development 18; practice, identification of different forms of 23–5; practice, value of 14; reading recommendations 29; research, evidence from 14–18; research, limitations of 18–20; theory to practice 20–5; training and performance, relationship between 15, 20–1
athletic experience, expert performance coaches and 100–2
Athletic Talent Development Environment (ATDE) model (Henriksen, K.) 48–9, 50
attention processes 198–9
augmented feedback, scheduling of 148–9
avoidance behavior, "choking" and 181–2

Baker, J., Cobley, S., and Schorer, J. 36
Baker, Joseph (Joe) xiii–xiv, 1–9, 13–29, 36, 83
Ballesteros, Severiano 165
Balyi, Istvan 48, 49, 50, 65, 66
Bandura, Albert 117–18
Baumeister, Roy 184–5
Becker, Boris 33
before movement, factors facilitating learning 137–41
behavior, motor skills and 134–5
Beilock, Sian L. xiv, 6, 177–94
Bernard, Gary xiv, 151–3
Bernstein, Nikolai 135–6, 259
biomechanical reps, role of 146
biomechanics, motor skills and 134–5
Bouchard, Claude 19
Bounce (Syed, M.) 13
brain, motor skills and 133–4; *see also* neural processes; neurological trauma
Brand, Ralf xiv–xv, 92–4

British Rowing World Class Start (WCS) 41–2
Bryan, William Lowe 14
Bullock, N. *et al.* 64

Cabrera, Ángel 151
Causer, Joe 200
Champley, Stéphane 140–1
Chase, William 14–16, 19–20
Chinn, Coner 218–19
"choking" 6, 177–94; avoidance behavior
    181–2; evidence for 178–9; expectational
    heightening 184–5; expert perspective
    on 191–4; explicit monitoring 180–1;
    failure, imaging of 184; fluency, priming
    for 188–9; heightened expectations
    184–5; imaging failure 184; individual
    differences 183; intervention strategies
    190; performers' experiences 179–80;
    practicing under pressure 185–6; pre-
    performance routine, optimization of 186–
    8; prevention of, techniques for 185–90;
    reading recommendations 194; research,
    evidence from 178–85; risk factors 182–5;
    self-regulation and avoidance 181–2; skill-
    focused attention 180–1; strategy, focus on
    189–90; task characteristics 183; theory to
    practice 185–90; triggers 182–5
"chunking" 164
coach–scientist relationship 1–9; coach,
    multi-faceted role of 8; deliberate practice
    2; environmental factors in development
    of expertise, importance of 2–3; film
    depictions of athletic development 1; key
    issues for 7; reading recommendations
    8–9; research teamwork 7; research topics
    8; sport science research, application of 3;
    theory to practice 3–4, 7–8; traditions and
    culture of sport 3–4; training and practice,
    role of 2–3
coaching contexts 96, 97; coaches'
    professional knowledge and 98–9
coaching effectiveness 97–8
coaching experience 102
coaching expertise in a performance
    environment, definition of 97–9
Coach's Corner 4; Adam Sachs, High
    Performance Manager, Gymnastics
    Australia 66–7; Eddie Jones, Japanese
    Rugby Union National Team 26–8; Gary
    Bernard, PGA Professional and CEO, PGA
    of Canada 151–3; Hayley Wickenheiser,
    Canadian ice hockey Olympian 206–9;
    Hernán E. Humaña, former Canadian
    Olympic beach volleyball coach 129–30;

John Keogh, Senior Women's Coach,
    Rowing Canada, Aviron 40–3; Neil
    Craig, Director of Football Performance,
    Melbourne FC 227–9; Norma Plummer,
    Head Coach, West Coast Fever Netball
    Team 244–6; Patrick Hunt, Applied
    Technical Advancement Coach, Australian
    Institute of Sport 109–12; Ralf Brand,
    12-year first league basketball referee
    92–4; Scott Draper, National Coach,
    Tennis Australia 191–4; Tom Wilmott,
    Head Coach, New Zealand's Winter
    Performance Park & Pipe Programme
    169–74; Tricia Heberle, High Performance
    Director, Hockey Australia 65–6
Cobley, Steve xv, 4–5, 13–29, 83
cognitive skills, development with expertise
    232–3, 241
collective understanding of athlete
    development, constraints on 52
Collina, Pierluigi 81
Colvin, Geoff 13
communication and personality: addressing
    challenges of 88–9; officials in research
    and practice 77–81
competitive play, provision of 27–8
computer-based analysis, tactics and 237–9
condition concepts 234
condition profiles 235
conditions for development of expertise 250,
    253–4
confidence in and of officials 77
conflict management styles 78
Confucius 165
Côté, J., Baker, J., and Abernethy, B. 18, 22,
    50
Côté, Jean xv, 5, 48, 96–112, 257, 258
Coyle, Daniel 13, 47
Craig, Cathy 220–1
Craig, Neil xv, 163, 227–9
creative choices in decision making 223
creative decision making, limitations on
    teaching 225–6
Crosby, Sydney 210
current event profiles 235, 241–2

Damisch, L., Mussweiler, T., and Plessner,
    H. 76
decision making, expertise in 6, 210–30;
    components of expert decision making
    212–13; creative choices 223; decision
    skills, development of 241; deliberate
    practice 214; developmental histories
    of expert decision makers 213–14;

266

coaching expertise 99–100; developmental milestones 105–8; education, formal and informal 102–3; European Coaching Council 96; expert perspective on 109–12; high-performance coach development, stages of 105–8; performance coach development, activities and experiences of 104; reading recommendations 112; research, evidence from 97–103; theory to practice 104–8

expert perspective on: athletes, development of expertise in 26–8; "choking" 191–4; decision making, expertise in 227–9; expert performance coaches, development of 109–12; functional sport expertise systems 65–6, 66–7; implicit motor learning 169–74; observation as instructional method 129–30; officials in research and practice 92–4; practice, organization of 151–3; prediction 40–3; tactics, development of 244–6; visual perception, expertise in 206–9

expert visual perception 6, 195–209

expertise: pathways to 46–55; realistic pathways to 46–7; underlying components of 33

expertise, development of 6–7, 256–64; adaptive behavior, mapping of 263; decision making, expertise in 259–60; decision making in talent identification 263; deliberate play, concept of 257; deliberate play, role in learning 257; deliberate practice 257, 263; difficulties of route towards 254–64; implicit motor learning 259; observation as instructional method 259; officials, development of expertise in 258–9, 264; optimal talent development 258; performance coaching, development of expertise in 258–9, 264; practice, can research be informed by it? 260–2; practice, organization of 259; practice hours, quality of 263; pressure, practice under 263; quiet eye (QE) 260; reading recommendations 264; research, can practice inform it? 260–2; research, informed practice and 256; research, integrated approach to 262; study of expertise 256; study of expertise, issues for 262–4; tactics, development of 260; talent development, research on 257–8; talent identification, decision making in 263; "Teaching Games for Understanding" framework 256, 261–2, 263; visual perception, expertise in

260; *see also* athletes, development of expertise in

experts' learning 249, 251–2

explicit monitoring, "choking" and 180–1

failure, imaging of 184

Farrow, Damian xvi–xvii, 1–9, 210–30

feedback: augmented feedback, scheduling of 148–9; error detection and correction, feedback schedules and 145; feedback training and 87, 90–1; practice, organization of 141–5; quiet eye (QE) and problem solving 203; tactical feedback 239; *see also* visual outcome feedback

FIFA (Fédération Internationale de Football Association) 81, 83–4, 85, 160, 218

film depictions of athletic development 1

Fischer, Bobby 14

flow, maintenance of 77

fluency, priming for 188–9

Framingham Heart Study 251

Fransen, J. *et al.* 257

FTEM (Foundations, Talent, Elite and Mastery) 65–6, 66–7; application 58–9; architecture 56, 57; elements 56–8; gap analysis and intervention 60–4; interactions between levels 60; levels, developmental needs and 59; transition between levels 60

functional magnetic resonance imaging (fMRI) 116, 252

functional sport expertise systems 4–5, 45–67; application of development models 55; *Athletic Talent Development Environment* (ATDE) model (Henriksen, K.) 48–9, 50; collective understanding of athlete development, constraints on 52; deliberate practice 47, 48, 50, 51, 58–9; development, conceptualization of 52–5; Developmental Model of Sport Participation (DMSP) 48, 50; *Differentiated Model of Giftedness and Talent* (DMGT, Gagné, F.) 48, 50, 54–5; *Environmental Success Factors* (ESF) model (Henriksen, K.) 48–9; expert perspective on 65–6, 66–7; expertise, pathways to 46–55; literature reviews 51; *Long-Term Athlete Development* (LTAD) model (Balyi, I.) 48, 49, 50, 65, 66; models related to development of expertise 50–1; qualitative and quantitative case studies (musicians) 51; reading recommendations 67; realistic pathways to expertise 46–7; research, evidence from 46–55; talent

Panchuk, Derek xxi, 6, 195–209
Pattern Plotter (Australian Institute of Sport) 237–8, 240
pattern recognition training 218–19
Patterson, Jae T. xxi, 6, 132–53
Pearson, Sally 45
perceptual-cognitive competences 14, 72–3, 201, 210, 211, 220
perceptual traps 238
performance characteristics 33–4
performance coach development 5, 8, 96–112; activities and experiences of 104; expertise, development of 258–9, 264
performance skills: "choking" experiences 179–80; periodical analysis of 241
Perry, Ellyse 45
physical demands and positioning: addressing challenges of 89; officials in research and practice 81–3
Pizzera, Alexandra 83, 84
play and practice: determination of amounts of 26–7; for specializing years, integration of 22
play patterns in context of game events 242
play versus practice in athlete development 18
"playmakers" and tactics 231
Plessner, Henning xxi, 5, 71–95
Plummer, Norma xxi–xxii, 244–6
postural cue training 216–17
practice: can research be informed by it? 260–2; design of activities 241; hours of, quality of 263; identification of different forms of 23–5; importance for officials of 91–2; physical practice, timing considerations 126–7; under pressure 185–6, 263; training and, role of 2–3; value of 14
practice, organization of 5–6, 132–53; after movement, factors facilitating learning 141–5; augmented feedback, scheduling of 148–9; behavior, motor skills and 134–5; biomechanical reps, role of 146; biomechanics, motor skills and 134–5; brain, motor skills and 133–4; error detection and correction, feedback schedules and 145; evidence-based methodology 150; expert perspective on 151–3; expertise, development of 259; feedback 141–5; motor planning, practice factors facilitating 146–8; before movement, factors facilitating learning 137–41; reading recommendations 153; repetitions ("reps") 132–3, 135, 136,

137–8, 139–40, 142–3, 144, 145, 146, 147, 148, 150; research, evidence from 135–7; theory to practice 146–9; verbal reports of perceived movement success 149
pre-performance routine, optimization of 186–8
prediction 4–5, 30–44; deliberate practice 33; *Differentiated Model of Giftedness and Talent* (DMGT, Gagné, F.) 32–3; elite youth, performance characteristics of 34–5; expert perspective on 40–3; expertise, underlying components of 33; individual talent profiles as current best practice 38–40; performance characteristics 33–4; reading recommendations 44; research, evidence from 31–2; talent definitions 31–2; talent development 32–3, 37, 38–40; talent formula, idea of 30; talent identification 32, 41–2; talent predictions, potential errors in 36–7; talent selection, recent approaches to 33–5; theory to practice 35–40
preventive refereeing 77
procedural knowledge 232
Pythagoras 161

qualitative and quantitative case studies (musicians) 51
quiet eye (QE): anxiety and 199–201; blocked, variable and random practice 203; decision making 203; expertise, development of 260; feedback and problem solving 203; follow-up and continued practice 204; identification of characteristics 202; importance of 195; modeling in training 203; perceptual-cognitive training 201–5; testing in training 202–3; training processes at work 204–5

Raab, Markus xxii, 6, 83, 84, 210–30
reactors 72–3
reading recommendations: athletes, development of expertise in 29; "choking" 194; coach–scientist relationship 8–9; decision making, expertise in 229–30; expert performance coaches, development of 112; expertise, development of 264; functional sport expertise systems 67; implicit motor learning 174; observation as instructional method 131; officials in research and practice 94–5; practice, organization of 153; prediction 44; research, informed practice and 254–5;

base, emergence of tactics from 234–6; tactical behavior, analysis of 242; tactical feedback 239; tactical knowledge and specialized processes, development with expertise 236, 241; tactical patterns, detection of 237–8; tactical skills development, types of practice and 240–3; technical knowledge, development with expertise 232–3; technology-based tools 231, 236–40, 242–3; "three-second rule" 240, 242

The Talent Code (Coyle, D.) 13, 47

talent definitions 31–2

talent development 32–3, 37, 38–40; research on 257–8

talent formula, idea of 30

talent identification 32, 41–2; decision making in 263

Talent Is Overrated: What Really Separates World-Class Performers from Everybody Else (Colvin, G.) 13

talent predictions, potential errors in 36–7

talent profiles 38–40

talent selection, recent approaches to 33–5

talent transfer 45

"Teaching Games for Understanding" framework 225, 256, 261–2, 263

technical knowledge, development with expertise 232–3

technology: exploitation to improve tactical performance 236–40, 242–3; technology-based tools, tactical developments and 231, 236–40, 242–3

Terman, Lewis 2

theory into practice: athletes, development of expertise in 20–5; "choking" 185–90; coach–scientist relationship 3–4, 7–8; decision making, expertise in 214–25; expert performance coaches, development of 104–8; functional sport expertise systems 56–64; implicit motor learning 160–1, 161–4; observation as instructional method 119–27; practice, organization of 146–9; prediction 35–40; theoretical pathways to expertise 47–9; visual perception, expertise in 201–5

"three-second rule" 240, 242

3D-AD conceptual model of expertise development 52, 53, 54, 55, 61

traditions and culture of sport 3–4

training: general visual versus sport-specific training 216; off-court training 215–21; off-court training, future directions for 219–21; on-field decision training 222–5; pattern recognition training 218–19;

performance and, relationship between 15, 20–1; postural cue training 216–17; practice and, role of 2–3; sport-specific decision-making training 216–19; video training 83–4, 85, 86–7; visual simulation training 218–19; *see also* quiet eye (QE)

triggers to "choking" 182–5

Trudel, Pierre 99, 102

Tua, David 171–2

Unkelbach, Christian 76

Vaeyens, Roel 251

van der Kamp, John 262

verbal reports of perceived movement success 149

Vickers, Joan N. xxiii, 6, 195–209

videotape, use of 82, 91, 115–16, 120–1, 125, 128, 129–30, 135, 151–2, 189, 201, 203, 207–8; decision making and 210, 216, 217–18, 219, 220, 221, 227, 228; self-modeling videos 123, 128, 259; tactical development and 231, 232–3, 236, 240, 241, 242, 243, 245–6; video "feedforward" 122; video training 83–4, 85, 86–7

viewing others 120

virtual reality (VR) immersive simulation 220–1

Vision-in-Action (VIA) system 196

Visscher, Chris 35

visual gaze tracking and occlusion studies 124–5

visual outcome feedback: removal of access to 166–7; subjective awareness and 167–9

visual perception, expertise in 6, 195–209; anxiety and quiet eye 199–201; attention processes 198–9; deliberate practice 207; expert perspective on 206–9; expertise, development of 260; neural processes 198–9; quiet eye (QE): anxiety and 199–201; blocked, variable and random practice 203; decision making 203; feedback and problem solving 203; follow-up and continued practice 204; identification of characteristics 202; importance of 195; modeling in training 203; perceptual-cognitive training 201–5; testing in training 202–3; training processes at work 204–5; reading recommendations 209; research, evidence from 196–201; theory to practice 201–5

visual simulation training 218–19

Waldner, Jan-Ove 36

Ward, Micky 1

274